T0226612

Type I Diabetes

Guest Editors

DESMOND A. SCHATZ, MD
MICHAEL J. HALLER, MD
MARK A. ATKINSON, PhD

ENDOCRINOLOGY AND METABOLISM CLINICS OF NORTH AMERICA

www.endo.theclinics.com

Consulting Editor
DEREK LEROITH, MD, PhD

September 2010 • Volume 39 • Number 3

SAUNDERS an imprint of ELSEVIER, Inc.

W.B. SAUNDERS COMPANY
A Division of Elsevier Inc.

1600 John F. Kennedy Boulevard • Suite 1800 • Philadelphia, Pennsylvania 19103-2899

http://www.theclinics.com

ENDOCRINOLOGY AND METABOLISM CLINICS OF NORTH AMERICA Volume 39, Number 3
September 2010 ISSN 0889-8529, ISBN-13: 978-1-4377-2446-2

Editor: Rachel Glover
Developmental Editor: Jessica Demetriou

© **2010 Elsevier Inc. All rights reserved.**

This journal and the individual contributions contained in it are protected under copyright by Elsevier, and the following terms and conditions apply to their use:

Photocopying
Single photocopies of single articles may be made for personal use as allowed by national copyright laws. Permission of the Publisher and payment of a fee is required for all other photocopying, including multiple or systematic copying, copying for advertising or promotional purposes, resale, and all forms of document delivery. Special rates are available for educational institutions that wish to make photocopies for non-profit educational classroom use. For information on how to seek permission visit www.elsevier.com/permissions or call: (+44) 1865 843830 (UK)/(+1) 215 239 3804 (USA).

Derivative Works
Subscribers may reproduce tables of contents or prepare lists of articles including abstracts for internal circulation within their institutions. Permission of the Publisher is required for resale or distribution outside the institution. Permission of the Publisher is required for all other derivative works, including compilations and translations (please consult www.elsevier.com/permissions).

Electronic Storage or Usage
Permission of the Publisher is required to store or use electronically any material contained in this journal, including any article or part of an article (please consult www.elsevier.com/permissions). Except as outlined above, no part of this publication may be reproduced, stored in a retrieval system or transmitted in any form or by any means, electronic, mechanical, photocopying, recording or otherwise, without prior written permission of the Publisher.

Notice
No responsibility is assumed by the Publisher for any injury and/or damage to persons or property as a matter of products liability, negligence or otherwise, or from any use or operation of any methods, products, instructions or ideas contained in the material herein. Because of rapid advances in the medical sciences, in particular, independent verification of diagnoses and drug dosages should be made.

Although all advertising material is expected to conform to ethical (medical) standards, inclusion in this publication does not constitute a guarantee or endorsement of the quality or value of such product or of the claims made of it by its manufacturer.

Endocrinology and Metabolism Clinics of North America (ISSN 0889-8529) is published quarterly by Elsevier Inc., 360 Park Avenue South, New York, NY 10010-1710. Months of issue are March, June, September, and December. Periodicals postage paid at New York, NY and additional mailing offices. Subscription prices are USD 271.00 per year for US individuals, USD 457.00 per year for US institutions, USD 139.00 per year for US students and residents, USD 340.00 per year for Canadian individuals, USD 560.00 per year for Canadian institutions, USD 394.00 per year for international individuals, USD 560.00 per year for international institutions, and USD 206.00 per year for international and Canadian and foreign students/residents. To receive student/resident rate, orders must be accompanied by name of affiliated institution, date of term, and the signature of program/residency coordinator on institution letterhead. Orders will be billed at individual rate until proof of status is received. Foreign air speed delivery is included in all *Clinics* subscription prices. All prices are subject to change without notice. **POSTMASTER:** Send address changes to *Endocrinology and Metabolism Clinics of North America*, Elsevier Health Sciences Division, Subscription Customer Service, 3251 Riverport Lane, Maryland Heights, MO 63043. **Customer Service: Telephone: 1-800-654-2452** (U.S. and Canada); **1-314-447-8871** (outside U.S. and Canada). **Fax: 1-314-447-8029. E-mail: journalscustomerservice-usa@elsevier.com** (for print support); **journalsonlinesupport-usa@elsevier.com** (for online support).

Reprints. For copies of 100 or more, of articles in this publication, please contact the Commercial Rights Department, Elsevier Inc., 360 Park Avenue South, New York, NY 10010-1710; phone: (+1) 212-633-3813; fax: (+1) 212-462-1935; e-mail: reprints@elsevier.com.

Endocrinology and Metabolism Clinics of North America is covered in *MEDLINE/PubMed (Index Medicus)*, *EMBASE/Excerpta Medica, Current Contents/Clinical Medicine, Current Contents/Life Sciences, Science Citation Index, ISI/BIOMED, BIOSIS,* and *Chemical Abstracts.*

Printed and bound by CPI Group (UK) Ltd, Croydon, CR0 4YY

Transferred to Digital Print 2011

Contributors

CONSULTING EDITOR

DEREK LEROITH, MD, PhD
Chief, Division of Endocrinology, Metabolism, and Bone Diseases, Department of Medicine, Mount Sinai School of Medicine, New York, New York

GUEST EDITORS

DESMOND A. SCHATZ, MD
Professor and Associate Chair, Division of Endocrinology, Department of Pediatrics, University of Florida, Gainesville, Florida

MICHAEL J. HALLER, MD
Assistant Professor, Division of Endocrinology, Department of Pediatrics, University of Florida, Gainesville, Florida

MARK A. ATKINSON, PhD
Professor, Department of Pathology, University of Florida, Gainesville, Florida

AUTHORS

MARK A. ATKINSON, PhD
Professor, Department of Pathology, University of Florida, Gainesville, Florida

TANDY AYE, MD
Assistant Professor of Pediatrics, Department of Pediatrics, Stanford Medical Center, Stanford, California

JEN BLOCK, RN, CDE
Department of Pediatrics, Stanford Medical Center, Stanford, California

EZIO BONIFACIO, PhD
Deutsche Forschungsgemeinschaft Center for Regenerative Therapies Dresden, Technische Universität Dresden, Dresden, Germany

BRUCE BUCKINGHAM, MD
Professor of Pediatric Endocrinology, Department of Pediatrics, Stanford Medical Center, Stanford, California

WILLIAM T. CEFALU, MD
Joint Program on Diabetes, Endocrinology and Metabolism, Louisiana State University Health Sciences Center School of Medicine, New Orleans; Pennington Biomedical Research Center, Baton Rouge, Louisiana

PHILIP E. CRYER, MD
Irene E. and Michael M. Karl Professor of Endocrinology and Metabolism in Medicine, Washington University School of Medicine; Physician, Barnes-Jewish Hospital, St Louis, Missouri

MICHAEL J. HALLER, MD
Assistant Professor, Division of Endocrinology, Department of Pediatrics, University of Florida, Gainesville, Florida

IRL B. HIRSCH, MD
Professor of Medicine, Division of Metabolism, Endocrinology and Nutrition, University of Washington, Seattle, Washington

SANDRA D.K. KINGMA, MD
VU University Medical Center, Amsterdam, The Netherlands

JEAN M. LAWRENCE, ScD, MPH, MSSA
Research Scientist/Epidemiologist, Department of Research and Evaluation, Kaiser Permanente, Southern California, Pasadena, California

GRACIELA LORCA, PhD
Department of Microbiology and Cell Science, University of Florida, Gainesville, Florida

DAVID M. MAAHS, MD, PhD
Assistant Professor of Pediatrics, Department of Pediatrics, Barbara Davis Center for Childhood Diabetes, University of Colorado Denver, Aurora, Colorado

CLAYTON E. MATHEWS, PhD
Associate Professor, Department of Pathology, Immunology, and Laboratory Medicine, The University of Florida College of Medicine, Gainesville, Florida

ELIZABETH J. MAYER-DAVIS, PhD
Professor, Departments of Nutrition and Medicine, University of North Carolina at Chapel Hill, Chapel Hill, North Carolina

SANJEEV N. MEHTA, MD, MPH
Instructor in Pediatrics, Harvard Medical School; Research Associate and Staff Physician, Pediatric, Adolescent and Young Adult Section, and Genetics and Epidemiology Section, Joslin Diabetes Center, Boston, Massachusetts

L. YVONNE MELENDEZ-RAMIREZ, MD
Joint Program on Diabetes, Endocrinology and Metabolism, Louisiana State University Health Sciences Center School of Medicine, New Orleans; Pennington Biomedical Research Center, Baton Rouge, Louisiana

JOSEF NEU, MD
Department of Pediatrics, University of Florida, Gainesville, Florida

ROBERT J. RICHARDS, MD
Joint Program on Diabetes, Endocrinology and Metabolism, Louisiana State University Health Sciences Center School of Medicine, New Orleans; Pennington Biomedical Research Center, Baton Rouge, Louisiana

R. PAUL ROBERTSON, MD
Clinical Professor of Medicine and Affiliated Professor of Pharmacology, Division of Endocrinology and Metabolism, Pacific Northwest Diabetes Research Institute, University of Washington, Seattle, Washington

DESMOND A. SCHATZ, MD
Professor and Associate Chair, Division of Endocrinology, Department of Pediatrics, University of Florida, Gainesville, Florida

BETTY T. TAO, PhD
Research Analyst, Center for Health Research and Policy, CNA, Alexandria, Virginia

DAVID G. TAYLOR, PhD
Research Team Leader, Office of the President, CNA, Alexandria, Virginia

TERRI C. THAYER, BA
Graduate Research Assistant, Department of Pathology, Immunology, and Laboratory Medicine, The University of Florida College of Medicine, Gainesville, Florida; The University of Pittsburgh School of Medicine, Pittsburgh, Pennsylvania

ANGELA H. TRIDGELL, MD
Pediatric Endocrinology Fellow, Division of Endocrinology and Diabetes, Seattle Children's Hospital, University of Washington, Seattle, Washington

DAVID M. TRIDGELL, MD
Endocrinology Fellow, Division of Metabolism, Endocrinology and Nutrition, University of Washington, Seattle, Washington

ERIC W. TRIPLETT, PhD
Department of Microbiology and Cell Science, University of Florida, Gainesville, Florida

NANCY A. WEST, PhD
Instructor, Department of Epidemiology, Colorado School of Public Health, University of Colorado Denver, Aurora, Colorado

S. BRIAN WILSON, MD, PhD
Associate Professor, Department of Pathology, Immunology, and Laboratory Medicine, The University of Florida College of Medicine, Gainesville, Florida

JOSEPH I. WOLFSDORF, MB, BCh
Professor of Pediatrics, Harvard Medical School; Clinical Director and Associate Chief, Division of Endocrinology, Children's Hospital Boston, Boston, Massachusetts

ANETTE G. ZIEGLER, MD
Forschergruppe Diabetes, Klinikum rechts der Isar, Technische Universität München, München, Germany

Contents

Foreword   xiii

Derek LeRoith

Preface   xvii

Desmond A. Schatz, Michael J. Haller, and Mark A. Atkinson

Epidemiology of Type 1 Diabetes   481

David M. Maahs, Nancy A. West, Jean M. Lawrence,
and Elizabeth J. Mayer-Davis

> This article describes the epidemiology of type 1 diabetes mellitus (T1D) around the world and across the lifespan. Epidemiologic patterns of T1D by demographic, geographic, biologic, cultural, and other factors in populations are presented to gain insight about the causes, natural history, risks, and complications of T1D. Data from large epidemiologic studies worldwide indicate that the incidence of T1D has been increasing by 2% to 5% worldwide and that the prevalence of T1D is approximately 1 in 300 in the United States by 18 years of age. Research on risk factors for T1D is an active area of research to identify genetic and environmental triggers that could potentially be targeted for intervention. Although significant advances have been made in the clinical care of T1D with resultant improvements in quality of life and clinical outcomes, much more needs to be done to improve care of, and ultimately find a cure for, T1D. Epidemiologic studies have an important ongoing role to investigate the complex causes, clinical care, prevention, and cure of T1D.

Economics of Type 1 Diabetes   499

Betty T. Tao and David G. Taylor

> This article reviews economic methodologies developed for estimating cost of illness, examines the current literature on diabetes costs, and presents the latest estimates of the economic impact of type 1 diabetes in terms of direct medical costs (ie, treatment costs) and indirect costs (eg, lost wages).

Advances in the Prediction and Natural History of Type 1 Diabetes   513

Ezio Bonifacio and Anette G. Ziegler

> Type 1 diabetes (T1D) has the hallmark characteristics of autoimmunity superimposed on genetic susceptibility. Both genes (HLA) and immune markers (autoantibodies) have been validated as predictive markers of the subsequent development of the disease in higher-risk relatives and the lower-risk general population. Over the last three decades, using a combination of genes, immune, and metabolic markers, clinicians are now able to quantify an individual's disease risk from 1 in 100,000 to more than 1 in 2. This article reviews these biomarkers and T1D prediction

strategies, and discusses potential implications of prediction and natural history for the pathogenesis of T1D.

Efforts to Prevent and Halt Autoimmune Beta Cell Destruction   527

Michael J. Haller, Mark A. Atkinson, and Desmond A. Schatz

> Despite improvements in understanding of the natural history of type 1 diabetes (T1D), an intervention capable of consistently and safely preventing or reversing the disease has not been developed. The inability to cure this disorder is largely because of the complex pathophysiology of T1D, continued struggles to identify its precise etiologic triggers, and voids in understanding of the immunologic mechanisms that specifically target pancreatic beta cells. Rapidly improving technologies for managing T1D require critical discussions about equipoise, especially when considering interventions deemed high risk in terms of their safety. This article reviews the conceptual basis for prevention versus intervention trials in settings of T1D, past experiences of clinical trials studying these purposes, and controversial issues regarding disease interdiction, and seeks to provide a roadmap for future efforts to cure this disorder.

Use of Nonobese Diabetic Mice to Understand Human Type 1 Diabetes   541

Terri C. Thayer, S. Brian Wilson, and Clayton E. Mathews

> In 1922, Leonard Thompson received the first injections of insulin prepared from the pancreas of canine test subjects. From pancreatectomized dogs to the more recent development of animal models that spontaneously develop autoimmune syndromes, animal models have played a meaningful role in furthering diabetes research. Of these animals, the nonobese diabetic (NOD) mouse is the most widely used for research in type 1 diabetes (T1D) because the NOD shares several genetic and immunologic traits with the human form of the disease. In this article, the authors discuss the similarities and differences in NOD and human T1D and the potential role of NOD mice in future preclinical studies, aiming to provide a better understanding of the genetic and immune defects that lead to T1D.

The Intestinal Microbiome: Relationship to Type 1 Diabetes   563

Josef Neu, Graciela Lorca, Sandra D.K. Kingma, and Eric W. Triplett

> This article discusses recent evidence that associates the developing intestinal microbiome to the pathogenesis of autoimmune T1D. It attempts to identify avenues that should be pursued that relate this new evidence to interventions that eventually could result in prevention.

Contemporary Management of Patients with Type 1 Diabetes   573

Sanjeev N. Mehta and Joseph I. Wolfsdorf

> The current standard of care for patients with type 1 diabetes (T1D) employs a system of intensive diabetes management aimed at near-normal glycemia, which reduces the risk of micro- and macrovascular complications. Optimal management is an ongoing process based on a patient-centered collaboration with a primary care clinician and a multidisciplinary

diabetes team that provides diabetes management, including education and psychosocial support. Intensive diabetes therapy attempts to mimic physiologic insulin replacement. Over the past 15 years, there has been widespread use of multiple-dose insulin regimens using a variety of insulin analogs, administered either by injection or insulin pump therapy, together with medical nutrition therapy, frequent self-monitoring of blood glucose and, more recently, continuous logo glucose monitoring. It is now possible to achieve previously unattainable levels of glycemic control with less risk of severe hypoglycemia, and yet only a minority of patients achieves target hemoglobin A1c values. This review discusses contemporary management of T1D with a focus on health outcomes.

Inpatient Management of Adults and Children with Type 1 Diabetes   595

David M. Tridgell, Angela H. Tridgell, and Irl B. Hirsch

Type 1 diabetes poses unique inpatient challenges because of the risks of diabetic ketoacidosis, uncontrolled hyperglycemia, and hypoglycemia. Although newer insulin analogs and insulin pumps provide means for improved glycemic control, they can be daunting for nonexperts. This article focuses on inpatient and perioperative insulin management of stable, nonketotic, nonpregnant adults and children with type 1 diabetes. These principles can also be applied to patients with steroid-induced hyperglycemia.

Toward Closing the Loop: An Update on Insulin Pumps and Continuous Glucose Monitoring Systems   609

Tandy Aye, Jen Block, and Bruce Buckingham

This article reviews current pump and continuous glucose monitoring therapy and what will be required to integrate these systems into closed-loop control. Issues with sensor accuracy, lag time, and calibration are discussed as well as issues with insulin pharmacodynamics, which result in a delayed onset of insulin action in a closed-loop system. A stepwise approach to closed-loop therapy is anticipated, where the first systems will suspend insulin delivery based on actual or predicted hypoglycemia. Subsequent systems may control to range, limiting the time spent in hyperglycemia by mitigating the effects of a missed food bolus or underestimate of consumed carbohydrates, while minimizing the risk of hypoglycemia.

Complications of Type 1 Diabetes   625

L. Yvonne Melendez-Ramirez, Robert J. Richards, and William T. Cefalu

The prevalence of diabetes is increasing worldwide and the concern regarding the number of new cases of diabetes relates to the development of chronic complications. It has been recognized for years that the complications are a cause of considerable morbidity and mortality worldwide and as such, negatively affect the quality of life in individuals with diabetes with an increase in disability and death. Specifically, the complications of diabetes have been classified as either microvascular (ie, retinopathy, nephropathy, and neuropathy) or macrovascular (ie, cardiovascular disease, cerebrovascular accidents, and peripheral vascular disease). For purposes of this article, the authors focus on a brief review of the major complications.

Hypoglycemia in Type 1 Diabetes Mellitus   641

Philip E. Cryer

Iatrogenic hypoglycemia, typically the result of the interplay of therapeutic hyperinsulinemia and compromised defenses resulting in hypoglycemia-associated autonomic failure (HAAF) in diabetes, is a problem for people with type 1 diabetes mellitus (T1DM). It causes recurrent morbidity is sometimes fatal, leads to recurrent hypoglycemia, and precludes euglycemia over a lifetime of T1DM. Risk factors include those that result in relative or absolute insulin excess and those indicative of HAAF in diabetes. Elimination of hypoglycemia from the lives of people with T1DM will likely be accomplished by new treatment methods that provide plasma glucose-regulated insulin replacement or secretion.

Update on Transplanting Beta Cells for Reversing Type 1 Diabetes   655

R. Paul Robertson

Whole pancreas has been used successfully for transplantation for more than 30 years, and islets have been used reproducibly with success for 10 years; both procedures require drugs for immunosuppression. Success is judged by discontinuation of exogenous insulin-based treatment and maintenance of normal or nearly normal hemoglobin A1c. Successful pancreas transplantation has beneficial effects on retinopathy, nephropathy, neuropathy, macrovascular disease, and quality of life. Such findings are suggested for islet transplantation, but insufficient information is available to draw firm conclusions. Because of the paucity of annual pancreas donations, research for human beta cell surrogates is essential to provide a transplantation approach to therapy for a greater number of recipients.

Index   669

FORTHCOMING ISSUES

December 2010
Gastroenteropancreatic System and Its Tumors: Part I
Aaron I. Vinik, MD, *Guest Editor*

March 2011
Gastroenteropancreatic System and Its Tumors: Part II
Aaron I. Vinik, MD, *Guest Editor*

June 2011
Endocrine Hypertension
Lawrence R. Krakoff, MD, *Guest Editor*

RECENT ISSUES

June 2010
Vitamin D
Sol Epstein, MD, *Guest Editor*

March 2010
Hormones and the Science of Athletic Performance
Primus-E. Mullis, MD, *Guest Editor*

December 2009
Pediatric Endocrinology: Part II
Robert Rapaport, MD, *Guest Editor*

FORTHCOMING RELATED INTEREST
Medical Clinics of North America Volume 95, Issue 2 (March 2011)
Prediabetes and Diabetes Prevention
Michael Bergman, MD, *Guest Editor*

THE CLINICS ARE NOW AVAILABLE ONLINE!

Access your subscription at:
www.theclinics.com

Foreword

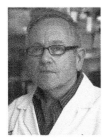

Derek LeRoith, MD, PhD
Consulting Editor

In this issue highlighting recent advances in type 1 diabetes, the editorial team has expertly compiled articles covering the entire spectrum of the disease. From pathophysiology to clinical management and ongoing bench and clinical research efforts, this edition represents a major contribution to academic and practicing physicians involved in type 1 diabetes research and management.

An article from Drs Maahs, West, Mayer-Davis, and Lawrence starts off this series and discusses the epidemiology of type 1 diabetes. These studies in various countries and ethnic populations are important for improving our understanding of the genetic and environmental factors that are causative for the disease. This improved understanding can lead to new ideas on prevention of the disease.

The article from Drs Tao and Taylor shines a much-needed light on the detailed costs of living with type 1 diabetes. Although type 1 diabetes represents 6% to 7% of the diabetic population, the economic burden for this disorder is much greater. Type 1 diabetes often starts early and the cost over years is cumulative. The costs of concomitant autoimmune disorders, the effect of type 1 diabetes on lifestyle, days off schooling and work, and the emotional toll of living with type 1 diabetes are substantial and are examined in detail in this important article.

In addition to an improved understanding of the genetic and environmental triggers of type 1 diabetes, the past 30 years have seen marked advances in our understanding of the natural history of "pre–type 1 diabetes." Drs Bonifacio and Ziegler continue this edition with a discussion of biomarkers used in the prediction of type 1 diabetes. In a very scholarly article, they point out the caveats involved in prediction models and emphasize the need for further research.

The pursuit of a "cure" for type 1 diabetes remains the ultimate dream for all involved in diabetes care and research. In a rather erudite article, Drs Haller, Atkinson, and Schatz discuss various therapeutic trials both completed as well as ongoing to achieve primary prevention, secondary prevention, or even reversal of autoimmunity. Using a "bench to the bedside" approach, the authors emphasize the many difficulties investigators and patients face in designing and participating in type 1 diabetes clinical trials.

Drs Thayer, Wilson, and Mathews describe the value of using the nonobese diabetic (NOD) mouse as a model that resembles human type 1 diabetes, including genetic and

Endocrinol Metab Clin N Am 39 (2010) xiii–xv
doi:10.1016/j.ecl.2010.05.013
0889-8529/10/$ – see front matter © 2010 Elsevier Inc. All rights reserved.

other pathogenic mechanisms. Although the NOD mouse shares many features of human type 1 diabetes and has been touted as representing an excellent model for studying "prevention" of the disorder, the authors correctly point out some important caveats, namely that the disease process is much more rapid in NOD mice, and their response to various manipulations does not always extrapolate to responses by type 1 patients.

Emerging evidence strongly supports the role of the gut microbiome in various human diseases. For example, the microbiome has been implicated as playing a significant role in obesity as well as inflammatory bowl disease. Drs Neu, Lorca, Kingma, and Triplett describe how the microbiome, through its interaction with gut mucosa, may affect the innate immune system, thereby adding to the potential environmental factors that are causative in the development of autoimmunity and, subsequently, type 1 diabetes.

Moving back from the research front to the patient's bedside, Drs Mehta and Wolfsdorf discuss insulin analogs and technology currently used in the management of type 1 diabetes. The past two decades have seen marked improvements in methods for insulin delivery and blood glucose monitoring, as well as better implementation of lifestyle change emphasis on medical nutritional therapy as a component of diabetes management. These advances have played a key role in our ability to control blood glucose and lower hemoglobin A_{1c}.

Given the advances in diabetes management, Drs Tridgell, Tridgell, and Hirsch make a strong case for good (albeit not overzealous) control given recent controversies surrounding intensive glycemic control of hyperglycemia in hospitalized patients. They discuss the benefits of glycemic control in reducing hospital complications and shortening admission while attempting to avoid the potential complications associated with hypoglycemia. In providing practical advice on insulin therapy, this article emphasizes that "sliding scale therapy" should not be considered standard of care. Instead, hospitalized patients with type 1 diabetes should be treated with insulin infusions or basal-bolus regimens using analog insulins.

Moving further along the pathway toward using technology in type 1 diabetes, Drs Aye, Block, and Buckingham explore the development of the artificial pancreas. The closed-loop system has long been considered the Holy Grail for health care professionals treating patients with type 1 diabetes. Although various devices have been developed and are improving at impressive speeds, there remain a number of important challenges. Accuracy of glucose monitoring, delay in insulin effects, and avoidance of hypoglycemia must be perfected before the artificial pancreas becomes a reality.

Despite the many improvements in diabetes management, the risk of complications remains a formidable opponent for patients living with type 1 diabetes. Complications of type 1 diabetes are discussed by Drs Melendez-Ramiraz, Richards, and Cefalu. Although the classic microvascular complications, such as retinopathy, nephropathy, and neuropathy, are clearly related to glycemic control, as shown by the Diabetes Control and Complications Trial, the follow-up study showed that delayed macrovascular effects may also be prevented in the patient with type 1 diabetes, by judicious glycemic control. The authors also discuss the evidence of genetics that may affect complications, such as the emerging studies on haptoglobin genes.

To avoid the complications associated with type 1 diabetes, the primary goal of therapy is to achieve the best possible level hemoglobin A_{1c} without causing recurrent severe hypoglycemia. Dr Cryer discusses the pathophysiology of hypoglycemia, hypoglycemia unawareness, and the fear of hypoglycemia that keep many patients from achieving optimal control. This article also reviews the morbidity and rare occurrence of mortality associated with hypoglycemia.

Recurrent hypoglycemia is often cited as a reason to consider pancreatic transplantation. As discussed by Dr Robertson in his article, pancreatic transplantation has a longer and more successful history than islet cell transplantation. Whole pancreas transplantation succeeds in more than 75% to 80% of cases and the patients often remain off insulin therapy and a reduction in microvascular complications has been demonstrated. The same cannot be said, as yet, for pancreatic islet cell transplantation, although there is hope for similar results assuming sufficient donor islets can be obtained in the future. In both cases, immunosuppression is required that in the past led to complications, although newer drug regimens offer the promise of successful transplantation with fewer side effects.

Reading the articles in this issue has been tremendously enlightening. This collection of articles provides a thorough discussion of the past and, more importantly, a glimpse at the future for diabetes research and care. On behalf of the editors, we hope you find this edition of *Endocrinology and Metabolism Clinics of North America* helpful in furthering your understanding of type 1 diabetes.

Derek LeRoith, MD, PhD
Division of Endocrinology, Metabolism, and Bone Diseases
Department of Medicine
Mount Sinai School of Medicine
One Gustave L. Levy Place
Box 1055, Altran 4-36
New York, NY 10029, USA

E-mail address:
derek.leroith@mssm.edu

Preface

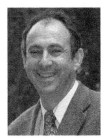 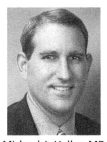 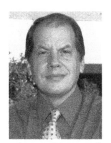

Desmond A. Schatz, MD   Michael J. Haller, MD   Mark A. Atkinson, PhD

Guest Editors

This timely edition of *Endocrinology and Metabolism Clinics of North America* focuses on type 1 diabetes mellitus (T1D). Featuring articles by the leaders in the field, we review state-of-the-art clinical care and research into the prevention and cure of this onerous disease. The broad spectrum of topics should be of interest to anyone involved in the care of affected patients or efforts aimed at the prevention and cure of T1D. As we reflect on advances in our understanding of the pathogenesis of this disease and the rapidly changing ways in which patients with T1D are managed, the "T1D glass" (depending on the eyes of the beholder) can be perceived as "half empty" or "half full."

The hallmark Diabetes Control and Complications Trial (DCCT) convincingly showed a clear relationship between tight glycemic control and a reduction in complications. As such, intensive management has become the accepted approach to management, and technologic advances in pumps and glucose monitoring systems have set the stage for development of the "artificial," albeit not biologic, pancreas. Hope should translate into reality in the next few years. Additionally, we now know that T1D is an autoimmune disease whose onset can be predicted using a combination of immunologic, genetic (HLA), and metabolic markers. As such, the stage is set for prevention. These advances have allowed investigators the opportunity to intervene at a variety of stages in the natural history of the disease process. Such efforts have accelerated with the formation of large networks of collaborating investigators (Diabetes Prevention Trial—Type 1 [DPT-1], TrialNet, European Nicotinamide Diabetes Intervention Trial [ENDIT], DCCT, Epidemiology of Diabetes Interventions and Complications Study [EDIC], and so forth). Recent trials to preserve beta-cell function in subjects at risk for T1D (oral insulin) and new-onset patients have shown promising results (eg, anti-CD3, Diamyd, and Rituximab). In addition, the past decade has seen a greater understanding of beta-cell biology leading to replacement of beta-cell function with pancreatic, islet, and stem cell transplants, all of which are small steps forward on the road to curing T1D.

Endocrinol Metab Clin N Am 39 (2010) xvii–xviii
doi:10.1016/j.ecl.2010.05.012
0889-8529/10/$ – see front matter © 2010 Elsevier Inc. All rights reserved.

Yet, even as these statements highlight research progress, they call attention to current challenges, areas of active investigation, and the need for additional discoveries. The potential benefits of improved glycemic control are reaching only a minority of patients and, as such, T1D continues to be a tremendous burden on the individual and on society. In addition, many of the "successful" immunosuppressive/immuno-regulatory interventions (noted previously) are of questionable translation to the general T1D population. Clearly, we still have much to learn. Improved knowledge of beta-cell development, the precise triggers and immune mechanisms leading to the disease, the genesis of complications, and barriers to implementation of the artificial pancreas will all rapidly "fill the glass."

Given the current state of affairs, we chose to consider the "T1D glass" as "half full" and look forward to a future edition of *Endocrinology and Metabolism Clinics of North America* that describes progress toward ensuring that our glass will eventually overflow.

Desmond A. Schatz, MD
Division of Endocrinology
Department of Pediatrics
University of Florida
PO Box 100296
Gainsville, FL 32610, USA

Michael J. Haller, MD
Division of Endocrinology
Department of Pediatrics
University of Florida
PO Box 100296
Gainsville, FL 32610, USA

Mark A. Atkinson, PhD
Department of Pathology
University of Florida
PO Box 100275
Gainsville, FL 32610, USA

E-mail addresses:
schatda@peds.ufl.edu (D.A. Schatz)
hallemj@peds.ufl.edu (M.J. Haller)
atkinson@ufl.edu (M.A. Atkinson)

Epidemiology of Type 1 Diabetes

David M. Maahs, MD, PhD[a],[*], Nancy A. West, PhD[b],
Jean M. Lawrence, ScD, MPH, MSSA[c], Elizabeth J. Mayer-Davis, PhD[d],[e]

KEYWORDS

- Type 1 diabetes • Epidemiology • Incidence
- Prevalence • Children

This article describes the epidemiology of type 1 diabetes mellitus (T1D) around the world and across the lifespan. Epidemiologic patterns of T1D by demographic, geographic, biologic, cultural, and other factors in populations are presented to gain insight about the causes, natural history, risks, and complications of T1D. Studies of the epidemiology of T1D in diverse populations are aimed at the identification of causal factors of the disease and its complications. The elucidation of the complex interaction between genetic and environmental factors leading to T1D should inform ongoing efforts to treat, prevent, and eventually cure T1D.

T1D is a heterogeneous disorder characterized by destruction of pancreatic beta cells, culminating in absolute insulin deficiency. Most cases are attributable to an autoimmune-mediated destruction of beta cells (type 1a) although a small minority of cases result from an idiopathic destruction or failure of beta cells (type 1b). T1D accounts for 5% to 10% of the total cases of diabetes worldwide.[1] A second and more prevalent category, type 2 diabetes (T2D), is characterized by a combination of resistance to insulin action and inadequate compensatory insulin secretory response.[1] T1D has been historically, and continues to be, the most common type of diabetes in children and adolescents, although type 2 diabetes (T2D) is increasingly diagnosed in youth.[2,3]

This work was supported in part by K23 DK075360 from the National Institutes of Health.

[a] Department of Pediatrics, Barbara Davis Center for Childhood Diabetes, University of Colorado Denver, PO Box 6511, Mail Stop A140, Aurora, CO 80045, USA

[b] Department of Epidemiology, Colorado School of Public Health, University of Colorado Denver, 13001 East 17th Avenue, Campus Box B-119, Aurora, CO 80045, USA

[c] Department of Research and Evaluation, Kaiser Permanente Southern California, 100 South Los Robles, 4th floor, Pasadena, CA 91101, USA

[d] Department of Nutrition, University of North Carolina at Chapel Hill, 2211 McGavran-Greenberg Hall, Campus Box 7461, Chapel Hill, NC 27599-7461, USA

[e] Department of Medicine, University of North Carolina at Chapel Hill, 2211 McGavran-Greenberg Hall, Campus Box 7461, Chapel Hill, NC 27599-7461, USA

* Corresponding author.
E-mail address: David.maahs@ucdenver.edu

Endocrinol Metab Clin N Am 39 (2010) 481–497
doi:10.1016/j.ecl.2010.05.011
0889-8529/10/$ – see front matter © 2010 Elsevier Inc. All rights reserved.

In this article, the authors review the epidemiology of T1D in the following order: incidence and prevalence, risk factors, clinical course, treatment and management, and complications. Other reviews of the epidemiology of T1D have been published recently[4] including a text on the epidemiology of diabetes in youth.[5] In addition, some topics in this article are reviewed in greater detail in later sections and references are provided.

INCIDENCE AND PREVALENCE OF T1D

The current prevailing paradigm on the cause of T1D hypothesizes that environmentally triggered autoimmune destruction of pancreatic beta cells occurs against the background of genetic risk,[6] although alternate hypotheses exist.[7,8] It follows that global variation in the incidence, prevalence, and temporal trends in T1D are reported. In this section, findings from large T1D registry studies such as the World Health Organization Multinational Project for Childhood Diabetes, known as the DIAMOND Project,[9,10] EURODIAB,[11,12] and the SEARCH for Diabetes in Youth (SEARCH) study are emphasized.[2,3] Reports on trends in T1D are more commonly available from countries with better established public health surveillance systems and diabetes research infrastructure. Data that allow for the study of T1D from the more developing world are a research priority.

The DIAMOND Project was initiated by the World Health Organization in 1990 to address the public health implications of T1D with a main objective to describe the incidence of T1D in children. An initial report in 2000 described the incidence of T1D in children 14 years of age or less in 50 countries worldwide totaling 19,164 cases from a population of 75.1 million children (an estimated 4.5% of the world's population in this age range) from 1990 to 1994.[9] A greater than 350-fold difference in the incidence of T1D among the 100 populations worldwide was reported with age-adjusted incidences ranging from a low of 0.1/100,000 per year in China and Venezuela to a high of 36.5/100,000 in Finland and 36.8/100,000 per year in Sardinia. The lowest incidence (<1/100,000 per year) was reported in the populations from China and South America and the highest incidence (>20/100,000 per year) was reported in Sardinia, Finland, Sweden, Norway, Portugal, the United Kingdom, Canada, and New Zealand. The US populations included in the DIAMOND study drawn from the states of Pennsylvania, Alabama, and Illinois reported incidences of 10 to 20/100,000 per year. Approximately half of the European populations reported incidence between 5 and 10/100,000 per year with the remainder having higher rates. The incidence of T1D increased with age in most populations with the highest incidence observed in children aged 10 to 14 years. Within-country variation was also reported with rates 3 to 5 times higher in Sardinia than in continental Italy, with similar variation reported within Portugal, New Zealand, and China. A statistically significant male-to-female excess in incidence was reported in 3 centers, but no populations reported a female excess. These investigators hypothesize that the explanation for the variation within ethnic groups may be caused by differences in genetic admixture or environmental/behavioral factors. They also reported that in countries undergoing rapid social change, population exposure to putative etiologic factors for T1D may change rapidly, highlighting the importance of such registries for the development and testing of genetic and environmental hypotheses on the pathogenesis of T1D.

In the United States, the SEARCH for Diabetes in Youth Study has been designed to identify incident and prevalent cases of diabetes among individuals less than 20 years of age in a multicenter study design with a goal of estimating the incidence and prevalence of diabetes in the United States by age, sex, and race/ethnicity.[3] In 2002 to

2003, 1905 youth with T1D were diagnosed in SEARCH from a population of more than 10 million person-years under surveillance. Rates were highest in non-Hispanic white youth compared with other race/ethnicities and were slightly higher in females compared with males (relative risk [RR], 1.028; 95% confidence interval [CI], 1.025–1.030). The incidence rate of T1D in 2002 to 2003 peaked in the age groups 5 to 9 years and 10 to 14 years and incidence per 100,000 person-years by age group was as follows: 0 to 4 years, 14.3; 5 to 9 years, 22.1; 10 to 14 years 25.9; 15 to 19 years, 13.1. Dabelea and colleagues[3] noted that the T1D incidence rates from the SEARCH study were higher than previous US reports from Allegheny County,[13] and from Philadelphia[14] for non-Hispanic white children but lower than for African American children[14]; the SEARCH rates for Hispanic youth were similar to those reported for Puerto Rican children in Philadelphia[14,15] but higher than those reported in Colorado in the 1980s.[16] For non-Hispanic whites, the incidence rate of T1D in SEARCH was greater than 20/100,000 person-years compared with 16.5/100,000 in Allegheny County in the early 1990s. However, ascertainment techniques differ by study and must be considered when comparing incidence rates by study.

In the SEARCH study, the prevalence of T1D was 2.28/1000 in youth less than age 20 years or 5399 cases in a population of ~3.5 million.[2] Among children less than 10 years of age, T1D accounted for almost all of the reported cases of diabetes, whereas in youth aged 10 to 19 years, the proportion with T2D out of the total sample of youth with diabetes ranged from 6% (in non-Hispanic whites) to 76% (in American Indians). The investigators estimated that 154,369 youth in the United States had diabetes (T1D, T2D or unspecified forms) in 2001.

INCIDENCE: TEMPORAL TRENDS

An updated report from the DIAMOND Project examined the trends in incidence of T1D from 1990 to 1999 in 114 populations from 57 countries. Based on 43,013 cases of T1D from a study population of 84 million children aged 14 years or less,[10] the average annual increase in incidence in this time period was 2.8% (95% CI 2.4%–3.2%) with a slightly higher rate in the period 1995 to 1999, 3.4% (95% CI 2.7%–4.3%) than in the period 1990 to 1994, 2.4% (95% CI 1.3%–3.4%). These trends for increased incidence of T1D were seen across the world in the populations studied (4.0% in Asia, 3.2% in Europe, and 5.3% in North America) with the exception of Central America and the West Indies, where T1D is less prevalent, and where the trend was a decrease of 3.6%. Such reported increases cannot be attributed to genetic shifts in such a short period of time and the investigators state that causative agents should be investigated in the environment or the gene-environment interaction. Furthermore, recent studies[17–19] demonstrate environmental factors have a stronger effect on individuals with lower risk genotypes compared with those at higher risk genetically.

Using US data from the Colorado IDDM study registry and the SEARCH study, the incidence of T1D was shown to increase in the past 3 decades.[20] The incidence of T1D was 14.8/100,000 per year (95% CI 14.0–15.6) in 1978 to 1988 and was 23.9/100,000 per year (95% CI 22.2–25.6) in 2002 to 2004 for the state of Colorado. During this 26-year period, the incidence of T1D increased by 2.3% (95% CI 1.6–3.1) per year with significant increases for both non-Hispanic white and Hispanic youth.

The EURODIAB ACE study group ascertained 16,362 cases of T1D in 44 centers throughout Europe and Israel covering a population of ~28 million children during the period 1989 to 1994.[11] As in the DIAMOND report, the standardized annual incidence rate varied greatly from 3.2/100,000 person-years in Macedonia to 40.2/100,000 person-years in 2 regions of Finland. In this time period, the annual increase in the incidence rate of T1D was 3.4% (95% CI 2.5%–4.4%) although the rate of increase was noted to be higher in some central European countries. The rates of increase were found to be the highest in the youngest age group: ages 0 to 4 years (6.3%, 95% CI 1.5%–8.5%), 5 to 9 years (3.1%, 95% CI 1.5%–4.8%), and 10 to 14 years (2.4%, 95% CI 1.0%–3.8%), with earlier onset implying a longer burden of disease as well as the more immediate challenge of caring for T1D in a toddler.

RISK FACTORS FOR DEVELOPMENT OF T1D

Various risk factors for development of T1D such as age, sex, race, genotype, geographic location, and seasonality are reviewed in this section.

Age

T1D is the major type of diabetes in youth, accounting for 85% or more of all diabetes cases in youth less than 20 years of age worldwide.[2,21,22] In general, the incidence rate increases from birth and peaks between the ages of 10 and 14 years during puberty.[3,10,11] The increasing incidence of T1D throughout the world is especially marked in young children.[10,23] Registries in Europe suggest that recent incident rates of T1D were highest in the youngest age group (0 to 4 years).[11] Incidence rates decline after puberty and seem to stabilize in young adulthood (15 to 29 years). The incidence of T1D in adults is lower than in children, although approximately one-fourth of persons with T1D are diagnosed as adults.[24] Clinical presentation occurs at all ages and as late as the ninth decade of life.[22] Up to 10% of adults initially believed to have type 2 diabetes are found to have antibodies associated with T1D[25] and beta cell destruction in adults seems to occur at a much slower rate than in young T1D cases, often delaying the need for insulin therapy after diagnosis. Individuals diagnosed with autoimmune diabetes when they are adults have been referred to as having latent autoimmune diabetes of adults.[26,27]

Gender

Although most common autoimmune diseases disproportionately affect females, on average girls and boys are equally affected with T1D in young populations.[28] A distinctive pattern has been observed such that regions with a high incidence of T1D (populations of European origin) have a male excess, whereas regions with a low incidence (populations of non-European origin) report a female excess.[29,30] Many reports indicate an excess of T1D cases in male adults after the pubertal years (male/female ratio ≥ 1.5) in populations of European origin.[31–34]

Race/Ethnicity

Worldwide differences in T1D by race/ethnicity are discussed earlier in this article where worldwide incidence rates and prevalence estimates are presented. In many of these reports, data are presented by comparisons within and between country or region, but not by race/ethnicity per se, in part because many of the countries either are relatively homogeneous with regard to race/ethnicity or lack the power based on their sample size to examine rates by race/ethnicity. However, the SEARCH study does provide specific data on the role of race/ethnicity within the United States.[35]

The SEARCH for Diabetes in Youth Study recently published a set of papers in a supplement to *Diabetes Care*[35] in which race- and ethnic-specific issues in diabetes in 9174 American youth are reviewed for 5 major race and ethnic groups in the United States, non-Hispanic white,[36] African American,[37] Hispanic,[38] Asian and Pacific Islander,[39] and Navajo[40] populations. In these papers, the investigators estimate the prevalence and incidence of diabetes in youth less than 20 years by age, sex, race/ethnicity, and diabetes type, as well as characterize key risk factors for diabetic complications by race/ethnicity and diabetes type (**Table 1** for incidence/prevalence data in the SEARCH study by age and race-ethnicity).

In the non-Hispanic white population the prevalence of T1D was 2.0/1000 and the incidence was 23.6/100,000 (with a slightly higher incidence rate for males than females [24.5 vs 22.7 per 100,000, respectively, $P = .04$]). The investigators conclude that these rates of T1D among non-Hispanic white youth are among the highest in the world. These youth had adverse cardiometabolic risk profiles (>40% with increased low-density lipoprotein [LDL], <3% met dietary recommendations for saturated fat, and among those ≥ 15 years of age 18% were current smokers) which put them at risk for future health complications related to diabetes.

In African American youth in the SEARCH study, the prevalence of T1D was 0.57/1000 (95% CI 0.47–0.69) for youth aged 0 to 9 years and 2.04/1000 (1.85–2.26) for youth aged 10 to 19 years. The incidence of T1D for those aged 0 to 9 years and 10 to 19 years during 2002 to 2005 was 15.7/100,000. Of the African American youth who attended the research visit with T1D, 50% of those aged 15 years or more had A1c greater than 9.5%, and 44.7% were either overweight or obese.

The incidence of T1D in Hispanic youth in the SEARCH study was 15.0/100,000 and 16.2/100,000 for girls and boys aged 0 to 14 years. Poor glycemic control as well as

Table 1
The SEARCH for Diabetes in Youth Study: prevalence (index year 2001) and incidence rates (incident years 2002–2005 combined) of type 1 diabetes among 5 race-ethnicity groups by age category

Race-Ethnicity		Age Category			
		0–4 Years	5–9 Years	10–14 Years	15–19 Years
NHW	Prevalence per 1000	0.38	1.63	2.56	3.22
	(95% CI)	(0.33, 0.44)	(1.53, 1.75)	(2.43, 2.70)	(3.07, 3.38)
	Incidence per 100,000	19.4	30.1	32.9	11.9
	(95% CI)	(17.8, 21.1)	(28.1, 32.2)	(30.9, 35.0)	(10.8, 13.2)
AA	Prevalence per 1000	0.22	0.90	1.79	2.32
	(95% CI)	(0.14, 0.34)	(0.72, 1.11)	(1.55, 2.08)	(2.02, 2.66)
	Incidence per 100,000	12.0	19.3	21.3	9.5
	(95% CI)	(9.6, 14.8)	(16.3, 22.9)	(18.3, 24.8)	(7.4, 12.0)
Hispanic	Prevalence per 1000	0.17	0.70	1.47	1.71
	(95% CI)	(0.12, 0.25)	(0.59, 0.84)	(1.30, 1.67)	(1.51, 1.94)
	Incidence per 100,000	10.2	18.2	18.4	8.7
	(95% CI)	(8.3, 12.6)	(15.5, 21.3)	(15.6, 21.5)	(6.8, 11.1)
API	Prevalence per 1000	0.18	0.34	0.62	0.93
	(95% CI)	(0.11, 0.30)	(0.23, 0.49)	(0.47, 0.81)	(0.74, 1.16)
	Incidence per 100,000	5.2	7.6	9.1	5.7
	(95% CI)	(3.3, 8.0)	(5.3, 10.9)	(6.6, 12.5)	(3.8, 8.6)
Navajo	Prevalence per 1000	0	0.16	0.15	0.43
	(95% CI)		(0.06, 0.41)	(0.06, 0.38)	(0.23, 0.79)
	Incidence per 100,000	1.15	3.28	1.95	4.03
	(95% CI)	(0.20, 6.49)	(1.11, 9.64)	(0.53, 7.10)	(1.57, 10.37)

Data from Mayer-Davis EJ, Bell RA, Dabelea D, et al. The many faces of diabetes in American youth: type 1 and type 2 diabetes in five race and ethnic populations: the SEARCH for Diabetes in Youth Study. Diabetes Care 2009;32(Suppl 2):S99–101.

high LDL-cholesterol and triglycerides were common and 44% of these youth with T1D were overweight or obese.

The incidence of T1D among Asian and Pacific Islander youth was 6.4 and 7.4/100,000 person-years in those aged 0 to 9 and 10 to 19 years, respectively. The Pacific Islanders were more likely to be obese compared with the Asian or Asian-Pacific Islanders (mean body mass index [calculated as weight in kilograms divided by the square of height in meters] 26 vs 20 kg/m^2, $P<.0001$).

Most Navajo youth who were identified as having diabetes were diagnosed with T2D (66/83 in the SEARCH paper). The investigators state that T1D is present in Navajos, but that it is infrequent and estimate that the prevalence of T1D in Navajo youth is less than 0.5/1000 and the incidence less than 5/100,000 per year. Regardless of type, Navajo youth were likely to have poor glycemic control and a high prevalence of unhealthy behaviors and depressed mood.

Genotype

Of the multiple genes implicated in susceptibility (and resistance) to T1D, the most important are the human leukocyte antigen (HLA) complex on chromosome 6, in particular the HLA class II. Two susceptibility haplotypes in the HLA class II region are now considered the principal susceptibility markers for T1D.[41] Although 90% to 95% of young children with T1D carry either or both susceptibility haplotypes, approximately 5% or fewer persons with HLA-conferred genetic susceptibility actually develop clinical disease.[42]

Approximately 40% to 50% familial clustering in T1D is attributable to allelic variation in the HLA region.[43] The remaining genetic risk is made up of many diverse genes, each having a small individual effect on genetic susceptibility.[41] Several reports suggest a recent temporal trend of fewer high-risk HLA genotypes in youth diagnosed with T1D, suggesting an increased influence of environmental factors in the development of T1D during the past few decades.[17,19,44]

Although most T1D cases occur in individuals without a family history of the disease, T1D is strongly influenced by genetic factors. In the United States, individuals with a first-degree relative with T1D have a 1 in 20 lifetime risk of developing T1D, compared with a 1 in 300 lifetime risk for the general population.[45] Monozygotic twins have a concordance rate of more than 60% if followed long enough,[46] whereas dizygotic twins have a concordance rate of 6% to 10%. Genetic susceptibility for T1D ranges from marked in childhood-onset T1D to a more modest effect in adult-onset T1D, with children having a higher identical twin concordance rate and a greater frequency of HLA genetic susceptibility.[47,48] Siblings of children with onset of T1D before the age of 5 years have a 3- to 5-fold greater cumulative risk of diabetes by age 20 years compared with siblings of children diagnosed between 5 and 15 years of age.[49] Diabetes with onset before age 5 years is a marker of high familial risk and suggests a major role for genetic factors. The offspring of affected mothers have a 2% to 3% risk, whereas offspring of affected fathers have a 7% risk.[50]

An association between T1D and other autoimmune diseases, such as autoimmune thyroid disease, Addison disease, celiac disease, and autoimmune gastritis, is well established.[51] The clustering of these autoimmune diseases is related to genes within the major histocompatibility complex.[52]

SEASONALITY OF ONSET AND BIRTH

Patterns in the seasonality for both the month of birth and the month of diagnosis of T1D have been reported. Although the seasonality of T1D diagnosis seems intuitively obvious given the well-documented environmental role in T1D's pathogenesis, it is also hypothesized that the seasonal environment at birth may have an influence on diabetes incidence later in life. Among 9737 youth with T1D in the SEARCH study, the percentage of observed to expected births differed across the months with a deficit of November-February births and an excess in April-July births. This birth month effect was not observed in youth recruited from the centers in the more southern locations (South Carolina, Hawaii, Southern California), but only in the more northern latitudes (Colorado, Washington, and Ohio).[53] A report from Ukraine also reported a strong seasonal birth pattern with the lowest rates of T1D in December and the highest in April.[54] Similar reports of higher rates of T1D among youth born in spring and lower rates among youth born in the fall have been published from Europe,[54–57] New Zealand,[58] and Israel,[59] but not in other studies from Europe, East Asia, or Cuba.[57,60–62]

One hypothesis to explain such seasonal variation in T1D by birth month is that of seasonal variation in maternal vitamin D levels and vitamin D's effect on both beta cells and immune cells. Vitamin D deficiency has been associated with T1D[63,64] and the use of cod liver oil (a rich source of vitamin D) during pregnancy[65] and the first year of life[66] has been associated with a lower risk of T1D. Recent reports suggest that vitamin D deficiency is common in the pediatric population in the United States,[67] even in solar-rich environments.[68]

A seasonal pattern in the onset of T1D with increased cases during late autumn, winter, and early spring has been well known and repeatedly confirmed in youth.[69] The seasonal variation in infections implicated to precipitate T1D is suspected to play a primary role in this observation. Reports on the seasonality of T1D in adults have been mixed, but a recent report from Sweden on more than 5800 patients aged 15 to 34 years found the higher incidence during January-March and the lowest during May-July with no difference by gender.[69] Although viral disease has long been proposed as a potential trigger of beta cell destruction, insufficient exposure to early infections might increase the risk of T1D as the maturation of immune regulation after birth is driven by exposure to microbes.[70] The evidence linking specific infections with T1D remains inconclusive.[71]

OTHER RISK FACTORS

Epidemiologic studies have identified that environmental factors operating early in life seem to trigger the immune-mediated process in genetically susceptible individuals. That nongenetic factors play a role in the development of T1D is shown by migration studies, increasing incidence within genetically stable populations, and twin studies. The environmental triggers that initiate pancreatic beta cell destruction remain largely unknown.

Nutritional factors that have been investigated include cow's milk, breastfeeding, wheat gluten, and vitamins D and E.[42] Evidence regarding early introduction of cow's milk (or protective effects of breast milk consumption) in infants contributing to the development of childhood T1D is equivocal[72–75] and may depend on genetic suscep-tibility.[76] Timing of introduction of cereals/gluten or other foods to the infant diet has been suggested to alter risk for autoimmunity and development of T1D.[77–79] Increased use of vitamin D supplementation during infancy has been associated with reduced risk for childhood T1D.[80] Increased maternal consumption of vitamin D during pregnancy has also been associated with decreased risk of islet autoimmunity in the offspring.[81] A protective association was observed for serum α-tocopherol in relation to T1D.[82] Despite these intriguing associations, there is little firm evidence of the significance of nutritional factors in the etiology of T1D.

CLINICAL COURSE

The clinical course of T1D is typically characterized by the acute onset of the classic symptoms of diabetes: polyuria, polydipsia, and weight loss. However, given the increased awareness of T1D as well as research studies in which at-risk children are screened for diabetes autoantibodies, some youth present with sufficient residual beta cell function to be maintained on low doses of insulin, often once daily, at the time of diagnosis. The course of autoimmune diabetes is characterized by ongoing beta cell destruction and increased need for exogenous insulin. Identification of patients at risk for T1D and interventions to slow or halt autoimmune beta cell destruction are the focus of intense investigation (see the article by Bonifacio and Ziegler elsewhere in this issue for further exploration of this topic). This general period with residual beta cell function and insulin secretion is referred to as the honeymoon period during which management of glycemia is greatly aided by residual autonomous insulin production. As residual beta cell function diminishes, as shown by unmeasurable levels of c-peptide in serum, the management of T1D becomes increasingly complex and challenging for the children, their parents, and health care professionals.

As the clinical onset of T1D follows an acute course in most cases, an important issue at the presentation of T1D is that of the symptoms and severity of T1D, in particular that of diabetic ketoacidosis (DKA). The EURODIAB group reported on the frequency, severity, and geographic variation of DKA at presentation of T1D across 24 centers in Europe that included 1260 children at diagnosis of T1D.[12] Polyuria was the most common presenting symptom (96%), followed by weight loss (61%), and fatigue (52%). Duration of symptoms was less than 2 weeks in only 25% of the children, although this was more common in children less than 5 years of age, suggesting that efforts to educate populations on T1D's classic symptoms could improve early diagnosis and reduce the severity of metabolic derangement at presentation. DKA, defined as pH less than 7.3, was reported in 42% of children, with 33% having a pH between 7.3 and 7.1, and 9% with severe DKA (<7.1). A strong inverse correlation between the background rate of T1D and proportion of newly diagnosed youth presenting with DKA was reported such that in centers with more T1D, children were more likely to be diagnosed with T1D before the development of this metabolic emergency.

TREATMENT AND MANAGEMENT

Several therapeutic options for persons with T1D currently exist and include multiple daily injections of rapid-acting insulin with meals combined with a daily basal insulin as well as continuous subcutaneous insulin infusion via an insulin pump. Other regimens such as premixed insulin are also used in certain clinical situations. Guidelines for the care of T1D in children[83] and adults[84] have been published. In addition, screening recommendations exist to monitor for the microvascular (retinopathy, neuropathy, and nephropathy) and macrovascular (cardiovascular) complications of T1D (Melendez-Ramirez, Richards, and Cefalu).

Glycemic control is the cornerstone of diabetes care. However, even in the Diabetes Control and Complications Trial (DCCT), the mean A1c for adolescents compared with adults was 1% to 2% higher in both the intensive and conventionally treated arms. Despite this, rates of hypoglycemia were higher in adolescents than in adults.[85] More recently, studies published since the DCCT have shown that mean levels of A1c have remained higher than current glycemic goals with the Hvidore study reporting a mean A1c of 8.6% in more than 2000 youth with T1D worldwide.[86] Similarly, data from the SEARCH study report a mean A1c of 8.2% in youth with T1D with 17% having an A1c of 9.5% or more.[87] These data from Hvidore and SEARCH are after DCCT in which it has been shown conclusively that intensive glycemic control improves vascular outcomes in T1D. Several factors have been suggested to play a role in poorer glycemic control in youth than in adults including insulin resistance of puberty, fear of hypoglycemia (especially in youth with hypoglycemic unawareness and the inability to effectively communicate to caregivers about this), and the psychological challenges of adolescence, among others.[88] In the SEARCH study, the statistically significant correlates of poorer glycemic control in the multivariate model for T1D were younger age, longer diabetes duration, weight less than 85th percentile (vs being obese), living in a single-parent household or other household structure (vs living in a 2-parent household), type of diabetes care provider (adult endocrinologist or none vs pediatric endocrinologist), race/ethnicity other than non-Hispanic white, being female, and lower parental education.[87]

Insulin pump (continuous subcutaneous insulin infusion [CSII]) therapy became more widely accepted for youth with T1D in the mid-1990s after the availability of rapid-acting insulin. Previously, pediatric diabetologists were cautious about pump use in children, particularly as a result of the threefold increase in severe hypoglycemia reported amongst intensively treated patients in DCCT.[89] Of those in the DCCT, two-thirds used an insulin pump at some time and all used regular insulin in their pumps. With advances in insulin development and in pump features, however, the fear of severe hypoglycemia associated with intensive diabetes management has diminished. Numerous reviews of insulin pump therapy exist.[90–92]

In the SEARCH study, sociodemographic characteristics were associated with insulin regimen. Insulin pump therapy was more frequently used by older youth, females, non-Hispanic whites, and families with higher income and education ($P = .02$ for females, $P<.001$ for others). Insulin pump use was associated with the lowest hemoglobin A1c levels in all age groups.[93]

There is great hope that technological advances will lead to improved glycemic outcomes. One such advance, the development of continuous glucose monitors (CGM), was evaluated in a recent clinical trial funded by the Juvenile Diabetes Research Foundation. Among children and adults with T1D with an A1c of 7.0% or more at enrollment in the study, a significant reduction in A1c was observed in adults (≥25 years) but not in participants aged 5 to 14 years or 15 to 24 years when subjects assigned to CGM use were compared with the controls.[94] However, when further stratified by CGM use, reductions in A1c were observed among children and young adults who wore the CGM for at least 6 days a week during the study period.[95] Among study participants whose A1c was less than 7.0% at enrollment in the trial, of which about half were less than 25 years of age, the CGM group was able to maintain A1c levels at baseline values with less biochemical hypoglycemia, whereas A1c levels rose with time in the control group.[96] Further research is needed to identify barriers and address challenges to improved care in youth with T1D.

PREVALENCE OF COMPLICATIONS

The DCCT showed that intensive glycemic control reduces the long-term vascular complications of hyperglycemia in T1D. Unfortunately, diabetic complications continue to be a major cause of morbidity and mortality in persons with T1D and cardiovascular disease (CVD) is the leading cause of death.[97] Moreover, intensively controlled blood glucose often comes at the cost of increased hypoglycemia compared with less intensive (or pre-DCCT conventional) management.[89,98] Specifically, improved glycemic control in the DCCT was associated with a 2- to 6-fold increase in severe hypoglycemia in intensively treated subjects compared with conventionally treated subjects.[99]

However, in the past few decades several advances have been made in the care of persons with T1D including home glucose monitoring,[100] development of insulin analogues,[101] demonstration of the benefit of intensive diabetes management on the prevention of microvascular[85,89] and macrovascular disease,[98,102] insulin pump therapy,[103] and more recently the advent of CGM.[104] Although hypoglycemia continues to be the most important barrier to tight glycemic control, the increased use of insulin pumps or nonpeaking basal insulin have decreased this risk[105] and consistent use of CGM technology has the potential for further reductions in hypoglycemic events.[95]

Furthermore, there are data to suggest that care for T1D has improved as shown by reduced rates of microvascular disease in the past decades,[106–108] whereas data on CVD suggest that substantially less progress has been made in reduction of macrovascular disease rates.[97,108,109] However, the DCCT/EDIC study has shown that intensive glycemic control over a mean of 6.5 years reduced CVD complications by 57% after a mean of 17 years of follow-up.[98] To address the increased morbidity and mortality caused by CVD in T1D, guidelines have been published[83,110–114] that address CVD risk factors in youth with T1D. All of these guidelines emphasize the importance of improved glycemic control to optimize cardiovascular health in youth with T1D, a topic the authors have reviewed recently with respect to dyslipidemia.[115]

In addition to glycemic control, hypertension and dyslipidemia are also important vascular disease risk factors with extensive data to support their role as targets to improve cardiovascular health in people with T1D.[116] Despite abundant data on the importance of control of blood pressure and dyslipidemia, adequate control of these vascular disease risk factors is frequently not achieved.[117,118] There are fewer data addressing these issues in children and adolescents.[115] Therefore, despite extensive data that support aggressive treatment of vascular disease risk factors (glycemia, blood pressure, and cholesterol, among others) in adults with T1D, the question arises as to how these data in adults apply to youth with T1D and furthermore how CVD risk factors should be treated in youth with T1D.

Unfortunately, although the clinical care and outcomes of T1D continue to improve, early mortality in T1D remains, as do questions on how to prevent this.[109] For patients diagnosed with T1D at less than 18 years of age between 1965 and 1979 and followed to 1994, the standardized mortality ratios (SMR) in Japan (n = 1408) and Finland (n = 5126) were 12.9 and 3.7, respectively.[119] A Norwegian cohort of 1906 patients with T1D diagnosed at less than 15 years of age between 1973 and 1982 (46,147 person-years) reported an SMR for all-cause mortality of 4.0 with an SMR of 20 for ischemic heart disease. Acute metabolic complications of T1D were the most common cause of death in those less than 30 years of age.[120] Similarly, data from the United Kingdom report a hazard ratio of 3.7 for annual mortality for people with T1D compared with nondiabetics (8.0 vs 2.4/100,000 person-years) with CVD as the predominant cause of death.[121] EURODIAB has reported an SMR of 2.0 in 12 European countries that followed 28,887 children with T1D (141 deaths during 219,061 person-years) with a range of SMR from 0 to 4.7 among the countries included in the study.[122] The complications of T1D (see the article by Melendez-Ramirez and colleagues) and hypoglycemia (see the article by Philip E. Cryer) are reviewed elsewhere in this issue.

SUMMARY

Data from large epidemiologic studies worldwide indicate that the incidence of T1D has been increasing by 2% to 5% worldwide and that the prevalence of

T1D is approximately 1 in 300 in the United States by 18 years of age. Research on risk factors for T1D is an active area of research to identify genetic and environmental triggers that could potentially be targeted for intervention. Although significant advances have been made in the clinical care of T1D with resultant improvements in quality of life and clinical outcomes, much more needs to be done to improve care of, and ultimately find a cure for T1D. Epidemiologic studies have an important ongoing role to investigate the complex causes, clinical care, prevention, and cure of T1D.

REFERENCES

1. American Diabetes Association. Diagnosis and classification of diabetes mellitus. Diabetes Care 2009;32(Suppl 1):S62–7.
2. Liese AD, D'Agostino RB Jr, Hamman RF, et al. The burden of diabetes mellitus among US youth: prevalence estimates from the SEARCH for Diabetes in Youth Study. Pediatrics 2006;118:1510–8.
3. Dabelea D, Bell RA, D'Agostino RB Jr, et al. Incidence of diabetes in youth in the United States. JAMA 2007;297:2716–24.
4. Rewers M, Norris J, Dabelea D. Epidemiology of type 1 diabetes mellitus. Adv Exp Med Biol 2004;552:219–46.
5. Dabelea D, Klingensmith GJ, editors. Epidemiology of pediatric and adolescent diabetes. New York (NY): Informa Healthcare USA Inc; 2008.
6. Eisenbarth GS. Type I diabetes mellitus. A chronic autoimmune disease. N Engl J Med 1986;314:1360–8.
7. Wilkin TJ. The accelerator hypothesis: weight gain as the missing link between type I and type II diabetes. Diabetologia 2001;44:914–22.
8. Gale EA. Declassifying diabetes. Diabetologia 2006;49:1989–95.
9. Karvonen M, Viik-Kajander M, Moltchanova E, et al. Incidence of childhood type 1 diabetes worldwide. Diabetes Mondiale (DiaMond) Project Group. Diabetes Care 2000;23:1516–26.
10. DIAMOND Project Group. Incidence and trends of childhood type 1 diabetes worldwide 1990–1999. Diabet Med 2006;23:857–66.
11. Variation and trends in incidence of childhood diabetes in Europe. EURODIAB ACE Study Group. Lancet 2000;355:873–6.
12. Levy-Marchal C, Patterson CC, Green A. Geographical variation of presentation at diagnosis of type I diabetes in children: the EURODIAB study. European and dibetes. Diabetologia 2001;44(Suppl 3):B75–80.
13. Libman IM, LaPorte RE, Becker D, et al. Was there an epidemic of diabetes in nonwhite adolescents in Allegheny County, Pennsylvania? Diabetes Care 1998; 21:1278–81.
14. Lipman TH, Jawad AF, Murphy KM, et al. Incidence of type 1 diabetes in Philadelphia is higher in black than white children from 1995 to 1999: epidemic or misclassification? Diabetes Care 2006;29:2391–5.
15. Lipman TH, Chang Y, Murphy KM. The epidemiology of type 1 diabetes in children in Philadelphia 1990–1994: evidence of an epidemic. Diabetes Care 2002; 25:1969–75.
16. Kostraba JN, Gay EC, Cai Y, et al. Incidence of insulin-dependent diabetes mellitus in Colorado. Epidemiology 1992;3:232–8.
17. Hermann R, Knip M, Veijola R, et al. Temporal changes in the frequencies of HLA genotypes in patients with type 1 diabetes–indication of an increased environmental pressure? Diabetologia 2003;46:420–5.

18. Kaila B, Dean HJ, Schroeder M, et al. HLA, day care attendance, and socio-economic status in young patients with type 1 diabetes. Diabet Med 2003;20:777–9.

19. Gillespie KM, Bain SC, Barnett AH, et al. The rising incidence of childhood type 1 diabetes and reduced contribution of high-risk HLA haplotypes. Lancet 2004;364:1699–700.

20. Vehik K, Hamman RF, Lezotte D, et al. Increasing incidence of type 1 diabetes in 0- to 17-year-old Colorado youth. Diabetes Care 2007;30:503–9.

21. Vandewalle CL, Coeckelberghs MI, De Leeuw IH, et al. Epidemiology, clinical aspects, and biology of IDDM patients under age 40 years. Comparison of data from Antwerp with complete ascertainment with data from Belgium with 40% ascertainment. The Belgian Diabetes Registry. Diabetes Care 1997;20:1556–61.

22. Thunander M, Petersson C, Jonzon K, et al. Incidence of type 1 and type 2 diabetes in adults and children in Kronoberg, Sweden. Diabetes Res Clin Pract 2008;82:247–55.

23. Patterson CC, Dahlquist GG, Gyurus E, et al. Incidence trends for childhood type 1 diabetes in Europe during 1989–2003 and predicted new cases 2005–20: a multicentre prospective registration study. Lancet 2009;373:2027–33.

24. Haller MJ, Atkinson MA, Schatz D. Type 1 diabetes mellitus: etiology, presentation, and management. Pediatr Clin North Am 2005;52:1553–78.

25. Turner R, Stratton I, Horton V, et al. UKPDS 25: autoantibodies to islet-cell cytoplasm and glutamic acid decarboxylase for prediction of insulin requirement in type 2 diabetes. UK Prospective Diabetes Study Group. Lancet 1997;350:1288–93.

26. Leslie RD, Williams R, Pozzilli P. Clinical review: type 1 diabetes and latent autoimmune diabetes in adults: one end of the rainbow. J Clin Endocrinol Metab 2006;91:1654–9.

27. Naik RG, Palmer JP. Latent autoimmune diabetes in adults (LADA). Rev Endocr Metab Disord 2003;4:233–41.

28. Soltesz G, Patterson CC, Dahlquist G. Worldwide childhood type 1 diabetes incidence–what can we learn from epidemiology? Pediatr Diabetes 2007;8(Suppl 6):6–14.

29. Green A, Gale EAM, Patterson CC. Incidence of childhood-onset insulin-dependent diabetes mellitus: the EURODIAB ACE Study. Lancet 1992;339:905–9.

30. Karvonen M, Pitkaniemi M, Pitkaniemi J, et al. Sex difference in the incidence of insulin-dependent diabetes mellitus: an analysis of the recent epidemiological data. World Health Organization DIAMOND Project Group. Diabetes Metab Rev 1997;13:275–91.

31. Gale EA, Gillespie KM. Diabetes and gender. Diabetologia 2001;44:3–15.

32. Weets I, De Leeuw IH, Du Caju MV, et al. The incidence of type 1 diabetes in the age group 0–39 years has not increased in Antwerp (Belgium) between 1989 and 2000: evidence for earlier disease manifestation. Diabetes Care 2002;25:840–6.

33. Pundziute-Lycka A, Dahlquist G, Nystrom L, et al. The incidence of type I diabetes has not increased but shifted to a younger age at diagnosis in the 0–34 years group in Sweden 1983–1998. Diabetologia 2002;45:783–91.

34. Kyvik KO, Nystrom L, Gorus F, et al. The epidemiology of type 1 diabetes mellitus is not the same in young adults as in children. Diabetologia 2004;47:377–84.

35. Mayer-Davis EJ, Bell RA, Dabelea D, et al. The many faces of diabetes in American youth: type 1 and type 2 diabetes in five race and ethnic populations: the SEARCH for Diabetes in Youth Study. Diabetes Care 2009;32(Suppl 2):S99–101.

36. Bell RA, Mayer-Davis EJ, Beyer JW, et al. Diabetes in non-Hispanic white youth: prevalence, incidence, and clinical characteristics: the SEARCH for Diabetes in Youth Study. Diabetes Care 2009;32(Suppl 2):S102–11.
37. Mayer-Davis EJ, Beyer J, Bell RA, et al. Diabetes in African American youth: prevalence, incidence, and clinical characteristics: the SEARCH for Diabetes in Youth Study. Diabetes Care 2009;32(Suppl 2):S112–22.
38. Lawrence JM, Mayer-Davis EJ, Reynolds K, et al. Diabetes in Hispanic American youth: prevalence, incidence, demographics, and clinical characteristics: the SEARCH for Diabetes in Youth Study. Diabetes Care 2009;32(Suppl 2):S123–32.
39. Liu LL, Yi JP, Beyer J, et al. Type 1 and type 2 diabetes in Asian and Pacific Islander U.S. youth: the SEARCH for Diabetes in Youth Study. Diabetes Care 2009;32(Suppl 2):S133–40.
40. Dabelea D, DeGroat J, Sorrelman C, et al. Diabetes in Navajo youth: prevalence, incidence, and clinical characteristics: the SEARCH for Diabetes in Youth Study. Diabetes Care 2009;32(Suppl 2):S141–7.
41. Mehers KL, Gillespie KM. The genetic basis for type 1 diabetes. Br Med Bull 2008;88:115–29.
42. Virtanen SM, Knip M. Nutritional risk predictors of beta cell autoimmunity and type 1 diabetes at a young age. Am J Clin Nutr 2003;78:1053–67.
43. Concannon P, Erlich HA, Julier C, et al. Type 1 diabetes: evidence for susceptibility loci from four genome-wide linkage scans in 1,435 multiplex families. Diabetes 2005;54:2995–3001.
44. Vehik K, Hamman RF, Lezotte D, et al. Trends in high-risk HLA susceptibility genes among Colorado youth with type 1 diabetes. Diabetes Care 2008;31: 1392–6.
45. Redondo MJ, Fain PR, Eisenbarth GS. Genetics of type 1A diabetes. Recent Prog Horm Res 2001;56:69–89.
46. Redondo MJ, Jeffrey J, Fain PR, et al. Concordance for islet autoimmunity among monozygotic twins. N Engl J Med 2008;359:2849–50.
47. Redondo MJ, Yu L, Hawa M, et al. Heterogeneity of type I diabetes: analysis of monozygotic twins in Great Britain and the United States. Diabetologia 2001;44: 354–62.
48. Fourlanos S, Dotta F, Greenbaum CJ, et al. Latent autoimmune diabetes in adults (LADA) should be less latent. Diabetologia 2005;48:2206–12.
49. Gillespie KM, Gale EA, Bingley PJ. High familial risk and genetic susceptibility in early onset childhood diabetes. Diabetes 2002;51:210–4.
50. Hamalainen AM, Knip M. Autoimmunity and familial risk of type 1 diabetes. Curr Diab Rep 2002;2:347–53.
51. Tsirogianni A, Pipi E, Soufleros K. Specificity of islet cell autoantibodies and coexistence with other organ specific autoantibodies in type 1 diabetes mellitus. Autoimmun Rev 2009;8:687–91.
52. Barker JM. Type 1 diabetes associated autoimmunity: natural history, genetic associations and screening. J Clin Endocrinol Metab 2006;91(4):1210–7.
53. Kahn HS, Morgan TM, Case LD, et al. Association of type 1 diabetes with month of birth among U.S. youth: The SEARCH for Diabetes in Youth Study. Diabetes Care 2009;32:2010–5.
54. Vaiserman AM, Carstensen B, Voitenko VP, et al. Seasonality of birth in children and young adults (0–29 years) with type 1 diabetes in Ukraine. Diabetologia 2007;50:32–5.
55. Jongbloet PH, Groenewoud HM, Hirasing RA, et al. Seasonality of birth in patients with childhood diabetes in The Netherlands. Diabetes Care 1998;21:190–1.

56. Samuelsson U, Johansson C, Ludvigsson J. Month of birth and risk of developing insulin dependent diabetes in south east Sweden. Arch Dis Child 1999; 81:143–6.

57. McKinney PA. Seasonality of birth in patients with childhood type I diabetes in 19 European regions. Diabetologia 2001;44(Suppl 3):B67–74.

58. Willis JA, Scott RS, Darlow BA, et al. Seasonality of birth and onset of clinical disease in children and adolescents (0–19 years) with type 1 diabetes mellitus in Canterbury, New Zealand. J Pediatr Endocrinol Metab 2002;15:645–7.

59. Laron Z, Shamis I, Nitzan-Kaluski D, et al. Month of birth and subsequent development of type I diabetes (IDDM). J Pediatr Endocrinol Metab 1999;12: 397–402.

60. Ye J, Chen RG, Ashkenazi I, et al. Lack of seasonality in the month of onset of childhood IDDM (0.7–15 years) in Shanghai, China. J Pediatr Endocrinol Metab 1998;11:461–4.

61. Kida K, Mimura G, Ito T, et al. Incidence of type 1 diabetes mellitus in children aged 0–14 in Japan, 1986–1990, including an analysis for seasonality of onset and month of birth: JDS study. The Data Committee for Childhood Diabetes of the Japan Diabetes Society (JDS). Diabet Med 2000;17:59–63.

62. Collado-Mesa F, Diaz-Diaz O, Ashkenazi I, et al. Seasonality of birth and type 1 diabetes onset in children (0–14 years) in Cuba. Diabet Med 2001;18:939–40.

63. Mathieu C, Gysemans C, Giulietti A, et al. Vitamin D and diabetes. Diabetologia 2005;48:1247–57.

64. Mohr SB, Garland CF, Gorham ED, et al. The association between ultraviolet B irradiance, vitamin D status and incidence rates of type 1 diabetes in 51 regions worldwide. Diabetologia 2008;51:1391–8.

65. Stene LC, Ulriksen J, Magnus P, et al. Use of cod liver oil during pregnancy associated with lower risk of type I diabetes in the offspring. Diabetologia 2000;43:1093–8.

66. Stene LC, Joner G. Use of cod liver oil during the first year of life is associated with lower risk of childhood-onset type 1 diabetes: a large, population-based, case-control study. Am J Clin Nutr 2003;78:1128–34.

67. Kumar J, Muntner P, Kaskel FJ, et al. Prevalence and associations of 25-hydroxyvitamin D deficiency in US children: NHANES 2001–2004. Pediatrics 2009; DOI: 10.1542/peds.2009-0051.

68. Bierschenk L, Alexander J, Wasserfall C, et al. Vitamin D levels in subjects with and without type 1 diabetes residing in a solar rich environment. Diabetes Care 2009;32:1977–9.

69. Ostman J, Lonnberg G, Arnqvist HJ, et al. Gender differences and temporal variation in the incidence of type 1 diabetes: results of 8012 cases in the nationwide Diabetes Incidence Study in Sweden 1983–2002. J Intern Med 2008;263: 386–94.

70. Pundziute-Lycka A, Urbonaite B, Dahlquist G. Infections and risk of type I (insulin-dependent) diabetes mellitus in Lithuanian children. Diabetologia 2000;43:1229–34.

71. Goldberg E, Krause I. Infection and type 1 diabetes mellitus – a two edged sword? Autoimmun Rev 2009;8:682–6.

72. Norris JM, Beaty B, Klingensmith G, et al. Lack of association between early exposure to cow's milk protein and beta-cell autoimmunity. Diabetes Autoimmunity Study in the Young (DAISY). JAMA 1996;276:609–14.

73. Virtanen SM, Hypponen E, Laara E, et al. Cow's milk consumption, disease-associated autoantibodies and type 1 diabetes mellitus: a follow-up study in

siblings of diabetic children. Childhood Diabetes in Finland Study Group. Diabet Med 1998;15:730–8.

74. Bodington MJ, McNally PG, Burden AC. Cow's milk and type 1 childhood diabetes: no increase in risk. Diabet Med 1994;11:663–5.

75. Mayer EJ, Hamman RF, Gay EC, et al. Reduced risk of IDDM among breast-fed children. The Colorado IDDM Registry. Diabetes 1988;37:1625–32.

76. Vaarala O, Knip M, Paronen J, et al. Cow's milk formula feeding induces primary immunization to insulin in infants at genetic risk for type 1 diabetes. Diabetes 1999;48:1389–94.

77. Norris JM, Barriga K, Klingensmith G, et al. Timing of initial cereal exposure in infancy and risk of islet autoimmunity. JAMA 2003;290:1713–20.

78. Ziegler AG, Schmid S, Huber D, et al. Early infant feeding and risk of developing type 1 diabetes-associated autoantibodies. JAMA 2003;290:1721–8.

79. Virtanen SM, Kenward MG, Erkkola M, et al. Age at introduction of new foods and advanced beta cell autoimmunity in young children with HLA-conferred susceptibility to type 1 diabetes. Diabetologia 2006;49:1512–21.

80. Hypponen E, Laara E, Reunanen A, et al. Intake of vitamin D and risk of type 1 diabetes: a birth-cohort study. Lancet 2001;358:1500–3.

81. Fronczak CM, Baron AE, Chase HP, et al. In utero dietary exposures and risk of islet autoimmunity in children. Diabetes Care 2003;26:3237–42.

82. Knekt P, Reunanen A, Marniemi J, et al. Low vitamin E status is a potential risk factor for insulin-dependent diabetes mellitus. J Intern Med 1999;245:99–102.

83. Silverstein J, Klingensmith G, Copeland K, et al. Care of children and adolescents with type 1 diabetes: a statement of the American Diabetes Association. Diabetes Care 2005;28:186–212.

84. American Diabetes Association. Standards of medical care in diabetes–2010. Diabetes Care 2010;33(Suppl 1):S11–61.

85. Effect of intensive diabetes treatment on the development and progression of long-term complications in adolescents with insulin-dependent diabetes mellitus: Diabetes Control and Complications Trial. Diabetes Control and Complications Trial Research Group. J Pediatr 1994;125:177–88.

86. Danne T, Mortensen HB, Hougaard P, et al. Persistent differences among centers over 3 years in glycemic control and hypoglycemia in a study of 3,805 children and adolescents with type 1 diabetes from the Hvidore Study Group. Diabetes Care 2001;24:1342–7.

87. Petitti DB, Klingensmith GJ, Bell RA, et al. Glycemic control in youth with diabetes: the SEARCH for Diabetes in Youth Study. J Pediatr 2009;155:668–72.

88. Chase HP. Understanding diabetes. 11th editon. Denver (CO): Paros Press; 2006.

89. The effect of intensive treatment of diabetes on the development and progression of long-term complications in insulin-dependent diabetes mellitus. The Diabetes Control and Complications Trial Research Group. N Engl J Med 1993;329:977–86.

90. Maahs DM, Horton LA, Chase HP. The use of insulin pumps in youth with type 1 diabetes. Diabetes Technol Ther 2010;12(Suppl 1):S59–65.

91. Chase H. Understanding insulin pumps and continuous glucose monitors. 1st edition. Denver (CO): The Children's Diabetes Foundation at Denver; 2010. p. 7.

92. Phillip M, Battelino T, Rodriguez H, et al. Use of insulin pump therapy in the pediatric age-group: consensus statement from the European Society for Paediatric Endocrinology, the Lawson Wilkins Pediatric Endocrine Society, and the International Society for Pediatric and Adolescent Diabetes, endorsed by the American

Diabetes Association and the European Association for the Study of Diabetes. Diabetes Care 2007;30:1653–62.

93. Paris CA, Imperatore G, Klingensmith G, et al. Predictors of insulin regimens and impact on outcomes in youth with type 1 diabetes: the SEARCH for Diabetes in Youth Study. J Pediatr 2009;155:183–9.

94. Tamborlane WV, Beck RW, Bode BW, et al. Continuous glucose monitoring and intensive treatment of type 1 diabetes. N Engl J Med 2008;359:1464–76.

95. Juvenile Diabetes Research Foundation Continuous Glucose Monitoring Study Group. Effectiveness of continuous glucose monitoring in a clinical care environment: evidence from the Juvenile Diabetes Research Foundation continuous glucose monitoring (JDRF-CGM) trial. Diabetes Care 2010;33:17–22.

96. Juvenile Diabetes Research Foundation Continuous Glucose Monitoring Study Group. The effect of continuous glucose monitoring in well-controlled type 1 diabetes. Diabetes Care 2009;32:1378–83.

97. Libby P, Nathan DM, Abraham K, et al. Report of the National Heart, Lung, and Blood Institute-National Institute of Diabetes and Digestive and Kidney Diseases Working Group on Cardiovascular Complications of Type 1 Diabetes Mellitus. Circulation 2005;111:3489–93.

98. Nathan DM, Cleary PA, Backlund JY, et al. Intensive diabetes treatment and cardiovascular disease in patients with type 1 diabetes. N Engl J Med 2005; 353:2643–53.

99. Epidemiology of severe hypoglycemia in the Diabetes Control and Complications Trial. The DCCT Research Group. Am J Med 1991;90:450–9.

100. Saudek CD, Derr RL, Kalyani RR. Assessing glycemia in diabetes using self-monitoring blood glucose and hemoglobin A1c. JAMA 2006;295:1688–97.

101. Hirsch IB. Insulin analogues. N Engl J Med 2005;352:174–83.

102. Nathan DM, Lachin J, Cleary P, et al. Intensive diabetes therapy and carotid intima-media thickness in type 1 diabetes mellitus. N Engl J Med 2003;348: 2294–303.

103. Tamborlane WV. Fulfilling the promise of insulin pump therapy in childhood diabetes. Pediatr Diabetes 2006;7(Suppl 4):4–10.

104. Klonoff DC. Continuous glucose monitoring: roadmap for 21st century diabetes therapy. Diabetes Care 2005;28:1231–9.

105. Chase HP, Dixon B, Pearson J, et al. Reduced hypoglycemic episodes and improved glycemic control in children with type 1 diabetes using insulin glargine and neutral protamine Hagedorn insulin. J Pediatr 2003;143:737–40.

106. Maahs DM, Rewers M. Editorial. Mortality and renal disease in type 1 diabetes mellitus–progress made, more to be done. J Clin Endocrinol Metab 2006;91:3757–9.

107. Hovind P, Tarnow L, Rossing K, et al. Decreasing incidence of severe diabetic microangiopathy in type 1 diabetes. Diabetes Care 2003;26:1258–64.

108. Pambianco G, Costacou T, Ellis D, et al. The 30-year natural history of type 1 diabetes complications: the Pittsburgh Epidemiology of Diabetes Complications Study experience. Diabetes 2006;55:1463–9.

109. Rewers M. Why do people with diabetes die too soon? More questions than answers. Diabetes Care 2008;31:830–2.

110. American Diabetes Association. Management of dyslipidemia in children and adolescents with diabetes. Diabetes Care 2003;26:2194–7.

111. Kavey RE, Allada V, Daniels SR, et al. Cardiovascular risk reduction in high-risk pediatric patients: a scientific statement from the American Heart Association Expert Panel on Population and Prevention Science; the Councils on Cardiovascular Disease in the Young, Epidemiology and Prevention, Nutrition, Physical

Activity and Metabolism, High Blood Pressure Research, Cardiovascular Nursing, and the Kidney in Heart Disease; and the Interdisciplinary Working Group on Quality of Care and Outcomes Research: endorsed by the American Academy of Pediatrics. Circulation 2006;114:2710–38.

112. McCrindle BW, Urbina EM, Dennison BA, et al. Drug therapy of high-risk lipid abnormalities in children and adolescents: a scientific statement from the American Heart Association Atherosclerosis, Hypertension, and Obesity in Youth Committee, Council of Cardiovascular Disease in the Young, with the Council on Cardiovascular Nursing. Circulation 2007;115:1948–67.

113. Daniels SR, Greer FR. Lipid screening and cardiovascular health in childhood. Pediatrics 2008;122:198–208.

114. Donaghue KC, Chiarelli F, Trotta D, et al. ISPAD clinical practice consensus guidelines 2006–2007. Microvascular and macrovascular complications. Pediatr Diabetes 2007;8:163–70.

115. Maahs DM, Wadwa RP, Bishop F, et al. Dyslipidemia in youth with diabetes: to treat or not to treat? J Pediatr 2008;153:458–65.

116. American Diabetes Association. Standards of medical care in diabetes–2008. Diabetes Care 2008;31(Suppl 1):S12–54.

117. Maahs DM, Kinney GL, Wadwa P, et al. Hypertension prevalence, awareness, treatment, and control in an adult type 1 diabetes population and a comparable general population. Diabetes Care 2005;28:301–6.

118. Wadwa RP, Kinney GL, Maahs DM, et al. Awareness and treatment of dyslipidemia in young adults with type 1 diabetes. Diabetes Care 2005;28:1051–6.

119. Asao K, Sarti C, Forsen T, et al. Long-term mortality in nationwide cohorts of childhood-onset type 1 diabetes in Japan and Finland. Diabetes Care 2003; 26:2037–42.

120. Skrivarhaug T, Bangstad HJ, Stene LC, et al. Long-term mortality in a nationwide cohort of childhood-onset type 1 diabetic patients in Norway. Diabetologia 2006; 49:298–305.

121. Soedamah-Muthu SS, Fuller JH, Mulnier HE, et al. All-cause mortality rates in patients with type 1 diabetes mellitus compared with a non-diabetic population from the UK general practice research database, 1992–1999. Diabetologia 2006;49:660–6.

122. Patterson CC, Dahlquist G, Harjutsalo V, et al. Early mortality in EURODIAB population-based cohorts of type 1 diabetes diagnosed in childhood since 1989. Diabetologia 2007;50:2439–42.

Economics of Type 1 Diabetes

Betty T. Tao, PhD[a],*, David G. Taylor, PhD[b]

KEYWORDS

- Cost of type 1 diabetes • Economics of type 1 diabetes
- Cost-of-illness analysis

Economic evaluation is used to weigh the relative merits of health care policies and programs by examining the costs and benefits associated with alternatives. In the case of diabetes, for example, an intervention that would delay the onset of type 1 diabetes (T1D) symptoms by a year cannot be adequately evaluated without knowing the full costs incurred by a patient in a year. It might be that a particular intervention is prohibitively expensive, whereas another equally effective therapy is much more affordable. Thus, estimating the costs of a disease, called cost-of-illness (COI) analysis, can help inform policy makers as to where scarce resources should be focused so that funded work has the highest potential impact. Because of the increasing number of patients and the high costs of care, in terms of maintenance and complications, diabetes has been the focus of several COI studies over the years because the epidemic has grown.[1–4]

Although many studies over the past few decades have examined the cost of diabetes, they typically combine T1D and type 2 diabetes (T2D), the 2 major forms of the disease. However, the underlying differences in the pathologic condition and expression of the 2 diseases imply that there is no basis for assuming that the costs associated with T1D are proportional to the share of T1D patients to total diabetic patients. With the increasing focus on obesity and the increase in the incidence of T2D, the impact of T1D is often overlooked. However, because large sums are spent on T1D research each year and T1D incidence rates continue to increase, accurate accounting of the societal costs of T1D would provide valuable information to the public, government, health care providers, and organizations focused on finding a cure for the disease.[5]

This article reviews methodologies developed for estimating COI, examines the current literature on diabetes costs, and presents the latest estimates of the economic impact of T1D in terms of both direct medical costs (ie, treatment costs) and indirect costs (eg, lost wages) resulting from the disease. The article discusses the methods

[a] Center for Health Research and Policy, CNA, 4825 Mark Center Drive, Alexandria, VA 22311, USA
[b] Office of the President, CNA, 4825 Mark Center Drive, Alexandria, VA 22311, USA
* Corresponding author. 1021 North Garfield Street, Apartment 512, Arlington, VA 22201.
E-mail address: betatao@gmail.com

Endocrinol Metab Clin N Am 39 (2010) 499–512
doi:10.1016/j.ecl.2010.05.004
0889-8529/10/$ – see front matter © 2010 Elsevier Inc. All rights reserved.

and data used in cost studies, reviews methods for separating T1D patients from all patients with diabetes in national representative datasets, and discusses the challenges in identifying T1D patients in large population surveys. The costs that are associated with T1D are examined and the various approaches for measuring them discussed. Finally, before drawing conclusions the authors discuss limitations of current studies and suggest future work.

COST OF ILLNESS: METHODS AND DATA

Economic evaluations consist of a comparison of the costs and consequences of alternative services or interventions. In general, full economic evaluations consist of the following: cost-effectiveness analysis (CEA), cost-utility analysis (CUA), and cost-benefit analysis (CBA). CEA and CUA evaluate the costs and effects of an intervention in terms of outcomes, such as dollars per life-years gained. CUA accounts for individuals' preferences, or utility levels, and would instead examine the effect of an intervention in terms of dollars per quality-adjusted life-years or disability-adjusted life-years. CBA evaluates all costs and benefits associated with an intervention in terms of dollars.[6]

COI analyses are thus a partial economic analysis because they examine the costs of a disease without any comparison with alternatives. However, a COI analysis is a necessary input in full economic evaluation of alternative programs that would affect disease prevention, or delay the onset of symptoms. COI studies provide health care policy makers and research funders with additional information that can be considered along with the medical science behind a particular disease to evaluate potential choices among policies or research funding decisions. Furthermore, COI studies provide information on disease costs that are important in understanding the relative impact among diseases. As is seen in this article, the indirect costs associated with T1D are disproportionate to the disease population. Thus, making policy decisions without considering COI results could lead to misinformed policy decisions for T1D care and research.

Methods

Estimating the economic impact of diseases requires examining medical and nonmedical costs. Medical costs include those directly related to the disease, doctor visits, and reoccurring consumable costs, such as insulin, syringes, or test strips for diabetes. Medical costs also medical treatment for complications or comorbidities related to diabetes. For example, if diabetic patients are more likely to suffer from cardiovascular disease, some of the costs associated with cardiovascular disease should be included in the cost of diabetes. However, cardiovascular diseases that would have occurred in a similar population of patients without diabetes should not be included. COI studies should provide a method for correctly apportioning these costs. Some researchers, in studies further described, have implemented specific methods to apportion costs related to comorbidities according to their prevalence in the patient and nonpatient population. Other medical costs may include costs related to transportation for medical visits and the research spent on investigating a cure, prevention, or delay of symptoms.

Nonmedical costs, frequently referred to as indirect costs, can be substantial, particularly for chronic diseases. In the case of T1D, which generally occurs at a young age, the accumulation of lost productivity can be particularly substantial because it occurs over a lifetime with the disease. Additional important factors that should be considered when calculating indirect costs include early mortality related to the disease and its impact on lost wages, disability related to the disease, and the lost productivity of informal caretakers (such as family members).

Estimating indirect costs can involve making difficult decisions on how to measure the value of human life.[1] The human capital approach to estimating indirect costs of early mortality or disability uses market earnings to measure the associated lost productivity. One difficulty in implementing this method is determining the wages associated with nonmarket activities, such as a homemaker's time. Researchers have approximated some of these costs by estimating how much it would cost to purchase equivalent services from the market.[6] Most studies use the human capital approach to estimating indirect costs.[1]

Another method for measuring the costs of early mortality examines the extra compensation workers require to take on additional risk in the work place. This method uses consumers' actual revealed preferences to estimate the value of additional life. For example, if 2 jobs are identical but the first job is associated with 1 more job-related death for every 10,000 workers and workers earn $500 more per year than the workers in the second job, then the implied value of a statistical life is $5 million for workers in the second job who are willing to forgo $500 for a 1 in 10,000 lower annual risk.[7] However, depending on the occupation or circumstance, the implied value of an additional year of life can vary greatly. Another way to value additional life is to actually ask individuals how much they are willing to pay for a particular cure or intervention that prolongs life by a certain period.[6]

The time frame for estimating costs may differ depending on the study. Many studies examine the total costs of a disease over a year using the estimated disease prevalence.[2,4] Another method examines an incidence-based calculation of the costs over an individual or a cohort's lifetime. Examples include the calculations of lifetime costs of smoking, stroke, and obesity.[8-11] For T1D, as is discussed, an incidence approach that considers lifetime costs is especially appropriate because of the disease's early onset and required lifetime maintenance.

Data

The availability of data is commonly the limiting factor for estimating disease costs. Ideally, a single dataset for a large, nationally representative population would provide detailed direct and indirect cost data for individuals with T1D. Medical claims databases provided detailed information on the medical care used by patients, costs of the medical care, and the diagnoses associated with each visit. However, claims data may be from one insurer or cover individuals residing in one state, and are usually not representative of the whole country. Furthermore, relying on insurance data limits the population to those individuals with insurance and can skew the data by omitting the costs for the uninsured population. In addition, claims data may lack the information needed to estimate the lost productivity associated with the disease of patients and informal caretakers.

The US government sponsors various large surveys related to health care. These surveys generally allow for nationally representative estimates of medical care use and disease prevalence rates (for the more prevalent diseases) in the United States and provide the most comprehensive and frequently used datasets for COI studies. Table A1 of an American Diabetes Association (ADA) 2007 study describes available data sources.[2] Three important nationally representative data sources that can be used to examine disease prevalence are summarized:

- The *Medical Expenditures Panel Survey (MEPS)*[12] collects data on medical care use, expenditure, and the sources of payment. The data contain health-status measures, use and expenditure by medical service, income, and demographic measures. Sample members are asked to recall medical conditions and events, with supplemental information collected from medical care providers identified by household respondents. Each year, MEPS collects data on approximately 30,000 individuals. MEPS administers the Diabetes Care Survey (DCS), a self-reported questionnaire to individuals who report having diabetes. The DCS collects information on health care use such as the use of insulin, oral medications, and even diet and exercise behavior of diabetic patients. However, it does not ask diabetic patients which type of diabetes they have.

- The *National Health Interview Survey (NHIS)*[13] interviews households to collect detailed information on the health status and conditions (including diabetes—not separated by type), behaviors, and access to care of a nationally representative large group of people. Although it collects some information on health care use, it does not contain health expenditure data. The NHIS sample consists of 100,000 persons surveyed annually.
- The *National Health and Nutrition Examination Survey (NHANES)*[14] was designed to monitor the health and nutritional status of adults and children in the United States. It collects information on medical, dental, and physiologic measurements, and laboratory testing by medical personnel. The laboratory component includes tests for blood glucose and c-peptide levels, which allow for estimating of undiagnosed patients and distinguishing between different types of diabetes, but sample sizes are limited—the survey only examines approximately 5000 individuals per year.

Other National Health Care Surveys include the National Ambulatory Health Care Survey, National Hospital Ambulatory Medical Care Survey, National Hospital Discharge Survey, National Survey of Ambulatory Surgery, National Home and Hospice Care Survey, National Home Health Aid Survey, National Nursing Home Survey, National Nursing Assistant Survey, National Survey of Residential Care Facilities, and others.[15] These surveys provide information on the use of a nationally representative sample of individuals, but do not collect information on expenditures or costs.

Identifying T1D Patients

Understanding the costs incurred by individuals with T1D requires accurately categorizing patients in the available datasets. The American Diabetes Association estimates that there are 17.9 million individuals diagnosed with diabetes (T1D and T2D combined) in the United States.[2] According to the Centers for Disease Control and Prevention (CDC), 5% to 10% of diabetes patients have T1D.[16] T1D patients incur costs throughout their lifetime, starting typically at a young age compared with T2D patients, who are usually diagnosed later in life. Further, because T1D is an autoimmune disease characterized by the destruction of the insulin-secreting cells in the pancreas, patients are dependent on injected insulin to survive. In comparison, T2D patients can generally control their symptoms with changes in diet and physical activity or by taking oral medications during the early stages of the disease. Given these differences in the characteristics of the patients and the distinct nature of the diseases, it is not appropriate to assume that T1D costs represent 5% to 10% of the total cost of diabetes simply because patients with T1D make up 5% to 10% of the total number of patients with diabetes.

For patients with diabetes, most COI studies do not distinguish between the 2 forms of the disease and combine T1D and T2D patients and costs. Most studies that specifically examine the T1D population frequently concentrate on children, are not nationally representative, are not United States based, or examine only the medical expenditures related to T1D.[17] Two recent exceptions by Dall and colleagues[18] and Tao and colleagues[19,20] examined the costs of T1D in the United States, and found the costs of T1D to be disproportional to the number of T1D patients compared with the number of T2D patients.

A likely cause of the small amount of T1D cost studies is the difficulty in distinguishing patients with T1D from those with T2D in secondary data. Most population surveys simply ask whether a person has ever been told by a physician that he or she has diabetes, and data with detailed medical tests are not nationally representative. An exception is the NHANES, in which c-peptide (in itself of limited usefulness to distinguish T1D from T2D) is measured in some survey participants. However, the survey collects information on 5000 individuals a year, and the resulting population of T1D patients would be too small for meaningful analysis.

Alternatively, researchers have used "clinically derived definitions" to identify individuals with T1D from the larger diabetes datasets using such characteristics as age of onset and usage of insulin therapy. For example, one study categorized T1D based on whether the individual used insulin within 6 months of the date that diabetes was identified and never used any oral medication within the time period of the study.[3] Another study used the age of onset and the exclusive use of insulin for therapy as criteria for categorizing T1D, and confirmed the validity of these criteria using c-peptide data available in the NHANES.[21] Prior and colleagues[22] found that clinically derived definitions generally work well to distinguish T1D and T2D.

Tao and colleagues[19,20] recognized that categorizing T1D using these characteristics could lead to overestimates or underestimates of the number of T1D patients. Overestimation occurs if T2D patients are misclassified with T1D, which is possible given that obesity rates have been on the increase, especially in children. Because a strong indicator of T2D in a child is being overweight or obese,[23,24] the investigators refined their definition of individuals with T1D by excluding children younger than 18 years who reported having diabetes and who were also considered obese or did not use insulin therapy. The number of T1D patients is underestimated by the number of individuals diagnosed with T1D more than the age cutoff used. This figure includes those who are misdiagnosed with T2D because of their age. For example, latent autoimmune diabetes of the adult (LADA) occurs in adults older than 30 years and is commonly misdiagnosed as T2D in the early stages of the disease.[25] However, it is likely a slowly progressing form of T1D. An estimated 10% of adults diagnosed with T2D are misdiagnosed and truly have T1D.[26,27] Because the typical LADA patient is nonobese, the investigators limited the sample to patients with a body mass index (calculated as the weight in kilograms divided by height in meters, squared) of 30 or less if they were diagnosed when they were older than 30 years.[28,29] Similarly, Cusick and colleagues[30] categorized patients with T1D by whether they began insulin therapy within the year if diagnosed at age 30 or younger, whether they began insulin therapy within the year, and whether they were within 20% of their desired weight, and whether they were diagnosed at age 40 or younger. Tao and colleagues found that 1.1 million individuals had T1D in the United States. To confirm the validity of the estimated T1D sample of 1.1 million patients in the MEPS, the investigators applied the same T1D clinically derived definitions that had been described to the NHANES data; they found a sample representing 1.4 million individuals nationwide who had T1D, slightly larger than the MEPS sample. In general, the numbers found by the 2 methods were similar.

Medical claims data from insurance databases or Medicare/Medicaid provide diagnosis codes, which can also be used to identify patients who have diabetes.

For example, Dall and colleagues[18] examined the claims files from the 2006 Ingenix MCURE database, which provides the medical claims data of more than 16 million insured individuals younger than 65 years, the Medicare 5% Sample File, which covers nearly 2 million people age 65 and older, and California's MediCal database, which provides claims data for more than a million individuals on Medicaid. The investigators were able to identify T1D patients in the databases by analyzing the International Classification of Diseases, Ninth Revision, Clinical Modification (ICD-9-CM) codes associated with each claim.[31] Using claims data requires further extrapolation to generalize to the population, especially the noninsured population. Dall and colleagues[18] estimated that 1.0 million individuals had T1D in the United States in 2007. **Table 1** shows the number of T1D patients by age group found by Dall and colleagues and Tao and colleagues in comparison with the number of total diabetic patients found by the ADA. Although the 2 studies used differing methodologies and data sets, the estimated number of T1D patients were similar. Dall and colleagues found that T1D patients comprised approximately 5.7% of the total diagnosed diabetic population, but comprised almost 79% of the diabetic population younger than 18 years. Although Tao and colleagues found that T1D patients comprise a lower percentage of the total diabetic population for those younger than 18 years (40% vs the 79% found by Dall and colleagues), the investigators found the overall percentage of T1D patients to be 6.5% of the total diabetic population, which is similar to the percentage estimated by Dall and colleagues.

T1D COSTS
Medical Costs

The Agency for Health Research Quality reported that $48 billion in health expenditures were related to diabetes (T1D and T2D) in 2006 according to data from the MEPS.[32] These costs include hospital inpatient services, ambulatory care including hospital outpatient services, emergency room visits, prescribed medicines, and home health care. This figure is calculated using the primary diagnosis of a health care encounter and does not include medical expenditures where diabetes is

Table 1
Number of T1D and T2D patients in the United States

Age	Number of Diabetic Patients (ADA 2008) (Thousands)	Number of T1D Patients (Tao et al) (Thousands)	Percent T1D Patients (Tao et al) (%)	Number of T1D Patients (Dall et al) (Thousands)	Percent T1D Patients (Dall et al) (%)
<18	157	63	40.1	124	79.0
18–34	964	231	24.0	253	26.2
35–44	1,686	197	11.7	143	8.5
45–54	3,443	239	6.9	158	4.6
55–59	2,307	140	6.1	81	3.5
60–64	2,261	93	4.1	81	3.6
65–69	1,879	48	2.6	45	2.4
≥70	4,788	132	2.8	120	2.5
Total	17,485	1,143	6.5	1,005	5.7

Data from Refs.[2,18–20]

indirectly related. For example, diabetes is associated with higher risks for neurologic disease, peripheral vascular disease, cardiovascular disease, renal disease, endocrine/metabolic complications, ophthalmic disease, and other chronic complications.[4] Including all medical costs associated with diabetes and its comorbidities, this figure grows to $116 billion as estimated by the ADA.[2] Note that the ADA included costs associated with a nursing home, which the MEPS did not.

As mentioned, the distinct nature of T1D suggests that knowing the combined cost of T1D and T2D does not necessarily inform the calculation of individual costs for the 2 diseases, even if the population proportions are known. Dall and colleagues[18] estimated the costs of T1D separately from T2D using various data sources. The investigators examined the excess medical costs for T1D patients compared with T2D patients and the general population associated with hospital inpatient and outpatient visits, physician visits, emergency room, nursing home, prescription drugs, and medical supplies. To ensure that medical costs included those associated with T1D comorbidities, Dall and colleagues[18] calculated etiologic fractions, which estimated the share of medical costs associated with T1D complications by age and gender using the prevalence of T1D in the population and rate ratios of the number of medical events associated with each complication for diabetes and the general population. Dall and colleagues calculated that more than $10.5 million per year was spent on direct medical costs related to T1D, or roughly 10% of all diabetes medical expenditures. Considering that the population of patients with T1D is approximately 6%, medical costs are somewhat disproportional to the population of patients with T1D (**Table 2**).

Tao and colleagues used a matching methodology to examine the costs associated with T1D.[19,20] The investigators used the MEPS to identify T1D patients, and examined direct medical expenditures and indirect costs associated with the disease by matching a T1D patient to a counterpart without diabetes. Because finding an exact match becomes increasingly difficult as more matching variables are used, they implemented a propensity score matching technique first introduced by Rosenbaum and Rubin that is frequently used in the program-evaluation literature.[33] To obtain an

Table 2					
Yearly medical costs attributed to diabetes					
Cost Component	Diabetes (ADA 2008) (Millions)	T1D (Dall et al) (Millions)	Percent T1D (Dall et al) (%)	T1D (Tao et al[a]) (Millions)	Percent T1D (Tao et al) (%)
	(1)	(2)	(3) = (2)/(1) × 100	(4)	(5) = (4)/(1) × 100
Hospital inpatient	58,344	3,322	5.7	2,514	4.3
Nursing/ residential facility	7,487	4,447	59.4	—	—
Outpatient care	22,743	1,237	5.4	1,410	6.2
Medications and supplies	27,684	1,541	5.6	2,319	8.4
Total	116,258	10,547	9.1	6,243	5.4

[a] Tao et al do not estimate the costs associated with nursing homes.
Data from Refs.[2,18–20]

unbiased and accurate measure of costs attributed to T1D, the matched control individuals must be as similar to the population with T1D as possible so that the only difference between the 2 can be attributed to T1D. Tao and colleagues used a range of variables to match T1D patients to individuals without diabetes. The matching method does not require detailed and accurate knowledge of the relationship between diabetes and its comorbidities,[2,4] but there is a trade-off; matching does not work well when important unobservable differences between those with and without the disease exist, as is true for T2D.[34] However, the investigators argue that T1D is a good candidate for matching because unlike T2D, the presence of unobservable factors that affects the probability of having the disease is minimal. They note that 80% of T1D patients do not have a family member with the disease, and behavioral and environmental causes are not definitively known.[25,35] MEPS does not survey those institutionalized individuals and thus, the investigators did not provide an estimate of the nursing home costs attributed to T1D. Excluding nursing home costs from the figures estimated by Dall and colleagues, the 2 studies found that more than $6 billion in medical costs was attributed to T1D annually. The 2 independent methodologies used the calculations of the medical costs associated with T1D and yielded similar results. The annual medical cost estimates for T1D by both groups are compared in **Table 2** along with the ADA figures on the overall costs of diabetes.

The first column of **Table 2** shows the costs of diabetes (both forms of the disease), as reported by the ADA in 2008.[2] The second column shows the costs estimated by Dall and colleagues[18] for T1D and the third column shows the share of T1D costs as a percentage diabetes costs. Although the investigators found that T1D patients comprise 5.7% of the total diagnosed diabetic population, these T1D patients incur 9.1% of medical costs attributed to diabetes. The fourth column of **Table 2** shows the medical costs for T1D estimated by Tao and colleagues. The fifth column shows the costs attributed to T1D as estimated by Tao and colleagues as a percentage of total diabetes costs. The study found that medications and medical supply costs attributed to T1D were more than 8.4% of the total diabetes costs, although T1D patients comprise 6.5% of the total number of diabetic patients. In general, the estimates by the 2 studies were similar.

As mentioned, diabetes is associated with a higher risk of other conditions and often leads to complications, which can drive up medical costs for that subgroup of T1D patients. Dall and colleagues[18] estimated the health care use associated with each complication for T1D patients compared with the nondiabetic population. The investigators found that T1D patients used, overall, 2 to 4 times more medical care related to each complication than an individual without T1D. Further, T1D patients used more of each type of care, except for emergency room care, than T2D patients. Tao and colleagues[19,20] found that T1D patients with complications, as estimated as those patients who have an inpatient hospital stay, spent on average $23,000 more in medical care annually than patients without diabetes, almost 4 times their estimate for average medical costs. Of that $23,000, the majority, $14,000, or more than 60%, was spent on hospital inpatient care. The remaining costs consisted of ambulatory visits, medications and supplies, and emergency room visits.

Indirect Costs

The indirect costs associated with diabetes can be substantial. Diabetes can affect the productivity of patients, leading to increased missed days of work or school, and decreased productivity when at work or school.[36] Patients with T1D must test their blood glucose levels and inject insulin several times a day. Without even including the discomfort and lifestyle changes associated with the disease, the indirect costs can be very high. Milton and colleagues[37] compiled and reviewed studies in the literature addressing the social consequences of T1D. These investigators found that children with T1D were more likely to miss school and that their employment outcomes were worse, but school performance and educational attainment remained unaffected.

Tao and colleagues[19,20] measured indirect costs by estimating the lost workdays, bed days, and missed schooldays attributed to T1D by comparing a T1D patient with a similar individual without diabetes. Their study provided an overall measure of lost productivity attributed to T1D by comparing the incomes of T1D patients with those of individuals without diabetes, for a cohort older than 18 years. **Table 3** compares the indirect cost components of T1D patients with those of their matched individuals without diabetes. T1D patients missed twice as many workdays and 9 times as many schooldays as those without diabetes. Furthermore, income levels of T1D patients were 80% of their counterparts with no diabetes.

Dall and colleagues[18] estimated indirect costs by calculating the proportion of days spent receiving medical services related to T1D by age and gender, whereby office and outpatient visits accounted for half days and emergency room and hospital visits accounted for full days. The investigators estimated the long-term disability costs associated with T1D by using the proportion of hospital inpatient days.[18] **Table 4** shows the total yearly indirect costs attributed to T1D for the T1D population and the total diabetes population in millions of dollars. Indirect costs attributed to T1D were 7.5% of total indirect diabetes costs.

The ADA 2008 study estimated the number of deaths attributed to diabetes by using data from the CDC on the cause of death and by applying the etiologic fractions mentioned.[2] The investigators found that 284,000 deaths were attributed to diabetes in 2007. To estimate the proportion that was specifically attributed to T1D, Dall and colleagues[18] used the proportion of diabetes-attributed emergency room visits associated with T1D by comorbidity. The investigators then estimated loss attributed to T1D-related premature death by calculating the present value of future productivity by gender and age for these individuals. As shown in **Table 4**, the investigators estimated that early mortality costs attributed to T1D were 3.3 billion and 8.5% of the early mortality costs attributed to diabetes of both types in 2008.

Table 5 summarizes the yearly per capita and total medical and indirect costs attributed to T1D from the 2 recent estimates. Dall and colleagues[18] and Tao and colleagues[19,20] found that T1D is associated with approximately $14,000 in additional medical and indirect expenditure per year for an individual and more than $14 billion in

Table 3
Yearly per capita indirect costs by T1D status

Cost Component	No Diabetes (1)	T1D (2)	Attributed to T1D (3) = (2) − (1)	Ratio of T1D to Non-T1D (4) = (2)/(1)
Missed work (days)	5.3	10.8	5.5	2.0
Bed days (days)	3.6	11.2	7.6	3.1
Missed school (days)	0.4	3.7	3.3	9.3
Individual income (dollars)	30,122	22,958	−7,164.0	0.8
Household income (dollars)	54,991	45,511	−9,480.0	0.8

Data from Tao B, Pietropaolo M, Atkinson M, et al. Estimating the cost of type 1 diabetes in the U.S.: a propensity score matching method. PLoS One, in press; and Tao B, Taylor D. Economic costs of type 1 diabetes in the U.S. CNA/IPR 12984. January 2009.

Table 4
Total yearly indirect costs attributed to diabetes

Cost Component	Diabetes (Millions)	T1D (Millions)	Percent T1D (%)
Absenteeism	2,597	127	4.9
Presenteeism	19,955	1,240	6.2
Inability to do work from disability	7,949	674	8.5
Premature mortality	26,902	2,298	8.5
Reduced productivity (not in labor force)	757	39	5.2
Total	58,160	4,378	7.5

Data from Dall TM, Mann SE, Zhang Y, et al. Distinguishing the economic costs associated with type 1 and type 2 diabetes. Popul Health Manag 2009;12(2):103–10.

total expenditures for all T1D patients. The differing composition of medical and indirect costs between the 2 studies is likely because of the differing methodologies used by the researchers. Dall and colleagues found a larger amount of medical costs associated with T1D and Tao and colleagues estimated greater indirect costs. However, the overall cost estimates were similar. The overall costs of T1D, between $14 billion and $15 billion per year, constituted roughly 8% of all diabetes costs for a population of approximately 1 million patients with T1D, who comprised roughly 5% of the population of patients with diabetes. Thus, costs attributed to T1D are disproportionately higher than what the number of T1D patients compared with T2D patients would imply.

Lifetime Costs

Incidence-based costs of T1D measure lifetime costs by estimating the savings associated with the total elimination of the disease. Yearly costs offer only a snapshot of the impact of a disease, but can be easier to implement. Following a large group of individuals over a long period to estimate lifetime incidence may not be practical. Thus, studies examining the lifetime costs of a disease have combined data on annual incidence and prevalence to model lifetime expenditures.[38–40]

Mainly because of the lack of a large enough longitudinal sample, there are few incidence studies examining the health costs of diseases and only a handful that attempt to examine lifetime costs for T1D. A study by Stern and Levy[39] examined the direct costs of a T1D patient in Israel over a 35-year span. The investigators constructed a hypothetical T1D patient and traced out the probability of complications and associated costs over the next 35 years. Another study used an incidence method to

Table 5
Total medical and indirect costs

Cost Component	Dall et al		Tao et al	
	Per Capita	Yearly (Billions)	Per Capita	Yearly (Billions)
Medical	10,495	10.5	6,243	6.9
Indirect	4,361	4.4	7,164	7.5
Total	14,856	14.9	13,407	14.4

Data from Refs.[18–20]

	Table 6 Lifetime costs of a new cohort of T1D patients			
Age of Onset	**Number of New Patients (Millions)**	**Medical (In Million Dollars)**	**Income Loss (In Million Dollars)**	**Total Costs (In Million Dollars)**
3–9	6,483	746	1,208	1,954
10–19	11,980	1,489	2,923	4,412
20–29	3,528	337	1,130	1,467
30–39	3,976	395	1,279	1,674
40–45	2,464	309	776	1,085
Total	28,430	3,276	7,316	10,592

Data from Tao B, Pietropaolo M, Atkinson M, et al. Estimating the cost of type 1 diabetes in the U.S.: a propensity score matching method. PLoS One, in press; and Tao B, Taylor D. Economic costs of type 1 diabetes in the U.S. CNA/IPR 12984. January 2009.

estimate the cost of T1D in England and Wales.[40] The investigators applied baseline estimates on the incidence of T1D by age to total population figures, estimates on the excess mortality faced by T1D patients, and the probability of complications and their associated health care costs to estimate the cost faced by T1D patients by age. The investigators also examined the indirect costs associated with T1D of early mortality on lifetime earnings.

Tao and colleagues[19,20] used 2 approaches for measuring lifetime costs. First, they estimated the lifetime costs of a cohort of newly diagnosed patients by generating a longitudinal profile of costs from the cross sections of patients in their sample stratified by age and age of diagnosis. Second, using this longitudinal profile they estimated the amount incurred by the current population over the rest of its lifetime. The first approach seeks to measure the amount saved by a future cohort of newly diagnosed patients if the onset of T1D could be prevented. The second method finds the savings by the current patient population if a cure (ie, means to prevent or reverse the disease) were discovered today. These calculations, however, neglect improvements in health care technology over time. **Table 6** shows the estimated lifetime costs of a new cohort of newly diagnosed T1D patients. The investigators showed that, over their lifetime, a new cohort of patients with T1D—roughly 30,000 individuals—spent over $3 billion on medical costs and incurred more than $7 billion in lost wages. The total, $10 billion, was for a single cohort. The current population of T1D patients, estimated to be 1.4 million, was projected to incur $400 billion over their lifetime.[14,15]

SUMMARY

Knowing the economic impact of T1D is important to various stakeholders across the community. Patients, caregivers, and doctors all benefit from a broader understanding of the true costs of the disease. The research community, companies who develop drugs, and the health care policy community can use this information to better apportion scarce resources and determine equitable policies for T1D patients.

This article provides an introduction to COI methodologies and reviews the work on the costs of diabetes with a focus on T1D, an often-neglected population in economic analyses. As highlighted, previous studies often made an assumption that costs of T1D were similar to the general diabetes costs and were proportional to the fraction of patients with T1D. Furthermore, those studies that did try and independently calculate T1D costs were limited to small groups and were not nationally representa-tive. However, 2 recent studies showed the disproportionate nature of the costs of T1D. Although the studies found that T1D patients compose approximately 5% to 6% of the total diagnosed diabetic population, the medical and indirect costs attrib-uted to T1D were approximately 8%. One study estimated a larger proportion of direct costs, the other a larger proportion of indirect costs. Further, one study demonstrated the long-term impact of T1D, a disease often diagnosed early in life that has economic consequences across the lifetimes of patients. Combined with the ongoing medical research on T1D, COI studies add to the body of knowledge and quantify, from an economic standpoint, the costs, well known to the community, that are associated with the disease.

Although these recent studies are among the first to compute the economic costs of T1D to the individual and society in the United States, they are not yet complete in several ways. Thus, the following recommendations represent some ways to improve research in this area. First and most important is to ensure that the nationally represen-tative datasets used in COI analyses include a field on the type of diabetes. This addi-tion would allow researchers to estimate costs without having to assume clinically derived definitions of T1D, or require the use of non-nationally representative insur-ance claims data with diagnosis codes to identify T1D patients. Further, there is no easy method for including the discomfort and suffering caused by the multiple daily insulin shots. The economic impact on informal care givers—likely an important cost for T1D patients who are often children—is not captured, nor do the surveys capture the costs of over-the-counter drugs. Improving the data collected in each of these areas would allow more accurate T1D costs to be computed. This list is not meant to detract from the contributions of the recent studies; rather, these limitations are highlighted as a call to continued research to better document the true costs of T1D.

Patients with T1D suffer from a unique, autoimmune form of diabetes that differs in its economic impact from T2D. As might be expected given the different etiologies of the 2 forms of diabetes, costs are disproportionately higher for T1D patients. With a typical diagnosis early in life, T1D patients suffer economic impact across a lifetime with the disease. These recent COI results increase knowledge about the impact of T1D in the scientific and public community at large. These results can be built on by other researchers looking to improve on current studies on the economic costs of T1D. Armed with these estimates, better-informed decisions can be made regarding the country's limited health care resources.

REFERENCES

1. Ettaro L, Songer TJ, Zhang P, et al. Cost-of-illness studies in diabetes mellitus. Pharmacoeconomics 2004;22(3):149–64.
2. American Diabetes Association. Economic costs of diabetes in the U.S. in 2007. Diabetes Care 2008;31(3):596–615.
3. Johnson JA, Pohar SL, Majumdar SR. Health care use and costs in the decade after identification of type 1 and type 2 diabetes: a population-based study. Dia-betes Care 2006;29(11):2403–8.
4. American Diabetes Association. Economic costs of diabetes in the U.S. in 2002. Diabetes Care 2003;26(3):917–32.
5. Thomas J. Type 1 diabetes research landscape: CNA\IPR 12779. 2008.
6. Drummond MF, Sculpher MJ, Torrance GW, et al. Methods for the economic eval-uation of health care programmes. Oxford; New York; Auckland: Oxford Univer-sity Press; 2005.

7. Fisher A, Chestnut LG, Violette DM. The value of reducing risks of death: a note on new evidence. J Policy Anal Manage 1989;8(1):88–100.
8. Hodgson TA. Cigarette smoking and lifetime medical expenditures. Milbank Q 1992;70(1):81–125.
9. Taylor TN, Davis PH, Torner JC, et al. Lifetime cost of stroke in the United States. Stroke 1996;27(9):1459–66.
10. Thompson D, Edelsberg J, Colditz GA, et al. Lifetime health and economic consequences of obesity. Arch Intern Med 1999;159(18):2177–83.
11. Rasmussen SR, Prescott E, Sorensen TI, et al. The total lifetime costs of smoking. Eur J Public Health 2004;14(1):95–100.
12. Agency for Healthcare Research and Quality. Medical expenditure panel survey (MEPS) [internet]. Available at: http://www.meps.ahrq.gov/mepsweb. Accessed September 23, 2009.
13. National Center for Health Statistics at the Centers for Disease Control and Prevention. National Health Interview Survey (NHIS) [internet]. Available at: http://www.cdc.gov/nchs/nhis.htm. Accessed May 13, 2010.
14. National Center for Health Statistics at the Centers for Disease Control and Prevention. National Health and Nutrition Examination Survey (NHANES) [internet]. Available at: http://www.cdc.gov/nchs/nhanes.htm. Accessed September 23, 2009.
15. Centers for Disease Control and Prevention. Surveys and data collection systems [internet]. Available at: http://www.cdc.gov/nchs/surveys.htm. Accessed May 13, 2010.
16. Centers for Disease Control and Prevention. National diabetes fact sheet, United States [internet]. Available at: www.cdc.gov/diabetes/pubs/pdf/ndfs_2005.pdf. 2005. Accessed September 23, 2009.
17. Icks A, Holl RW, Giani G. Economics in pediatric type 1 diabetes—results from recently published studies. Exp Clin Endocrinol Diabetes 2007;115:448–54.
18. Dall TM, Mann SE, Zhang Y, et al. Distinguishing the economic costs associated with type 1 and type 2 diabetes. Popul Health Manag 2009;12(2):103–10.
19. Tao B, Pietropaolo M, Atkinson M, et al. Estimating the cost of type 1 diabetes in the U.S.: a propensity score matching method. PLoS One, in press.
20. Tao B, Taylor D. Economic costs of type 1 diabetes in the U.S. CNA/IPR 12984. 2009 Jan.
21. Koopman R, Mainous A, Diaz V, et al. Changes in age at diagnosis of type 2 diabetes mellitus in the United States, 1988 to 2000. Ann Fam Med 2005;3:60–3.
22. Prior MJ, Prout T, Miller D, et al. C-peptide and the classification of diabetes mellitus patients in the early treatment diabetic retinopathy study. Report number 6. The ETDRS Research Group. Ann Epidemiol 1993;3(1):9–17.
23. American Diabetes Association. Type 2 diabetes in children and adolescents. Diabetes Care 2000;23(3):381–9.
24. American Diabetes Association. Diagnosis and classification of diabetes mellitus. Diabetes Care 2008;31(Suppl 1):S55–60.
25. Dorman JS, McCarthy BJ, O'Leary LA, et al. Risk factors for insulin dependent diabetes. In: Harris MI, Cowie CC, Stern MP, et al, editors. Diabetes in America. 2nd edition. National Institute of Health NIDDK, no. 95–1468. Bethesda (MD): The National Diabetes Information Clearinghouse; 1995. p. 165–77, chapter 8.
26. Landin-Olsson M. Latent autoimmune diabetes in adults. Ann N Y Acad Sci 2002; 958:112–6.
27. Fourlanos S, Perry C, Stein MS, et al. A clinical screening tool identifies autoimmune diabetes in adults. Diabetes Care 2006;29(5):970–5.

28. Naik RG, Palmer JP. Latent autoimmune diabetes in adults (LADA). Rev Endocr Metab Disord 2003;4(3):233–41.
29. Prando R, Cheli V, Melga P, et al. Is type 2 diabetes a different disease in obese and nonobese patients? Diabetes Care 1998;21(10):1680–5.
30. Cusick M, Meleth A, Agron E, et al. Associations of mortality and diabetes complications in patients with type 1 and type 2 diabetes. Diabetes Care 2005;28: 617–25.
31. Centers for Disease Control and Prevention. Classification of diseases, functioning, and disability [internet]. Available at: http://www.cdc.gov/nchs/icd/icd9cm.htm. Accessed June 16, 2010.
32. Agency for Healthcare Research and Quality. Total expenses for selected conditions by type of service: United States 2005, Medical Expenditure Panel Survey Component Data 2005.
33. Rosenbaum PR, Rubin DB. The central role of the propensity score in observational studies for causal effects. Biometrika 1983;70(1):41–55.
34. Akobundu E, Ju J, Blatt L, et al. Cost-of-illness studies: a review of current methods. Pharmacoeconomics 2006;24(9):869–90.
35. Peng H, Hagopian W. Environmental factors in the development of type 1 diabetes. Rev Endocr Metab Disord 2006;7(3):149–62.
36. Kahn ME. Health and labor market performance: the case of diabetes. J Labor Econ 1998;16(4):878–99.
37. Milton B, Holland P, Whitehead M. The social and economic consequences of childhood-onset type 1 diabetes mellitus across the lifecourse: a systematic review. Diabet Med 2006;23(8):821–9.
38. Huang ES, Basu A, O'Grady M, et al. Projecting the future diabetes population size and related costs for the U.S. Diabetes Care 2009;32(12):2225–9.
39. Stern Z, Levy R. Analysis of direct cost of standard compared with intensive insulin treatment of insulin-dependent diabetes mellitus and cost of complications. Acta Diabetol 1996;33(1):48–52.
40. Gray A, Fenn P, McGuire A. The cost of insulin-dependent diabetes mellitus (IDDM) in England and Wales. Diabet Med 1995;12(12):1068–76.

Advances in the Prediction and Natural History of Type 1 Diabetes

Ezio Bonifacio, PhD[a],*, Anette G. Ziegler, MD[b]

KEYWORDS

- Type 1 diabetes • Autoantibodies • Islet autoimmunity

When making predictions, a number of specific assumptions should be noted from the very start. First, what is true of the past may not be true for the future. For example, type 1 diabetes (T1D) risk in Finland now is twice as high as it was 30 years ago and previous algorithms may no longer provide accurate predictions of future disease. Second, much of the data obtained regarding T1D comes from very select cohorts. Whites and individuals who have a family history of T1D represent most studies. Because much of what is presented in this article refers to data gathered from whites, it should be acknowledged that sometimes incorrect assumptions will be made about T1D in patients from all ethnicities because of the relative lack of data in those groups. Third, knowledge is gained mainly from studying children who are at risk for T1D. The biomarkers are relatively abundant in at-risk children compared with at-risk adults, and clinicians are still a long way from being able to predict T1D in adults. Fourth, and very importantly, risk estimates are an average rate, meaning that in a set of 100 individuals with the ascribed characteristics, an average of 50 will develop diabetes within 10 years. Some of the 100, however, will develop diabetes within a few weeks, some will never develop diabetes, and sadly there is still a lack of knowledge to say who will and who will not get the disease. Furthermore, the risks are described with gaussian confidence intervals, but for the individual who develops T1D it is an all-or-nothing event (not at all gaussian). If one accepts these caveats and limitations from the outset, one can use currently available genetic, immune, and metabolic biomarkers to provide risk estimates for individuals within the available data set.[1]

[a] Deutsche Forschungsgemeinschaft Center for Regenerative Therapies Dresden, Technische Universität Dresden, Tatzberg 47/49, 01307 Dresden, Germany
[b] Forschergruppe Diabetes, Klinikum rechts der Isar, Technische Universität München, Kölner Platz 1, 80804 München, Germany
* Corresponding author.
E-mail address: ezio.bonifacio@crt-dresden.de

Endocrinol Metab Clin N Am 39 (2010) 513–525
doi:10.1016/j.ecl.2010.05.007
0889-8529/10/$ – see front matter © 2010 Elsevier Inc. All rights reserved.

GENETIC MARKERS OF T1D RISK
Family History and Its Implications

Nearly 1 in every 250 United States children will be born into a family already affected by T1D.[2] Children with an affected family member have a 5% T1D risk by age 20, whereas children with no family history have a risk of only 0.3%. Risk in the children with a family history of diabetes can be further stratified on the basis of which affected family member has T1D (**Table 1**). A rare few may have an identical twin with T1D, in which case risk is nearly 50%.[3] A minority of the children with affected family members have two affected first-degree relatives and have a 20% risk. Most have one affected sibling (approximately 7% risk); father (approximately 5% risk); or mother (approximately 3% risk).[4] Despite the increased relative risk seen in children with an affected family member, most cases of T1D still come from the unaffected general population because of their far greater absolute number. Implications for the pathogenesis of T1D are that genetic load is substantial, but not absolute in determining disease. With respect to environment, a substantial amount of information has been published,[5] yet most of these data are based on association and should not be used to make firm conclusions. Moreover, environmental factors are often viewed simplistically

Table 1
Empiric risks[a] of autoantibodies and approximate risks of type 1 diabetes[b] on the basis of genetic markers

Genetic Marker	Number Per 100,000 Births	Any Islet Autoantibody Risk (%)	Multiple Islet Autoantibody Risk (%)	T1D Risk (%)
General population child	99,600	4.3	0.4	0.39
Protective HLA	73,700	4	0.03	0.04
High-risk HLA (3/4, 4/4)	2988	9.6	4.9	6
Relative of patient with T1D	400	9.4	4.8	6
Daughter	120	6.7	2.5	3
Son	120	8.5	4.1	5
Sibling	120	10.5	5.6	7
Multiple first-degree relatives	40	22	16	20
Monozygotic twin	Few	51	40	50
Protective HLA	80	4	0.1	0.1
High-risk HLA (3/4, 4/4)	28	27	20	25

Specificity of each of four islet autoantibody tests of 99%.

Protective HLA genotypes found in 74% of population, 20% of first-degree relatives, and 7% of T1D.[10,53]

High-risk HLA genotypes found in 3% of population, 7% of first-degree relatives, and 50% of T1D.[10,53]

The risks differ when these assumptions change as is the case in different populations. Islet auto-antibody risk depends on the definition of positivity (specificity and confirmation in second sample) and whether single or multiple samples are measured.

To be noticed is that as the T1D risk increases in the starting population, the likelihood that an autoantibody.

[a] Autoantibody risks are estimated empirically on the basis of the following assumptions: T1D risk in the population of 0.4%.

[b] T1D risk is approximate from the literature.[3,4,8]

with the question of whether they are causal or protective. In view of the substantial genetic load, it may be more informative to look at associations with environment as indicating genetic pathways of immune mediated beta cell loss. For example, a relationship between virus exposure and T1D could mean that immune activation against antigen, including virus, differs in T1D compared with people without chronic immune-mediated diseases so that chronic immune activation and infection are features rather than causes of T1D. Some novel functional genetic studies are potentially providing new insights into how environment is viewed.[6]

It is worth discussing chance in T1D prediction. Chance is all around, but there is a need to attribute an explanation to everything so that there is a reluctance to accept the possibility that the forces governing the outcome of the role of a dice (ie, the mathematics of chance) may also be selecting who develops T1D from within a group of individuals with similar genetic risk. "Penetrance" is the term given to the chance of genetic variation leading to disease. In the case of identical twins, it is indeed possible that chance alone rather than environment is the prime reason why immune activation against the beta cell in one of two identical twins ends up in sustained immune memory, and eventually diabetes, and in the other it is resolved without further consequences or even autoantibodies. It is not known whether the same twin will develop diabetes if the same experiment of nature could be performed again and again or if 50% of the time it will be the other twin, sometimes both, and sometimes none. One should not question the importance of environment in the current rise in T1D incidence (although by the ability to observe only a 30- to 40-year period in history one is potentially being narrow sighted), but caution is suggested in invoking environment as a determinant of T1D in one individual or groups of individuals.

The Major Genes for Prediction

HLA genotype provides most genetic risk for T1D (see **Table 1**). This fits well with an immune-mediated pathogenesis because HLA genes affect the diversity and specificity of immune responses. The HLA DR and DQ loci harbor alleles that are the most useful determinants of inherited risk.[7] T1D risk can be stratified 100-fold on the basis of HLA DR-DQ genotype.[8] If the a priori risk determined from family history is 7% (ie, a sibling), the risk can be further stratified from 0.3% up to 30% by considering HLA DR-DQ genotype. Similarly, T1D risk in children without a family history of T1D can be stratified from around 0.01% to over 5%.[9] Risk can be estimated empirically on the basis of the frequency of the HLA genotype of the child in the nondiabetic population, and in those who have T1D. For example, the HLA DR3, DR4-DQ8 genotype, which confers the highest T1D risk, is present in 2.3% of United States born white children[9] and 39% of patients who develop T1D before age 20 years. The risk of developing diabetes is approximately 7%. In comparison, the risk in children who have a T1D relative and have the DR3, DR4-DQ8 genotype is around 25%.[10] Extreme T1D risk (up to 50%) is present in a child with the DR3, DR4-DQ8 genotype who is born into a family with two or more affected family members.[11] Similar extreme risks were reported for children who are HLA DR3, DR4-DQ8 and are identical by descent to their affected sibling at these loci.[12] Finally, T1D is special with respect to genetic susceptibility in that there are HLA haplotypes that confer strong dominant protection.[7] T1D risk in a child with a T1D family history and with protective DRB1-DQB1 alleles, such as HLA DRB1∗1602-DQB1∗0602, DRB1∗07-DQB1∗0303, DRB1∗13-DQB1∗0603, and DRB1∗14-DQB1∗0503, is around 100-fold less than that in a child with similar family history but without these haplotypes.[8] Alleles at HLA class II DP loci[13] and class I loci, such as HLA A24, B38, and B39, also contribute to T1D risk,[14] but they have not yet been implemented in risk prediction models. Other genes or chromosome regions have been shown to confer T1D risk,[15] but their use in T1D prediction may not be high, and as such their incorporation into risk models has only been academic.

ISLET AUTOANTIBODIES: FORENSIC PREDICTION

The T1D risk status of a child changes markedly when islet autoantibodies develop. Autoantibodies are not thought to play a direct pathologic role in beta cell destruction, but they provide strong evidence that killing has and probably will take place again. Islet cell antibodies are the historical marker from which the earliest prediction strategies were based.[16] Autoantibodies to four major groups of islet proteins have been identified and used in predictive models: (1) insulin/proinsulin; (2) GAD65/67; (3) IA-2 (or ICA512)/IA-2β (or PHOGRIN); and (4) ZnT8.[17–21] Antibodies to other islet antigens exist,[22] but for the purposes of prediction, the four previously mentioned are currently adequate in children.[23–26]

Quantifiable Signals and Diverse Analytes that Require High-quality Assays

An important consideration of islet autoantibodies that differs from the use of genetic risk markers is that they are not present or absent categorical traits. They are measured by immunoassay and are defined by a quantifiable signal that is dependent on the strength and titer of immunoglobulin binding to antigen. Accuracy in identifying true disease-relevant signals depends on the quality of the assay used to distinguish true autoantibodies from disease-irrelevant binding. As such, substantial efforts in standardizing islet autoantibody measurement have occurred,[27,28] including the development of harmonized assays and reference units for large multicenter studies.[29] Although these have been exceptional achievements, there are still some impediments to the use and interpretation of autoantibodies. Autoantibodies to GAD65 and IA-2 are standardized and can be measured using commercial kits using radiobinding methods. Similarly, GAD antibodies can be measured with a commercially available enzyme-linked immunosorbent assay kit. Results from assays for insulin autoantibodies (IAA), however, are variable between laboratories with enormous differences in the sensitivity achieved. As yet, no commercial IAA assay is available that can achieve high sensitivity, and a select few research assays achieve high sensitivity (but importantly there are some). The ZnT8 antibodies have been recently identified and are not yet widespread in their use. There is currently only a handful of laboratories worldwide that have access to high-quality assays for the four antibodies that can be used for prediction. The early indirect immunofluorescent assay for islet cell autoantibodies is not commonly used.

Interpreting autoantibody results requires some knowledge of the assay and B cell responses because not all autoantibody-positive samples signal disease. B cell responses generally have the purpose of providing high-affinity multivalent antibodies through a selection and edit process that gives rise to multiple B cell clones that can persist throughout life.[30] Almost every B cell clone that is generated in the immune response to an organism or antigen produces a slightly different antibody even if they are directed against the same antigen or even epitope region. Most autoantibodies in T1D are of IgG isotype and the major subclass is IgG1.[31] The unique feature of an autoantibody is the antigen-binding site, which varies between each B cell clone in an individual. The specificity of every antibody is determined by a unique sequence of amino acids in its variable region.[32] At correct conformation and conditions, the antibody should bind tightly and specifically and only to its cognate antigen. The cognate antigen itself is often a complex structure and contains many sites to which autoantibodies could bind. These sites are characterized by their shape and physical interactions that occur between their exposed amino acids and those in the binding region of the autoantibody.[33] It should also be considered that autoantigens can themselves vary because of polymorphism within coding regions and the same antigenic site could differ between individuals.[34] When one talks about autoantibodies to even a single antigen, one is talking about highly diverse analytes. The job is to identify those autoantibody signals that are disease relevant and these are likely to be the ones with perfect antibody-autoantigen fit.

Considerations on the Target or Cognate Autoantigen

One should remember that the autoantibodies arise in vivo. Although the exact form and conformation of cognate antigen that the B cells see is not known, there are some clues that point to the likelihood that T1D-relevant autoreactive B cells see native or near native antigen in vivo. The original description of islet cell autoantibodies used frozen sections of human pancreas as substrate,[35] and fixation of the pancreas abolished binding of some islet cell autoantibodies. Detailed study of the autoantibody epitopes of known autoantigens shows that most need to be conformational for binding (ie, require tertiary shape).[36] In the case of IAA in humans, even the attachment of insulin to a solid phase is sufficient to disturb antibody antigen binding and results in low sensitivity and low specificity.[37] When trying to identify disease-relevant autoantibodies, it is perhaps wise not to tamper with antigen, and avoid the use of denatured proteins. It also seems unwise randomly to chop whole proteins or make peptide fragments to unveil or identify epitopes. A more sensible approach when designing antigens for autoantibody detection is to consider conformational domains of the antigen, natural processing, and potential degradation products of the antigen that may occur in vivo.

Assay Specificity and Disease Relevance: The Need for Multiple Islet Autoantibodies

Having established antigen and assay, we still need to consider probability. Bayes' theorem forms the basis of clinical diagnosis and describes the relationship between three parameters fundamental to diagnostic tests: (1) the sensitivity for disease, (2) the specificity in health or confounding disease, and (3) the a priori probability of disease in the subject being tested. In situations where the a priori probability of disease is relatively low, such as in children without a family history of T1D, the specificity of the test has a profound effect on the diagnostic use. Specificity is a function of true autoantibody signals versus nonspecific signals in the assay and how frequent the true autoantibodies are present in health. The threshold of positivity is often defined on the basis of a percentile of controls, which is at best the 99th percentile. Moreover, up to four autoantibodies are used in T1D. By chance alone there are a few percent of healthy individuals that are identified as autoantibody positive. The mathematically inclined see that most individuals in a population with single autoantibodies do not have autoimmune disease.[38–40] The detection of single autoantibodies, therefore, can rarely diagnose disease in the absence of corroborating clinical or laboratory evidence. Indeed, the presence of a single islet autoantibody in persons without clinical diabetes has rarely if ever been associated with pancreatic insulitis.[41]

T1D risk is markedly increased when islet autoantibodies to two or more of the antigen groups are found in a child.[42–47] Risk is incremental in relation to whether antibodies are against two, three, or four of the antigen groups, and among those without the full complement of four islet autoantibodies, T1D risk can vary in relation to which of the islet autoantibodies are present (**Fig. 1**). In particular, the presence of antibodies to IA-2 (or ICA512)/IA-2β (or PHOGRIN) is associated with highest risk.[44,48] Similar to

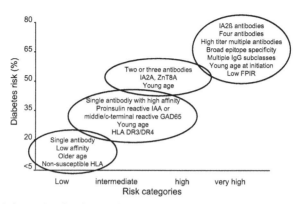

Fig. 1. Type 1 diabetes (T1D) risk stratification by islet autoantibody characteristics. Characteristics associated with low, intermediate, high, and very high risk are grouped from left to right on the abscissa with corresponding T1D risks on the ordinate. Increase in T1D risk is associated with progression of islet autoantibodies from single to multiple autoantibodies. HLA genotype discriminates risk in single antibody–positive children, but multiple antibody–positive children have high risk regardless of HLA genotype.

the number of islet autoantibodies, greater titer,[16,44] affinity,[49,50] and broadness of epitope reactivity[44] are features of islet autoantibodies that are associated with high T1D risk. The more islet autoantibodies one has and the stronger they are, the higher the T1D risk. Finally, islet autoantibodies can be transient,[51] but high titer islet autoantibodies to multiple islet antigens rarely if ever disappear before diabetes onset.

Combining Risk Biomarkers

T1D risk is a combination of the likelihood of developing disease and the rate at which it will develop. Considerable effort is made to determine risk on the basis of genes and autoantibodies, and to stage the prediabetes period using markers of beta cell function. Various combinations can be used to obtain similar overall risk, and for most combinations the risk can be calculated empirically. Risk can be stratified from less than 0.1% to greater than 70%. Current approaches use a stepwise decision tree[52] in which genetic risk is usually the first applied in the form of family history or HLA DR-DQ genotype. Autoantibodies are measured in those individuals who are considered to have sufficient genetic risk to warrant autoantibody testing. Because the risk of developing multiple islet autoantibodies is strongly linked to major histocompatibility complex (MHC) class II genotypes,[53] further typing is unlikely to be helpful in a child who has an armada of islet autoantibodies. Finally, beta cell function is measured in islet autoantibody–positive individuals using either the ability of the beta cell to secrete insulin in response to an intravenous glucose challenge or the ability of the individual to clear glucose after a meal challenge where low insulin secretion (eg, less than the first percentile) or impaired glucose tolerance are indicators of late-stage preclinical T1D.[54] More recently it has also been recognized that insulin demand from the body is also likely to affect the timing of clinical diabetes whereby increased demand as seen in obese and insulin-resistant individuals may bring forward clinical manifestation of diabetes.[55–57] A complete measure of insulin production together with insulin sensitivity may be a better measure of beta cell function for the purposes of T1D prediction.

Although the decision tree approach is logical, it may be expected that once effective preventative therapies become available, the decision tree approach could be replaced by the population-wide application of all the previously mentioned markers in a public health prevention manner. Clinicians may eventually move toward introducing a risk score based on the combination of all markers. This would represent a paradigm shift after years of increasingly complex layers of decisions in screening.

Finally, the T1D risk of an individual is not static throughout life. This is true even for genetically defined risk. Risk in a child who has no family history of T1D at birth increases more than 10-fold if his or her sibling develops T1D, and if the child has an identical twin who develops T1D, risk immediately increases 100-fold to around 50%.[3] Risk calculated from the autoantibody status usually increases over time as autoantibodies appear and their number rises. Younger age is associated with increased risk than older age. Beta cell function measures are expected to show decrease the closer someone is to disease onset. Over the lifespan of an individual, the calculated T1D risk on the basis of genes, autoantibody, age, and beta cell function change.

NATURAL HISTORY OF ISLET AUTOIMMUNITY
Early Immunization

Two characteristics are present in most children who develop T1D. Over 90% have at least one susceptible HLA class II haplotype and over 90% have islet autoantibodies. Regardless of the etiologic factors that may favor the development of islet autoimmunity in a child, it remains highly probable that the initiation of the disease process is the effector immune response to islet beta cell antigens and that the appearance of islet autoantibodies is the first detectable sign of this process.

Islet autoantibodies rarely appear before age 6 months and in children there is a peak incidence at around 1 to 2 years of age.[58,59] This suggests either that the events leading to islet autoimmunity are encountered after 6 months of age and potentially at increased frequency in early infancy or that the immune system does not have the propensity to manifest autoimmunity in the first 6 months of life. Because it has been demonstrated that neonates have deficiencies in antigen presentation and immune response,[60] and mammalian immune defense is at least partially taken care of by maternal transfer of protection against infection until weaning, it is certainly possible that the manifestation of IgG autoantibodies is impeded until late in the first year of life.

Early autoimmunization to islet antigens has a particular phenotype. Antibodies to the insulin-proinsulin antigen group are often among the first to appear,[58] and they have a strong association with HLA-DR4-DQ8 within pre-T1D children.[60] HLA DR4-DQ8–associated immune activation of insulin-reactive B and T cells is a frequent characteristic of the initial disease process of childhood diabetes. The IAA that are detected are of high-affinity IgG1 class at first detection suggesting rapid affinity maturation.[49] The high-affinity IAA bind to both insulin and proinsulin, and the intermediate products DES-(31–32)-proinsulin and DES-(64–65)-proinsulin (Adler, unpublished, 2006). These IAA probably recognize a common epitope.[49] Spreading of the immune response to other islet antigens is frequent and can be rapid (ie, acute response to all islet antigen groups) but in many cases spreading occurs at distinct time points almost as a series of new immune activation episodes.[31] This has been previously referred to as "chronic autoimmunity with remitting and relapsing activity."

The early insulin-proinsulin start and spread of autoimmunity to disease is a common autoimmunization phenotype in young prediabetic children, but it is not universal. Some prediabetic children have an acute explosive antibody response to all antigen groups with rapid progression to disease suggesting uncontrolled rapid beta cell destruction. In addition, a few young infants progress to diabetes after developing an early high-affinity autoantibody response to GAD65 before IAA. In contrast, antibodies to the IA-2/IA-2β and the ZnT8 antigen groups very rarely appear on their own or before IAA or GAD65/67 antibodies.[26] Whether the insulin, GAD, and explosive antibody phenotypes of pre-T1D represent immune response gene-associated variants or are consequences of different etiology is unknown.

Late Immunization

Although there may be a peak period of islet autoimmunization before age 2 years, islet autoantibodies can appear at any age.[59] Preliminary data from our BABYDIAB cohort shows a second peak incidence period around puberty. What is becoming more and more obvious is that the characteristics of the islet autoantibody profiles seen in these older antibody-positive children are heterogeneous and that the typical profile is different from that seen in the 1 to 2 year olds. Autoantibodies to single antigen groups, typically insulin or GAD65, without spreading is common. Lower-affinity IAA or GAD65 antibodies are also more common, as are antibodies directed against atypical epitopes. These late-appearing antibodies, even if persistent, often develop in the absence of the typical T1D and antigen-associated HLA alleles, which may explain why they appear atypical and do not often spread to multiple antibodies or disease. As with autoantibodies that develop early in life, however, the late appearance of antibodies in children with high-risk T1D genotypes is associated with progression to diabetes.

SPECULATIONS FROM THE NATURAL HISTORY FINDINGS
Immunization

Early islet autoantibody profiles suggest that the immune response occurs at the beta cell because the major targets are preferentially or exclusively expressed in the beta cell. The response against the beta cell–specific ZnT8 antigen is particularly informative because there is an exquisite specificity of autoantibodies to self-polymorphic variants of the protein. ZnT8 residue 325 lies within a major epitope of ZnT8 autoantibodies.[26,34] Children who are homozygous for the 325R variant make antibodies to the epitope that expresses 325R and not to the epitope expressing 325W, and vice versa, suggesting autoimmunization as a result of physiologic beta cell death or an event associated with induced beta cell death (eg, cytopathic virus). Also intriguing is the fact that more ubiquitous beta cell proteins, such as actin, and nuclear proteins targeted in systemic autoimmune diseases are not prominent autoantigens in T1D indicating that there must be more to antigen specificity than simply beta cell death. It is likely, therefore, that the precise target specificity of the response is favored by protein abundance in the beta cell, location within secretory structures, and preferential presentation of its peptides by the T1D-associated HLA class molecules. The right constellation to reach the threshold needed for a sustained effector immune response is likely also to include alleles at other immune response genes that lower immune activation threshold and an inflammatory cytokine milieu.

The different immunization profiles seen at early and late childhood are also potentially informative. They suggest that etiology could be heterogeneous (ie, events that lead to an insulin-dominant spreading autoimmunity at age 1 year are different from those that lead to a GAD65 restricted autoimmunity at age 11 years). It is also possible that immune activation thresholds differ with age. At very young age, an MHC-associated immunization process is predominant so that environment must provide an MHC-dependent predisposition or protection. As for any single environmental agent that causes islet autoimmunity, the evidence is still thin. Foods, viruses, vitamins, toxins, and the like have been associated, but only a few studies have looked at relationships to the appearance of islet autoimmunity, and proposed mechanisms are speculative and not entirely consistent with the autoantibody appearance findings described previously. It is hoped that the large number of cases that will be obtained by The Environmental Determinants of Diabetes in the Young study[61] will provide confirmation for some of the proposed associations so that mechanism can then be investigated.

Progression

There is no typical progression from the appearance of islet autoantibodies to clinical diabetes. It can be a matter of weeks to decades. Weeks is consistent with aggressive sustained islet beta cell destruction, whereas decades could represent either a series of waxing and waning episodes of beta cell destruction or a constant slow beta cell loss. The acute clinical onset suggests that a long prediabetes period is unlikely to have a constant rate of beta cell loss, but to include more and less active periods. Similarly, the observation that autoantibody responses spread to new islet antigens and epitopes at irregular intervals strongly suggests that active immunization is occurring at several occasions during the prediabetic period. Finally, although measureable loss of beta cell function down to below the first percentile of the normal population represents a biomarker of impending clinical disease, some islet autoantibody-positive subjects can stay at this level of function for years before clinical disease. All these observations point to the fact that beta cell destruction is under some sort of regulatory control.

A Few Missing Pieces

There are many missing pieces. The autoantibody and genetic biomarkers suggest pathways involved in susceptibility and pathogenesis, but there is little in the way of cell-mediated immunity in prediction and natural history, and there has been no discussion here of processes at and around the islet beta cell. Both of these areas of research are not yet consolidated with substantial reliable data. It is now accepted that autoreactive T cells may be present in both patients and healthy individuals. What distinguishes the autoreactive T cells in disease from those in health may be that those active in causing T1D have been activated and converted to memory T cells.[62–64] Focusing measurement on the memory T cell response and through the use of novel epitope-specific T-cell assays[65,66] is likely to provide the means to apply autoreactive T-cell measurements to prediction and a better understanding of the natural history of T1D.

SUMMARY

Although there are now better tools to measure an individual's genetic risk and document their autoantibody status, the objective measurement of ongoing beta cell death remains a major limitation in prediction of T1D. There is now sufficient evidence to state that insulitis occurs through the prediabetic period, but this may be sporadic and seems to be nowhere near as florid as what is see in rodent models of autoimmune diabetes.[67] Although it is assumed that insulitis is the causative factor in beta cell death, this has yet to be proved in human samples. It is hoped that with the renewed burst of activity in obtaining pancreas from diabetic and prediabetic individuals (Pancreatic Organ Donation Program),[67] and intensive research on this material, clinicians will be able to convert speculation from the natural history of autoantibodies into a clearer picture of disease mechanisms and pathogenesis.

ACKNOWLEDGMENTS

The authors are supported by funding from the National Institute of Diabetes and Digestive and Kidney Diseases; Juvenile Diabetes Research Foundation; the Kompetenznetz Diabetes Mellitus (Federal Ministry of Education and Research in Germany, FKZ 01GI0805-07); and the Deutsche Forschungsgemeinschaft (FZ111).

REFERENCES

1. Atkinson MA, Eisenbarth GS. Type 1 diabetes: new perspectives on disease pathogenesis and treatment. Lancet 2001;358:221–9.
2. Dabelea D, Bell RA, D'Agostino RB Jr, et al. Incidence of diabetes in youth in the United States. JAMA 2007;297:2716–24.
3. Redondo MJ, Jeffrey J, Fain PR, et al. Concordance for islet autoimmunity among monozygotic twins. N Engl J Med 2008;359:2849–50.
4. Hemminki K, Li X, Sundquist J, et al. Familial association between type 1 diabetes and other autoimmune and related diseases. Diabetologia 2009;52:1820–8.
5. Peng H, Hagopian W. Environmental factors in the development of type 1 diabetes. Rev Endocr Metab Disord 2006;7(3):149–62.
6. Dendrou CA, Plagnol V, Fung E, et al. Cell-specific protein phenotypes for the autoimmune locus IL2RA using a genotype-selectable human bioresource. Nat Genet 2009;41(9):1011–5.
7. Baisch JM, Weeks T, Giles R, et al. Analysis of HLA-DQ genotypes and susceptibility in insulin-dependent diabetes mellitus. N Engl J Med 1990;322:1836–41.
8. Lambert AP, Gillespie KM, Thomson G, et al. Absolute risk of childhood-onset type 1 diabetes defined by human leukocyte antigen class II genotype: a population-based study in the United Kingdom. J Clin Endocrinol Metab 2004;89: 4037–43.
9. Emery LM, Babu S, Bugawan TL, et al. Newborn HLA-DR, DQ genotype screening: age- and ethnicity-specific type 1 diabetes risk estimates. Pediatr Diabetes 2005;6:136–44.
10. Schenker M, Hummel M, Ferber K, et al. Early expression and high prevalence of islet autoantibodies for DR3/4 heterozygous and DR4/4 homozygous offspring of parents with type I diabetes: the German BABYDIAB study. Diabetologia 1999; 42:671–7.
11. Bonifacio E, Hummel M, Walter M, et al. IDDM1 and multiple family history of type 1 diabetes combine to identify neonates at high risk for type 1 diabetes. Diabetes Care 2004;27:2695–700.
12. Aly TA, Ide A, Jahromi MM, et al. Extreme genetic risk for type 1A diabetes. Proc Natl Acad Sci U S A 2006;103:14074–9.
13. Baschal EE, Aly TA, Babu SR, et al. HLA-DPB1∗0402 protects against type 1A diabetes autoimmunity in the highest risk DR3-DQB1∗0201/DR4-DQB1∗0302 DAISY population. Diabetes 2007;56(9):2405–9.
14. Nejentsev S, Howson JM, Walker NM, et al. Localization of type 1 diabetes susceptibility to the MHC class I genes HLA-B and HLA-A. Nature 2007; 450(7171):887–92.
15. Wellcome Trust Case Control Consortium. Genome-wide association study of 14,000 cases of seven common diseases and 3,000 shared controls. Nature 2007;447:661–78.
16. Bonifacio E, Bingley PJ, Shattock M, et al. Quantification of islet-cell antibodies and prediction of insulin-dependent diabetes. Lancet 1990;335:147–9.

17. Palmer JP, Asplin CM, Clemons P, et al. Insulin antibodies in insulin-dependent diabetics before insulin treatment. Science 1983;222:1337–9.
18. Baekkeskov S, Aanstoot HJ, Christgau S, et al. Identification of the 64K autoantigen in insulin-dependent diabetes as the GABA-synthesizing enzyme glutamic acid decarboxylase. Nature 1990;347:151–6.
19. Rabin DU, Pleasic SM, Shapiro JA, et al. Islet cell antigen 512 is a diabetes-specific islet autoantigen related to protein tyrosine phosphatases. J Immunol 1994;152:3183–8.
20. Lu J, Li Q, Xie H, et al. Identification of a second transmembrane protein tyrosine phosphatase, IA-2beta, as an autoantigen in insulin-dependent diabetes mellitus: precursor of the 37-kDa tryptic fragment. Proc Natl Acad Sci U S A 1996;93: 2307–11.
21. Wenzlau JM, Juhl K, Yu L, et al. The cation efflux transporter ZnT8 (Slc30A8) is a major autoantigen in human type 1 diabetes. Proc Natl Acad Sci U S A 2007; 104:17040–5.
22. Lieberman SM, DiLorenzo TP. A comprehensive guide to antibody and T-cell responses in type 1 diabetes. Tissue Antigens 2003;62:359–77.
23. Kulmala P, Savola K, Petersen JS, et al. Prediction of insulin-dependent diabetes mellitus in siblings of children with diabetes: a population-based study. The Childhood Diabetes in Finland Study Group. J Clin Invest 1998;101:327–36.
24. LaGasse JM, Brantley MS, Leech NJ, et al. Successful prospective prediction of type 1 diabetes in schoolchildren through multiple defined autoantibodies: an 8-year follow-up of the Washington State Diabetes Prediction Study. Diabetes Care 2002;25:505–11.
25. Barker JM, Barriga KJ, Yu L, et al. Prediction of autoantibody positivity and progression to type 1 diabetes: Diabetes Autoimmunity Study in the Young (DAISY). J Clin Endocrinol Metab 2004;89:3896–902.
26. Achenbach P, Lampasona V, Landherr U, et al. Autoantibodies to zinc transporter 8 and SLC30A8 genotype stratify type 1 diabetes risk. Diabetologia 2009;52:1881–8.
27. Bingley PJ, Bonifacio E, Mueller PW. Diabetes antibody standardization program: first assay proficiency evaluation. Diabetes 2003;52:1128–36.
28. Törn C, Mueller P, Schlosser M, et al. Diabetes antibody standardization program: evaluation of assays for autoantibodies to glutamic acid decarboxylase and islet antigen-2. Diabetologia 2008;51:846–52.
29. Bonifacio E, Yu L, Williams AK, et al. Harmonization of glutamic acid decarboxylase and islet antigen-2 autoantibody assays for National Institute of Diabetes and Digestive and Kidney Diseases Consortia. J Clin Endocrinol Metab, in press. DOI: 10.1210/jc.2010.030.
30. Lanzavecchia A, Sallusto F. Human B cell memory. Curr Opin Immunol 2009;21: 298–304.
31. Bonifacio E, Scirpoli M, Kredel K, et al. Early autoantibody responses in prediabetes are IgG1 dominated and suggest antigen-specific regulation. J Immunol 1999;163:525–32.
32. Chitarra V, Alzari PM, Bentley GA, et al. Three-dimensional structure of a heteroclitic antigen-antibody cross-reaction complex. Proc Natl Acad Sci U S A 1993; 90:7711–5.
33. Benjamin DC, Berzofsky JA, East IJ, et al. The antigenic structure of proteins: a reappraisal. Annu Rev Immunol 1984;2:67–101.
34. Wenzlau JM, Liu Y, Yu L, et al. A common non-synonymous single nucleotide polymorphism in the SLC30A8 gene determines ZnT8 autoantibody specificity in type 1 diabetes. Diabetes 2008;57:2693–7.

35. Bottazzo GF, Florin-Christensen A, Doniach D. Islet-cell antibodies in diabetes mellitus with autoimmune polyendocrine deficiencies. Lancet 1974;2:1279–83.
36. Binder KA, Banga JP, Madec A, et al. Epitope analysis of GAD65Ab using fusion proteins and rFab. J Immunol Methods 2004;295:101–9.
37. Greenbaum C, Palmer J, Kuglin B, et al. Insulin autoantibodies measured by radioimmunoassay methodology are more related to insulin-dependent diabetes mellitus than those measured by enzyme-linked immunosorbent assay: results of the Fourth International Workshop on the Standardization of Insulin Autoantibody Measurement. J Clin Endocrinol Metab 1992;74:1040–4.
38. Bingley PJ, Bonifacio E, Shattock M, et al. Can islet cell antibodies predict IDDM in the general population? Diabetes Care 1993;16:45–50.
39. Bingley PJ, Bonifacio E, Williams AJ, et al. Prediction of IDDM in the general population: strategies based on combinations of autoantibody markers. Diabetes 1997;46:1701–10.
40. Hagopian WA, Sanjeevi CB, Kockum I, et al. Glutamate decarboxylase-, insulin-, and islet cell-antibodies and HLA typing to detect diabetes in a general population-based study of Swedish children. J Clin Invest 1995;95:1505–11.
41. In't Veld P, Lievens D, De Grijse J, et al. Screening for insulitis in adult autoantibody-positive organ donors. Diabetes 2007;56:2400–4.
42. Bingley PJ, Christie MR, Bonifacio E, et al. Combined analysis of autoantibodies improves prediction of IDDM in islet cell antibody-positive relatives. Diabetes 1994;43:1304–10.
43. Verge CF, Gianani R, Kawasaki E, et al. Prediction of type I diabetes in first-degree relatives using a combination of insulin, GAD, and ICA512bdc/IA-2 auto-antibodies. Diabetes 1996;45:926–33.
44. Achenbach P, Warncke K, Reiter J, et al. Stratification of type 1 diabetes risk on the basis of islet autoantibody characteristics. Diabetes 2004;53:384–92.
45. Bingley PJ, Gale EA, European Nicotinamide Diabetes Intervention Trial (ENDIT) Group. Progression to type 1 diabetes in islet cell antibody-positive relatives in the European Nicotinamide Diabetes Intervention Trial: the role of additional immune, genetic and metabolic markers of risk. Diabetologia 2006;49(5): 881–90.
46. Orban T, Sosenko JM, Cuthbertson D, et al. Pancreatic islet autoantibodies as predictors of type 1 diabetes in the Diabetes Prevention Trial-Type 1. Diabetes Care 2009;32(12):2269–74.
47. Siljander HT, Veijola R, Reunanen A, et al. Prediction of type 1 diabetes among siblings of affected children and in the general population. Diabetologia 2007; 50(11):2272–5.
48. Decochez K, De Leeuw IH, Keymeulen B, et al. IA-2 autoantibodies predict impending type I diabetes in siblings of patients. Diabetologia 2002;45: 1658–66.
49. Achenbach P, Koczwara K, Knopff A, et al. Mature high-affinity immune responses to (pro)insulin anticipate the autoimmune cascade that leads to type 1 diabetes. J Clin Invest 2004;114:589–97.
50. Schlosser M, Koczwara K, Kenk H, et al. In insulin-autoantibody-positive children from the general population, antibody affinity identifies those at high and low risk. Diabetologia 2005;48:1830–2.
51. Yu J, Yu L, Bugawan TL, et al. Transient antiislet autoantibodies: infrequent occur-rence and lack of association with genetic risk factors. J Clin Endocrinol Metab 2000;85:2421–8.

52. Krischer JP, Cuthbertson DD, Yu L, et al. Screening strategies for the identification of multiple antibody-positive relatives of individuals with type 1 diabetes. J Clin Endocrinol Metab 2003;88:103–8.
53. Walter M, Albert E, Conrad M, et al. IDDM2/insulin VNTR modifies risk conferred by IDDM1/HLA for development of type 1 diabetes and associated autoimmunity. Diabetologia 2003;46(5):712–20.
54. Srikanta S, Ganda OP, Rabizadeh A, et al. First-degree relatives of patients with type I diabetes mellitus. Islet-cell antibodies and abnormal insulin secretion. N Engl J Med 1985;313:461–4.
55. Fourlanos S, Narendran P, Byrnes GB, et al. Insulin resistance is a risk factor for progression to type 1 diabetes. Diabetologia 2004;47:1661–7.
56. Bingley PJ, Mahon JL, Gale EA, et al. Insulin resistance and progression to type 1 diabetes in the European Nicotinamide Diabetes Intervention Trial (ENDIT). Diabetes Care 2008;31(1):146–50.
57. Xu P, Cuthbertson D, Greenbaum C, et al. Role of insulin resistance in predicting progression to type 1 diabetes. Diabetes Care 2007;30(9):2314–20.
58. Hummel M, Bonifacio E, Schmid S, et al. Brief communication: early appearance of islet autoantibodies predicts childhood type 1 diabetes in offspring of diabetic parents. Ann Intern Med 2004;140:882–6.
59. Siljander HT, Simell S, Hekkala A, et al. Predictive characteristics of diabetes-associated autoantibodies among children with HLA-conferred disease susceptibility in the general population. Diabetes 2009;58(12):2835–42.
60. Ziegler AG, Standl E, Albert E, et al. HLA-associated insulin autoantibody formation in newly diagnosed type I diabetic patients. Diabetes 1991;40:1146–9.
61. Hagopian WA, Lernmark A, Rewers MJ, et al. TEDDY–The Environmental Determinants of Diabetes in the Young: an observational clinical trial. Ann N Y Acad Sci 2006;1079:320–6.
62. Monti P, Scirpoli M, Rigamonti A, et al. Evidence for in vivo primed and expanded autoreactive T cells as a specific feature of patients with type 1 diabetes. J Immunol 2007;179:5785–92.
63. Danke NA, Yang J, Greenbaum C, et al. Comparative study of GAD65-specific CD4+ T cells in healthy and type 1 diabetic subjects. J Autoimmun 2005;25:303–11.
64. Endl J, Rosinger S, Schwarz B, et al. Coexpression of CD25 and OX40 (CD134) receptors delineates autoreactive T-cells in type 1 diabetes. Diabetes 2006;55(1):50–60.
65. Reijonen H, Mallone R, Heninger AK, et al. GAD65-specific CD4+ T-cells with high antigen avidity are prevalent in peripheral blood of patients with type 1 diabetes. Diabetes 2004;53(8):1987–94.
66. Velthuis JH, Unger WW, Abreu JR, et al. Simultaneous detection of circulating autoreactive CD8+ T-cells specific for different islet cell-associated epitopes using combinatorial MHC-multimers. Diabetes, in press. DOI:10.2337/db09-148.
67. Atkinson MA, Gianani R. The pancreas in human type 1 diabetes: providing new answers to age-old questions. Curr Opin Endocrinol Diabetes Obes 2009;16(4):279–85.

Efforts to Prevent and Halt Autoimmune Beta Cell Destruction

Michael J. Haller, MD[a],*, Mark A. Atkinson, PhD[b],
Desmond A. Schatz, MD[a]

KEYWORDS

- Type 1 diabetes • Intervention • Prevention
- Combination therapy

PREVENTION VERSUS INTERVENTION

One of the greatest philosophical and logistical challenges in designing studies aimed at interdicting T1D is deciding whether to focus the major effort on prevention or intervention.[1] To some, this may be considered a semantic argument surrounding the use of the terms *prevention* and *intervention*; but in fact, primary prevention (ie, prevention of autoimmunity), secondary prevention (ie, prevention of overt hyperglycemia in subjects with established autoimmunity), and intervention studies (ie, those aimed at preserving C-peptide rather than true reversal) are each unique. When one attempts to design studies aimed at interdicting T1D, each of the aforementioned windows of opportunity possesses a particular set of strengths and weaknesses. Perhaps more telling of the ongoing struggle to choose a central paradigm for T1D interdiction is the fact that primary prevention, secondary prevention, and intervention studies are all currently being performed as part of large multicenter trials.

Despite ongoing debate regarding optimal study design, consensus exists that acting early (ie, primary prevention) likely represents the best opportunity for effectively eradicating T1D.[2] However, the ability to accurately predict those destined to develop T1D improves as the presumed capability to effectively intervene declines (**Fig. 1**).[3] Therefore, potential therapies for primary prevention of T1D must be extremely safe, because they would be provided to subjects who may never actually develop the disease.

The ability to perform prevention studies, as they are currently conceived, is also hindered in that they require complex and massive screening efforts to identify subjects who are potentially eligible. For all of these reasons, prevention studies are

---

[a] Division of Endocrinology, Department of Pediatrics, University of Florida, PO Box 100296, Gainesville, FL 32610, USA
[b] Department of Pathology, University of Florida, PO Box 100275, Gainesville, FL 32610, USA
* Corresponding author.
E-mail address: hallemj@peds.ufl.edu

Endocrinol Metab Clin N Am 39 (2010) 527–539
doi:10.1016/j.ecl.2010.05.006
0889-8529/10/$ – see front matter © 2010 Elsevier Inc. All rights reserved.

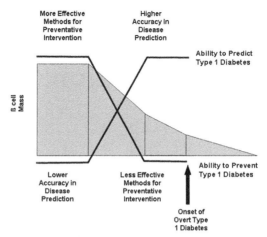

Fig. 1. The treatment dilemma for type 1 diabetes. Many studies from animal models of type 1 diabetes in combination with a much more limited series of investigations in humans suggest that early intervention not only is more effective in terms of disease prevention but also often requires more benign forms of therapy. In contrast, the ability to identify an individual who will truly develop type 1 diabetes increases as the individual approaches onset of overt disease. (*Adapted from* Atkinson MA, Eisenbarth GS. Type 1 diabetes: new perspectives on disease pathogenesis and treatment. Lancet 2001;358(9277):222; with permission.)

inherently difficult to plan and costly to execute. Were one to eliminate screening and move to a model of universal prevention, the difficulties of screening would be markedly reduced, but concerns over equipoise would, once again, be raised to levels beyond those in which individuals of elevated risk are identified and subjected to intervention.

In contrast to these considerations, informing patients with newly diagnosed T1D about opportunities to participate in intervention trials provides a far higher yield and lower cost paradigm for identifying and enrolling subjects in clinical trials. However, these trial designs have less likelihood of success, given the reduction of existing ß cell mass and established and aggressive autoimmunity in patients already diagnosed with T1D.

Ultimately, attempts to interdict the disease process at almost any point can logically be defended as long as the therapeutic agents are chosen with a thorough appreciation of relative risk and benefit. With this in mind, low-risk therapies can ethically be tested in prevention studies with large numbers of subjects, but are expensive and require many years to document effect. Conversely, high-risk therapies are more rightly reserved for intervention studies with smaller numbers of subjects who have T1D, and require only 1 to 2 years to document potential efficacy. To ensure a state of equipoise between risk and benefit, intervention studies in patients with recent onset of T1D have emerged as the model for studying immunomodulatory and immunosuppressive therapies with potentially significant side-effect profiles. Conversely, prevention studies remain focused on lower-risk therapies that can be applied to larger populations.

Although space limits an extensive discussion of every agent previously used and those currently in use in T1D prevention and intervention studies, this article details several therapies being investigated and briefly mentions several that have provided important lessons in the quest for developing a cure. The prevention of recurrent autoimmunity is key for a sustained disease reversal, should effective means to replace islet cell function be developed.

PREVENTION STRATEGIES

Improvements in understanding of the natural history of T1D, combined with markers identifying stages of "pre-type 1" diabetes, have led to the development of different windows of opportunity to interdict the disease process (see **Fig. 1**). Still, to implement effective prevention strategies, a far greater understanding of the immunologic, genetic, and environmental mechanisms leading to T1D are clearly required. Previous and ongoing prevention efforts have focused primarily on the use of low-risk antigen-specific therapies. Although these efforts have been unsuccessful in achieving their primary goal of prevention, they have undoubtedly succeeded in establishing international multicenter T1D research collaborations and have markedly improved understanding of the disease's natural history.

Insulin

Insulin has long been investigated as an autoantigen that might be manipulated to augment the natural history of T1D. Based on early studies in the nonobese diabetic (NOD) mouse[4] showing that early exposure to oral insulin in these high-risk animals was effective in preventing diabetes, and promising pilot studies in other autoimmune diseases showing oral tolerance, the Diabetes Prevention Trial–Type 1 (DPT-1) (NCT00004984) was organized to determine if either subcutaneous or oral insulin could prevent or delay the onset of T1D through the immunomodulatory effects of recurrent exposure to insulin. Performed in the late 1980s and early 1990s, DPT-1 was one of the first large multicenter, randomized, placebo-controlled trials to attempt prevention of T1D in high-risk patients. The DPT-1 screened more than 100,000 first- and second-degree relatives of patients with T1D to identify fewer than 3500 subjects who were positive for islet cell cytoplasmic autoantibody (ICA) +/- insulin autoantibody (IAA). Of these, 339 were enrolled in the parenteral arm and 372 in the oral insulin arm.

Although both oral and parenteral insulin showed excellent safety profiles, the DPT-1 failed to show therapeutic benefit for either investigational approach. However, the study proved that a large multicenter T1D collaborative was feasible and, as a result, the predominantly National Institutes of Health (NIH)–funded TrialNet was established. However, a post-hoc review of DPT-1 data showed that at-risk patients (ie, 5-year risk, 25%–50%) who received oral insulin and had high IAA levels experienced a considerable delay in the onset of T1D.[5] Therefore, TrialNet designed an appropriately powered follow-up study to determine if oral insulin can delay the onset of T1D in intermediate-risk individuals with two or more islet autoantibodies, one of which is IAA (NCT00419562). Relatives of patients with T1D are currently being screened to determine if they qualify for participation in the oral insulin study by participating in the TrialNet Natural History Study, which aims to identify and track patients at risk for developing T1D (NCT00097292).

Because insulin is a likely target autoantigen in the disease, similar studies focusing on achieving tolerance through alternative mechanisms of insulin delivery have been explored by other study groups. The Finnish Diabetes Prediction and Prevention Project (DIPP), in which intranasal insulin was administered to genetically at-risk auto-antibody positive subjects, failed to show a benefit[5] (NCT00223613). The Australian Intranasal Insulin Trial (INIT I), a safety study performed in adults, documented immune changes consistent with mucosal tolerance to insulin.[6] INIT II is now underway and is evaluating a larger population through determining the effect of different doses of intranasal insulin in preventing or slowing the onset of T1D[7] (NCT00336674). In addition, the Primary Oral/Intranasal Insulin Trial (Pre-POINT) will be attempting primary prevention in a dose-finding study to provide oral or intranasal insulin to genetically at-risk infants who have not yet developed T1D-associated autoantibodies.[8] Recently, interventional efforts using insulin B-chain immunotherapy in patients with newly diagnosed T1D were reported to show specific T-cell responses to the nonmetabolically active insulin, but no effect on C-peptide, when compared with placebo.[9]

Glutamic Acid Decarboxylase 65

Glutamic acid decarboxylase 65 (GAD65) is another autoantigen that has been targeted for potential therapeutic use in T1D. Similar to insulin, strong preclinical data from the NOD mouse[10] suggest that prevention after vaccination with GAD65 is possible. Early safety and dose-finding studies of GAD65 (Diamyd) were performed in adult patients with latent autoimmune diabetes, with subjects receiving two subcutaneous doses of GAD65 (4, 20, 100, or 500 μg) or placebo. Patients were followed up for 24 weeks, with no adverse events noted. In addition, the 20-ug dose seemed to show preservation of endogenous β cell function. A follow-up phase II trial, this time involving 70 children (10–18 years) with T1D, showed preservation of β cell function with no treatment-related adverse events[11] (NCT00435981). Patients with T1D who received 20 μg of GAD65 had fasting C-peptide levels at 24 weeks that were increased compared with placebo, and increased fasting and stimulated C-peptide levels from baseline to 24 weeks.[11] Earlier administration (ie, within 6 months of disease onset) appeared more efficacious, albeit the number of these subjects were limited. Based on these encouraging phase I and II data, TrialNet is performing a phase III placebo-controlled randomized trial of GAD65 in patients with newly diagnosed T1D (NCT00529399). Similar industry sponsored studies are being conducted concurrently in Europe and the United States. A GAD65 prevention study is being planned in individuals screened through the TrialNet Natural History Study who are found to be GAD autoantibody–positive.

INTERVENTION STRATEGIES

As opposed to the antigen-specific efforts noted in prevention trials, most early T1D intervention strategies have used immunosuppressive regimens to control autoimmunity and preserve β cell function. These studies were performed with relatively few patients with new-onset T1D and, when undertaken, were performed using drugs such as azathioprine,[12] cyclosporine,[13,14] and antithymocyte globulin along with prednisone.[15] Many of these immunosuppressive agents showed initial promise in preserving C-peptide but were nonetheless abandoned because of intolerable side-effect profiles and limited efficacy. In contrast, agents such as nicotinamide,[16] ketotifen,[17] and Bacille Calmette-Guérin (BCG),[18] all proved to be low-risk but also failed to show benefit in preserving β cell function. Additional low-risk non–antigen-specific therapies are currently being investigated, such as α-1 antitrypsin,[19] autologous umbilical cord blood infusion plus docosahexaenoic acid (DHA) and vitamin D_3 supplemementation,[20] heat shock protein–derived DiaPep227,[21] and avoidance of cow milk proteins (TRIGR).[22] Nevertheless, as experts struggle to develop both safe and effective therapies, they may be forced to accept the paradox that therapies with the immunologic power to effectively reverse T1D may already exist but may only succeed at the cost of inducing potential short-and long-term side effects that are worse than living with diabetes.

Anti-CD3

Depletion of autoreactive T cells is a logical approach to interdicting the disease process in T1D. Preclinical data from the NOD mouse have shown that monoclonal antibodies to CD3 are capable of preventing and reversing diabetes.[23,24] Two different anti-CD3 products, hOKT3gl (Ala-Ala/Teplizumab) and ChAglyCD3 (TRX4/Otelixizumab), have recently been used in human intervention studies (NCT00378508 and NCT00451321, respectively). While leading to short-term T-cell depletion after administration, anti-CD3 antibodies may selectively increase the production of regulatory T cells thought to counter the effector T-cell response responsible for islet destruction in settings of T1D. Published studies of anti-CD3 therapy have been promising and suggest C-peptide may be preserved for as long as 18 to 24 months after therapy.[25,26] However, depending on the protocol, current dosing regimens require a 6- to 14-day intravenous infusion, a requirement that may limit patient enrollment and possible widescale use of this agent.

Safety issues include the commonly occurring cytokine release syndrome after initial dosing; rashes; reactivation of Epstein-Barr virus; potential formation of antibodies to anti-CD3; and unknown long-term side effects. Larger studies of anti-CD3 are currently being performed by the two manufacturers of these monoclonal antibodies. In addition, TrialNet is implementing an anti-CD3 prevention study in very–high-risk nondiabetic relatives (ie, those with two or more islet autoantibodies plus evidence of impaired glucose tolerance).

Anti-CD20

The anti-CD20 monoclonal antibody Rituximab (Rituxan) down-regulates B-lymphocyte signaling of T cells, and therefore may reduce the ability of cytotoxic T cells to induce islet injury in settings of T1D. Rituximab is one of several agents chosen as part of the aforementioned paradigm, which focuses on agents that have already shown benefit in other human autoimmune disease. However, preclinical data with anti–B-lymphocyte activities have also shown efficacy in preventing and reversing diabetes in the NOD mouse.[27,28]

Now part of the standard therapeutic armamentarium for rheumatoid arthritis, non-Hodgkin's lymphoma, and transplant rejection, Rituximab has also shown recent promise in the treatment of lupus and multiple sclerosis. Within TrialNet, Rituximab was administered to patients with new-onset T1D within 100 days of diagnosis in a randomized placebo-controlled trial to determine of if four weekly intravenous infusions safely preserve C-peptide. Preservation of C-peptide was noted 1 year after Rituximab was administered (mean area under the curve [AUC]: 0.56 pmol/mL vs 0.47 pmol/mL for C-peptide and placebo, respectively) (NCT00279305). Although adverse events were also more common in the drug-treated patients, most events were grade 1 or 2 infusion reactions that were observed primarily during the first infusion. No increase in infection rates or neutropenia was observed in those who received Rituximab.

Although these data are encouraging in their support of the notion that B lymphocytes can be augmented to partially interdict the autoimmune process, data from the 2-year time point are eagerly awaited and will have to be carefully considered in determining future therapies.

Mycofenolate Mofetil and Anti-CD25

No single agent has shown an ability to indefinitely preserve C-peptide production in patients with new-onset T1D. Guided by the successes seen in cancer and HIV, combination or "cocktail therapy" that simultaneously uses multiple agents at lower doses has been proposed as a model to improve efficacy while limiting likelihood of therapeutic side effects. One of the first examples of combination therapy to treat T1D was recently investigated as part of the TrialNet consortium; Mycofenolate Mofetil (MMF) and Daclizumab (DZB/Zenapax) (NCT00100178). Both agents were previously used successfully in other human autoimmune settings and also have shown efficacy in animal models of T1D.[29] The rationale for the selection of these agents was based partly on safety profiles along with their presumed mechanisms of action. Specifically, the immunosuppressive profile of MMF combined with the depletion of activated T cells provided by DZB.

The MMF/DZB combination tested within the TrialNet involved a single intravenous infusion of the DZB antibody and daily oral therapy with MMF administered to patients with new-onset T1D. The study included three arms: MMF and DZB combination therapy, MMF monotherapy, and placebo. Unfortunately, neither MMF alone nor MMF in combination with DZB had an effect on the loss of C-peptide in patients with new-onset T1D.[30]

Cytotoxic T-Lymphocyte Antigen-4 Immunoglobulin

Cytotoxic T-lymphocyte antigen-4 (CTLA-4) is expressed on the surface of T-helper cells and transmits an inhibitory signal to T cells by blocking the stimulatory effect of CD28 binding.[31,32] In addition, CTLA-4 may play an important role in the function of tolerance-inducing regulatory T cells. Furthermore, polymorphisms in the CLTA-4 gene are known to associate with autoimmune diseases, including T1D.[32] Therefore, CTLA-4–Ig is a selective T-cell co-stimulation modulator and has been extensively investigated and already gained FDA approval for the treatment of rheumatoid arthritis (Abatacept/Orencia). Using a similar rationale, CTLA-4–Ig was proposed as another potential non–antigen-specific therapy for T1D. The TrialNet consortium is performing a randomized, double-blind, placebo-controlled trial of CTLA-4-Ig/placebo in patients with recently diagnosed T1D (NCT00505375). Because CTLA-4–Ig is administered as a monthly intravenous infusion, participation in this study required considerable commitment from patients, their families, and research staff. Nevertheless, the side-effect profile is well described and reasonably tolerable, and enrollment for the Trial-Net effort was completed in 2009. Data on safety and efficacy in patients with T1D are expected in 2011.

Anti-Thymocyte Globulin

Anti-thymocyte globulin (ATG) is a polyclonal anti–human T-cell antibody preparation produced by inoculating rabbits or horses with human thymocytes.[33] ATG has long been a critical part of preparative regimens for transplantation and cancer therapy because it results in nonspecific T-cell depletion.[34] Recovery from T-cell depletion after ATG therapy has been associated with a rebalance of the number of effector versus regulatory T-cells, and therefore it offers a potential advantage in resetting the immune system in patients with autoimmunity.[35] ATG represents another example of a powerful non–antigen-specific agent, and has been used either alone or in combination for treating various autoimmune conditions, including Wegner's granulomatosis, lupus, rheumatoid arthritis, multiple sclerosis, scleroderma, aplastic anemia and myelodysplastic syndromes, and even T1D.[36–45]

In terms of side effects, ATG therapy has been associated with cytokine release syndrome and serum sickness. Although not trivial, these side effects are tolerable, especially when ATG is administered at lower doses than those typically used in transplantation and cancer therapies. Definitive data are still awaited, but a small European study using one commercial form of ATG (ATG-Fresenius) showed potential efficacy and tolerance of ATG-related side effects.[45] In addition, an ongoing study of a second commercial form of ATG (Thymoglubulin) is being performed by the National Institutes of Health Immune Tolerance Network using patients with recently diagnosed T1D (NCT00515099).

ATG and Granulocyte Colony-Stimulating Factor (GCSF)

Although ATG monotherapy seems promising, consistent with the concept supporting combination therapy, an ATG-based protocol that includes a second agent, granulo-cyte colony–stimulating factor (GCSF), is likely to have even greater potential for preserving ß cell mass. Perhaps the best support for this assertion comes from data generated in a study in Brazil, in which young adults with very–recent-onset T1D received cyclophosphamide, GCSF, and ATG in what was termed a nonmyeloablative autotransplantation[46] (NCT00315133). The idea of immune depletion followed by regulatory T-cell mobilization or reinfusion, a mechanism deemed likely to result from this therapy, has strong preclinical data supporting the assertion that this approach may be able to ameliorate autoimmunity.[47] Although patients who received this combination therapy experienced considerable morbidity (eg, neutropenia, alopecia, testicular dysfunction), they also benefited from a remarkable degree of ther-apeutic efficacy. Of 23 treated subjects, 20 experienced at least 1 month of insulin independence, with most being insulin-free for more than a year. This study also repre-sents one of the first reports of a sustained increase in the stimulated C-peptide values in patients with T1D.[46,48] Although the results are undeniably proof of the potential for aggressive immunoablative therapy in treating T1D, the side-effect profile of this particular combination is unacceptable to most physicians caring for children with T1D.[49]

As our group has long supported the concept of safe combination therapies, we have attempted to deconstruct the Brazilian combination using the NOD mouse model to guide development of a lower-risk therapy for humans. By excluding cyclophosphamide and relying on a combination of only low-dose ATG and GCSF, we were recently able to show a durable reversal of diabetes in more than 75% of NOD mice, although ATG alone was only able to reverse disease in 33% of animals.[47] In addition, we showed that the combination therapy provided the most robust increase in regulatory T cells and, perhaps more impor-tantly for clinical application, enabled reversal of diabetes at higher initial glucose values than ATG alone. Given these exciting preclinical data, our group recently began planning for an analogous human trial designed to study the safety and potential efficacy of low-dose ATG (2.5 mg/kg total dose) and 12 weeks of pegy-lated GCSF therapy (Neulasta, 6 mg, every 2 weeks).

Cell Therapies

The concept of using cell therapies to provide a quantity of islet cells capable of restoring euglycemia in patients with T1D has long been thought to be a potential panacea for ameliorating the disease. However, this notion remains largely unfulfilled, because of the pronounced shortage of cadaveric islets combined with the inability to overcome the primary autoimmunity underlying the disorder, a step one would deem necessary before this approach could even be conceptually feasible.

However, over the past few years, the term *cell therapies* has undergone significant change in the T1D research arena as several groups have expanded this terminology away from exclusive reference to cell therapies designed to provide ß cell replacement (ie, islet transplantation and stem cell differentiation) toward the concept of using cell therapies as a means to provide direct immunoregulatory therapy. Clinical trials designed to test the potential of several cell types with the capacity to modulate the immune response are currently underway in patients with T1D.

Based on the observation that umbilical cord blood contains a dense population of highly potent regulatory T cells, our group recently completed a phase I study investigating the potential for a single autologous cord blood infusion to preserve C-peptide in young children with T1D. Although preliminary results regarding efficacy were inconclusive after 1 year, those studies showed that the approach was safe and resulted in short-term increases in regulatory T-cell frequencies.[20,50] Based on these results, a phase II study was recently initiated to determine the efficacy of a single autologous umbilical cord blood infusion, followed by 1 year of supplementation with high-dose vitamin D and omega 3 fatty acids to preserve C-peptide (NCT00873925).

Another cell-type of great interest for its potential to provide immune regulation is the dendritic cell (DC).[51] A primary function of DCs is to process antigenic material and present it on their cellular surface in a form recognized by other cells of the immune system. As such, they are a very logical target for designing cell-based immune therapies. Preclinical data from the NOD mouse have already shown proof of concept that manipulated DCs can effectively prevent T1D.[52] Based on this concept and preclinical data, a phase I study was initiated to determine if the injection of autologous modified DCs in subjects with T1D is safe and to look for any signals of tolerogenic immune response[53] (NCT00445913).

Mesenchymal stem cells (MSC) have also piqued the interest of T1D researchers, given recent data suggesting their pronounced ability to afford immunoregulation in various settings, ranging from autoimmune disease to graft-versus-host disease.[54] MSCs are a unique form of cell therapy in that most believe they have little to no known allosensitivity. Therefore, in theory, MSCs from any donor can be provided to any recipient. Because MSCs are thought to localize suppression of immune response in areas of inflammation with a degree of functional activity that is quantitatively controlled by the severity of tissue inflammation, they are another logical choice for cell-based immune therapy.

Although MSCs have a limited lifespan in vivo, this is potentially advantageous given concerns regarding the long-term risk of immortalized stem cells. In addition, MSCs can easily be re-dosed, because of their lack of inducing alloimmunity. Preclinical data from animal models of T1D have already shown the ability of MSC infusion to promote ß-cell repair, enhance insulin secretion, and facilitate islet allograft tolerance.[55,56] Enrollment for a phase II study using a commercially available MSC preparation (Prochymal) in patients with new-onset T1D was recently completed and safety and efficacy data are eagerly awaited (NCT00690066).

Beyond umbilical cord blood, DC, and MSC, other forms of cell-based therapies are being actively considered for T1D, including polyclonal regulatory T cells, antigen-specific regulatory T cells, and T cells modulated in vitro to produce anti-inflammatory cytokines in vivo.[57] None of these efforts has been actually applied in therapeutic settings of T1D, but these trials likely will be undertaken if concerns over safety and feasibility are overcome. The preclinical findings mentioned earlier, together with support from efforts in NOD mice, suggest that regulatory T cells are able to modulate T1D development.[55,56]

Learning from the Past to Predict the Challenges of the Future

Despite the formation of several dozen clinical trials seeking to prevent or reverse T1D, the past 30 years have been characterized by the inability of these efforts to provide substantial prolonged benefit to patients. This lack of an effective intervention has also delayed population-based screening for T1D because the ability to predict the disease in both higher-risk relatives and the general population has seen marked improvement over this same period (see the article by Bonifacio and Ziegler elsewhere in this issue for further exploration of this topic).

These trial "failures" are not without benefit, because they have shown that a phase-specific intervention, based on stage in the natural history of T1D, will likely be required for successfully interdicting in T1D. Many recently developed prevention and intervention studies exemplify another newly considered paradigm under which agents are not selected simply because of their therapeutic benefit in the NOD mouse model but also because of their providing established benefit in other human disorders considered of autoimmune origin. For example, drugs used to treat disorders such as rheumatoid arthritis, lupus, and multiple sclerosis can rationally be applied to T1D, with the additional benefit of having known safety and side-effect profiles. Similarly, the paradigm or concept of combination therapy has emerged as the growing number of monotherapy failures suggests that the complexity of autoimmunity underlying T1D is far too complicated to control with single agents. We believe that the simultaneous application of agents that individually provide immunosuppression, immunomodulation, and islet regeneration should improve future efforts seeking to intervene in T1D (**Fig. 2**).

One recent charge from both the T1D research and lay communities has been to improve the pace of efforts seeking to identify a cure for T1D. Although this motivation is laudatory, the potential for side effects must continually be balanced against the benefits of prevention and intervention strategies as the field moves forward to test agents (especially combination therapies). Furthermore, as the number of potential therapies subject to therapeutic trial continues to grow, an additional emerging challenge will be to decide how to choose agents for future interventional studies. In other words, agents with equally strong rationale for inclusion have recently been suggested (eg, anti-CD3, anti-CD20), but finite monetary and human resources limit the ability to use every agent with solid rationale in a timely manner. Although T1D is not an uncommon disease, the number of available subjects for prevention and interventional studies is not so large that studies can simply be designed and every one fully enrolled. Thus, additional factors, such as ease of delivery, agent cost, previous experience in

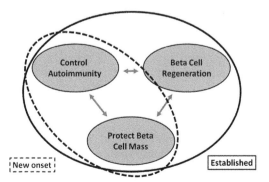

Fig. 2. Combination therapies for the reversal of type 1 diabetes. The reversal of type 1 diabetes will likely require a combination of agents providing immunomodulation, immunosuppression, and ß-cell regeneration. Patients with newly diagnosed type 1 diabetes may achieve cure through combination approaches that control autoimmunity and protect remaining ß cells. Addition of agents that stimulate ß-cell regeneration likely will be required to accomplish reversal in patients requiring long-term care.

other autoimmune disease, need for screening (in cases of T1D prevention), and applicability to large numbers of patients, must all be considered in appropriately rank-ordering potential interventions.

Finally, one of the greatest challenges that effects past, current, and future prevention and intervention studies is the proper interpretation of study data and comparison of outcomes between studies. Although recent studies have improved to the point that statistically significant changes in C-peptide are increasingly seen over time (ie, preservation), experts must continue to question whether these changes are, in fact, clinically significant. Without the ability to specify clinically significant end points, we believe that patients likely will not show continued interest in these forms of therapy, especially if delivery is onerous. Therefore, experts must also continue to search for clinically meaningful end points. Although the outright reversal or prevention of T1D is an easily understood end point, measurements of incremental metabolic improvements that guide one to that goal are less-easily agreed on. Peak, basal, and AUC C-peptide are common metabolic end points, but ones that do not adequately reflect complex changes in islet function. Interpretation of interventional data must also account for the age of enrolled subjects. Many interventional studies enroll young adults in whom T1D has a very different natural history from the that observed in children diagnosed with T1D at a younger age. Thus, application of even the most successful research interventions may not translate into similar clinical benefit for most patients with new-onset T1D who eagerly await proven interventions.

SUMMARY

The past 50 years have seen a rapid increase in knowledge of the epidemiologic patterns and natural history of T1D, insights that were anticipated to accelerate efforts seeking disease prevention and to allow for the development of a cure.[58] Although the clinical care for patients with T1D has dramatically improved, failure to adequately understand the precise mechanisms leading to clinical disease and to develop a suitable intervention to prevent or reverse this disease has left open the goal of finding a cure for T1D.

Future prevention and intervention studies must be designed with an appreciation of the lessons learned from previous efforts that have failed to provide a cure. One example is that single-agent therapies with drugs chosen largely based on their efficacy in animal models have failed to produce meaningful results. Rationally designed combination therapies with agents targeting immunosuppression, immunomodulation, and islet regeneration may more logically represent the future of successful prevention and intervention trials. In addition, as diabetes management techniques continue to improve, the safety and efficacy of future interventions must be balanced with the real costs (eg, physical, emotional, monetary) of living with T1D.

REFERENCES

1. Staeva-Vieira T, Peakman M, von Herrath M. Translational mini-review series on type 1 diabetes: Immune-based therapeutic approaches for type 1 diabetes. Clin Exp Immunol 2007;148(1):17–31.
2. Haller MJ, Atkinson MA, Schatz D. Type 1 diabetes mellitus: etiology, presentation, and management. Pediatr Clin North Am 2005;52(6):1553–78.
3. Atkinson MA, Eisenbarth GS. Type 1 diabetes: new perspectives on disease pathogenesis and treatment. Lancet 2001;358(9277):221–9.
4. Atkinson MA, Maclaren NK, Luchetta R. Insulitis and diabetes in NOD mice reduced by prophylactic insulin therapy. Diabetes 1990;39(8):933–7.

5. Kupila A, Sipila J, Keskinen P, et al. Intranasally administered insulin intended for prevention of type 1 diabetes–a safety study in healthy adults. Diabetes Metab Res Rev 2003;19(5):415–20.

6. Harrison LC, Honeyman MC, Steele CE, et al. Pancreatic beta-cell function and immune responses to insulin after administration of intranasal insulin to humans at risk for type 1 diabetes. Diabetes Care 2004;27(10):2348–55.

7. Harrison L. INIT II study web site. 2010. Available at: http://www.diabetestrials. org/initii.html. Accessed January 20, 2010.

8. Bonifacio E. JDRF funded research: pre-point. 2010. Available at: http:// onlineapps.jdfcure.org/AbstractReport.cfm?grant_id=26014&abs_type=LAY. Accessed January 20, 2009.

9. Orban T, Farkas K, Jalahej H, et al. Autoantigen-specific regulatory T cells induced in patients with type 1 diabetes mellitus by insulin B-chain immunotherapy. J Autoimmun 2010;34(4):408–15.

10. Tisch R, Yang XD, Liblau RS, et al. Administering glutamic acid decarboxylase to NOD mice prevents diabetes. J Autoimmun 1994;7(6):845–50.

11. Ludvigsson J, Faresjo M, Hjorth M, et al. GAD treatment and insulin secretion in recent-onset type 1 diabetes. N Engl J Med 2008;359(18):1909–20.

12. Silverstein J, Maclaren N, Riley W, et al. Immunosuppression with azathioprine and prednisone in recent-onset insulin-dependent diabetes mellitus. N Engl J Med 1988;319(10):599–604.

13. Bougneres PF, Carel JC, Castano L, et al. [Cyclosporin and childhood diabetes: preliminary findings of the Saint Vincent de Paul trial]. Journ Annu Diabetol Hotel Dieu 1987;181–6 [in French].

14. Carel JC, Boitard C, Eisenbarth G, et al. Cyclosporine delays but does not prevent clinical onset in glucose intolerant pre-type 1 diabetic children. J Autoimmun 1996;9(6):739–45.

15. Eisenbarth GS, Srikanta S, Jackson R, et al. Anti-thymocyte globulin and prednisone immunotherapy of recent onset type 1 diabetes mellitus. Diabetes Res 1985;2(6):271–6.

16. Gale EAM. European Nicotinamide Diabetes Intervention Trial (ENDIT): a randomised controlled trial of intervention before the onset of type 1 diabetes. Lancet 2004;363(9413):925–31.

17. Bohmer KP, Kolb H, Kuglin B, et al. Linear loss of insulin secretory capacity during the last six months preceding IDDM. No effect of antiedematous therapy with ketotifen. Diabetes Care 1994;17(2):138–41.

18. Huppmann M, Baumgarten A, Ziegler AG, et al. Neonatal Bacille Calmette-Guerin vaccination and type 1 diabetes. Diabetes Care 2005;28(5):1204–6.

19. Zhang B, Lu Y, Campbell-Thompson M, et al. Alpha1-antitrypsin protects beta-cells from apoptosis. Diabetes 2007;56(5):1316–23.

20. Haller MJ, Wasserfall CH, McGrail KM, et al. Autologous umbilical cord blood transfusion in very young children with type 1 diabetes. Diabetes Care 2009; 32(11):2041–6.

21. Huurman VA, van der Meide PE, Duinkerken G, et al. Immunological efficacy of heat shock protein 60 peptide DiaPep277 therapy in clinical type I diabetes. Clin Exp Immunol 2008;152(3):488–97.

22. TRIGR Study Group. Study design of the trial to reduce IDDM in the genetically at risk (TRIGR). Pediatr Diabetes 2007;8(3):117–37.

23. Herold KC, Bluestone JA, Montag AG, et al. Prevention of autoimmune diabetes with nonactivating anti-CD3 monoclonal antibody. Diabetes 1992;41(3): 385–91.

24. Sherry NA, Chen W, Kushner JA, et al. Exendin-4 improves reversal of diabetes in NOD mice treated with anti-CD3 monoclonal antibody by enhancing recovery of beta-cells. Endocrinology 2007;148(11):5136–44.

25. Keymeulen B, Vandemeulebroucke E, Ziegler AG, et al. Insulin needs after CD3-antibody therapy in new-onset type 1 diabetes. N Engl J Med 2005;352(25): 2598–608.

26. Haller MJ, Schatz DA. CD3-antibody therapy in new-onset type 1 diabetes mellitus. N Engl J Med 2005;353(19):2086–7 [author reply: 2086–7].

27. Xiu Y, Wong CP, Bouaziz JD, et al. B lymphocyte depletion by CD20 monoclonal antibody prevents diabetes in nonobese diabetic mice despite isotype-specific differences in Fc gamma R effector functions. J Immunol 2008;180(5):2863–75.

28. Fiorina P, Vergani A, Dada S, et al. Targeting CD22 reprograms B-cells and reverses autoimmune diabetes. Diabetes 2008;57(11):3013–24.

29. Ugrasbul F, Moore WV, Tong PY, et al. Prevention of diabetes: effect of mycophenolate mofetil and anti-CD25 on onset of diabetes in the DRBB rat. Pediatr Diabetes 2008;9(6):596–601.

30. Gottlieb PA, Quinlan S, Krause-Steinrauf H, et al. Failure to preserve beta-cell function with mycophenolate mofetil and daclizumab combined therapy in patients with new onset type 1 diabetes. Diabetes Care 2010;33(4):826–32.

31. Rudd CE, Taylor A, Schneider H. CD28 and CTLA-4 coreceptor expression and signal transduction. Immunol Rev 2009;229(1):12–26.

32. Korolija M, Renar IP, Hadzija M, et al. Association of PTPN22 C1858T and CTLA-4 A49G polymorphisms with type 1 diabetes in Croatians. Diabetes Res Clin Pract 2009;86(3):e54–7.

33. Feng X, Kajigaya S, Solomou EE, et al. Rabbit ATG but not horse ATG promotes expansion of functional CD4+CD25highFOXP3+ regulatory T cells in vitro. Blood 2008;111(7):3675–83.

34. Mohty M. Mechanisms of action of antithymocyte globulin: T-cell depletion and beyond. Leukemia 2007;21(7):1387–94.

35. Saccardi R, Kozak T, Bocelli-Tyndall C, et al. Autologous stem cell transplantation for progressive multiple sclerosis: update of the European Group for Blood and Marrow Transplantation autoimmune diseases working party database. Mult Scler 2006;12(6):814–23.

36. Fassas A, Anagnostopoulos A, Kazis A, et al. Peripheral blood stem cell transplantation in the treatment of progressive multiple sclerosis: first results of a pilot study. Bone Marrow Transplant 1997;20(8):631–8.

37. Frickhofen N, Heimpel H, Kaltwasser JP, et al. Antithymocyte globulin with or without cyclosporin A: 11-year follow-up of a randomized trial comparing treatments of aplastic anemia. Blood 2003;101(4):1236–42.

38. Kool J, de Keizer RJ, Siegert CE. Antithymocyte globulin treatment of orbital Wegener granulomatosis: a follow-up study. Am J Ophthalmol 1999;127(6):738–9.

39. McSweeney PA, Nash RA, Sullivan KM, et al. High-dose immunosuppressive therapy for severe systemic sclerosis: initial outcomes. Blood 2002;100(5): 1602–10.

40. Molldrem JJ, Leifer E, Bahceci E, et al. Antithymocyte globulin for treatment of the bone marrow failure associated with myelodysplastic syndromes. Ann Intern Med 2002;137(3):156–63.

41. Musso M, Porretto F, Crescimanno A, et al. Intense immunosuppressive therapy followed by autologous peripheral blood selected progenitor cell reinfusion for severe autoimmune disease. Am J Hematol 2001;66(2):75–9.

42. Rosenfeld S, Follmann D, Nunez O, et al. Antithymocyte globulin and cyclosporine for severe aplastic anemia: association between hematologic response and long-term outcome. JAMA 2003;289(9):1130–5.
43. Stratton RJ, Wilson H, Black CM. Pilot study of anti-thymocyte globulin plus mycophenolate mofetil in recent-onset diffuse scleroderma. Rheumatology (Oxford) 2001;40(1):84–8.
44. Schatz DA, Riley WJ, Silverstein JH, et al. Long-term immunoregulatory effects of therapy with corticosteroids and anti-thymocyte globulin. Immunopharmacol Immunotoxicol 1989;11(2–3):269–87.
45. Saudek F, Havrdova T, Boucek P, et al. Polyclonal anti-T-cell therapy for type 1 diabetes mellitus of recent onset. Rev Diabet Stud 2004;1(2):80–8.
46. Couri CE, Oliveira MC, Stracieri AB, et al. C-peptide levels and insulin independence following autologous nonmyeloablative hematopoietic stem cell transplantation in newly diagnosed type 1 diabetes mellitus. JAMA 2009;301(15):1573–9.
47. Parker MJ, Xue S, Alexander JJ, et al. Immune depletion with cellular mobilization imparts immunoregulation and reverses autoimmune diabetes in nonobese diabetic mice. Diabetes 2009;58(10):2277–84.
48. Voltarelli JC, Couri CE, Stracieri AB, et al. Autologous nonmyeloablative hematopoietic stem cell transplantation in newly diagnosed type 1 diabetes mellitus. JAMA 2007;297(14):1568–76.
49. Gitelman SE, Haller MJ, Schatz D. Autologous nonmyeloablative hematopoietic stem cell transplantation in newly diagnosed type 1 diabetes mellitus. JAMA 2009;302(6):624 [author reply: 624–5].
50. Haller MJ, Viener HL, Wasserfall C, et al. Autologous umbilical cord blood infusion for type 1 diabetes. Exp Hematol 2008;36(6):710–5.
51. Lande R, Gilliet M. Plasmacytoid dendritic cells: key players in the initiation and regulation of immune responses. Ann N Y Acad Sci 2010;1183:89–103.
52. Ma L, Qian S, Liang X, et al. Prevention of diabetes in NOD mice by administration of dendritic cells deficient in nuclear transcription factor-kappaB activity. Diabetes 2003;52(8):1976–85.
53. Phillips BE, Giannoukakis N, Trucco M. Dendritic cell mediated therapy for immunoregulation of type 1 diabetes mellitus. Pediatr Endocrinol Rev 2008;5(4):873–9.
54. Tyndall A, Uccelli A. Multipotent mesenchymal stromal cells for autoimmune diseases: teaching new dogs old tricks. Bone Marrow Transplant 2009;43(11):821–8.
55. Fiorina P, Jurewicz M, Augello A, et al. Immunomodulatory function of bone marrow-derived mesenchymal stem cells in experimental autoimmune type 1 diabetes. J Immunol 2009;183(2):993–1004.
56. Madec AM, Mallone R, Afonso G, et al. Mesenchymal stem cells protect NOD mice from diabetes by inducing regulatory T cells. Diabetologia 2009;52(7):1391–9.
57. Tang Q, Bluestone JA. The Foxp3+ regulatory T cell: a jack of all trades, master of regulation. Nat Immunol 2008;9(3):239–44.
58. Atkinson MA. Thirty years of investigating the autoimmune basis for type 1 diabetes: why can't we prevent or reverse this disease? Diabetes 2005;54(5):1253–63.

Use of Nonobese Diabetic Mice to Understand Human Type 1 Diabetes

Terri C. Thayer, BA[a,b], S. Brian Wilson, MD, PhD[a],
Clayton E. Mathews, PhD[a,*]

KEYWORDS

• NOD mouse • Genetics • Immunology • Type 1 diabetes

The use of animal models to study diseases is fundamental to the advancement of the understanding of basic biologic mechanisms and disease-specific dysfunctions and to the development and testing of therapeutics. When specifically considering diabetes, animal models have been used throughout the past century and a half for major advances in patient care, such as the discovery of insulin. More recently, mouse models, specifically the autoimmune diabetes-prone nonobese diabetic (NOD) mouse, have played an increasing role in the discovery of disease mechanisms, identification of autoantigens, and the development of a better understanding of the genetic pathogenesis of T1D. In the postgenomic era, the NOD model continues to serve essential roles in defining disease-associated alleles and identifying potential therapeutic interventions.

Initial descriptions of the diabetes-prone biobreeding rat[1,2] and the NOD mouse[3] were published approximately 40 years ago. However, continued technological advances in genetic manipulation, transgenic development, knockout and knockin vectors, and conditional knockout and expression technologies for the mouse genome have led to the wider use of the NOD mouse in T1D research. In addition, pathogenic (**Table 1**) and genetic (**Table 2**) similarities to the human condition theoretically make the NOD a more useful tool to study the cause, pathology, and progression of the disease. Although the NOD model is not without fault,[4–6] this model is

Grant Numbers and Sources of Support: Juvenile Diabetes Research Foundation, the National Institutes of Health grant R01 DK74656, and the Sebastian Family Endowment for Diabetes Research.
[a] Department of Pathology, Immunology, and Laboratory Medicine, The University of Florida College of Medicine, Gainesville, FL 32610, USA
[b] The University of Pittsburgh School of Medicine, One Children's Hospital Drive, 4401 Penn Avenue, Pittsburgh, PA 15224, USA
* Corresponding author. 1600 SW Archer Road, PO Box 100275, Room J597, Gainesville, FL 32610-0275.
E-mail address: clayton.mathews@pathology.ufl.edu

Table 1
Similarities between human T1D and NOD mice

	Human	NOD
Age at Onset	Most often diagnosed in children/young adults	3–6 mo
Insulitis	CD8+ T cells, macrophages, B cells, and CD4+ T cells. Very few NK cells	CD4+ T cells, B cells, CD8+ T cells, macrophages, and dendritic cells
Ketoacidosis	Controlled with insulin	Mild until late stages
Potential Autoantigens	INS, GAD 65, HSP60, IAPP, Slc30a8 (ZnT8), CPE, G6PC2 (IGRP), PDX-1, PTPRN (IA2), HSP90AB1, PTPRN2 (IA2β), REG3A, ICA1 (ICA69), IMO38 (MRPS31), PRPH, and SOX13	INS, GAD65, G6PC2 (IGRP), PDX-1, ICA69, IA2, DMPK,[a] and chromogranin A[a]
MHC Linked	Alleles of class HLA-II DR/DQ and class I HLA-A/B	MHC class II Ab^g/Ea^{null}, class I K^d/D^b
Reported Non-MHC Linkages	>50	>40
Lymphopenia	No	No
T Lymphoaccumulative	Yes	Yes
Role of T Regulatory Cells	No change in numbers, functional differences yet to be conclusive	No decrease in numbers, potential decrease in suppressive function
B Cells Required	Likely required for most cases[b]	Required for most cases[c]
NK Cell Number	No correlation found	Absent
NK Cell Function	No correlations found	Poor
NKT Cell Number	Deficiencies linked with susceptibility	Low
Hemolytic Complement	Dysregulation linked with complications	C5 deficient

Abbreviations: CPE, carboxypeptidase E; DMPK, dystrophia myotonica–protein kinase; G6PC2 or IGRP, glucose-6-phosphatase 2; GAD2 or GAD65, glutamic acid decarboxylase 65; HSP 60, heat shock protein 60; HSP90AB1, heat shock protein 90-beta; IAPP, islet amyloid polypeptide; ICA1 or ICA69, islet cell autoantigen 1; INS, insulin; NK, natural killer; PDX-1, pancreatic and duodenal homeobox 1; PRPH, peripherin; PTPRN or IA2, protein tyrosine phosphatase receptor type N; PTPRN2 or IA2β, receptor-type tyrosine-protein phosphatase N2; REG3A, regenerating islet-derived protein 3 alpha; Slc30a8 or ZnT8, solute-like carrier 30A8; SOX13, SRY-related HMG-box 13.

[a] DMPK and chromogranin A have not yet been identified as autoantigens in humans.

[b] Case report of an individual with X-linked agammaglobulinemia developed diabetes with T-cell reactivity to GAD65 and IA2.

[c] Although B-cell–deficient NOD mice are strongly resistant to spontaneous autoimmune diabetes, these mice are susceptible to mild insulitis and, on treatment with cyclophosphamide, develop diabetes.

particularly useful because it allows the isolation, study, and manipulation of specific genes, polymorphisms, and other genetic factors, to identify how a specific gene may function deleteriously and to understand how specific combinations of normal alleles result in immune dysregulation and autoimmune disease.

IMMUNOLOGY AND PATHOLOGY OF T1D: COMPARING MICE AND MEN

Trying to understand the pathology of diabetes using human samples is complex. Critical information has been derived through the study of organs procured from deceased human patients with T1D. The insulitic infiltrates of cadaveric pancreata demonstrate the presence of CD8[+] cytotoxic T lymphocytes (CTLs), macrophages (MΦs), B cells, and CD4[+] helper T cells.[7] In recent-onset cases in which insulitis was present, infiltrates affect insulin-positive islets as opposed to insulin-deficient endocrine clusters.[8] Analysis of beta and alpha cells shows only significant decreases of beta cells, with persisting insulitis and increased expression of major histocompatibility complex (MHC) I and Fas.[9] These data support the hypothesis that specific immune reactivity to beta-cell antigens is central to diabetes progression. However, even with newer programs, such as the Network for Pancreatic Organ Donors with Diabetes, human samples have been scarce; therefore, much of the knowledge delineating the pathogenesis of T1D has been extrapolated from studies using NOD mice.

In the NOD mouse, diabetes develops after infiltration of leukocytes into the pancreatic insulin-producing beta cells. Lymphocytic infiltration in the islet can be seen at around 3 weeks of age.[10,11] The infiltration in the islets of the NOD mouse initiates with dendritic cells (DCs) and MΦs followed by CD4[+] and CD8[+] T cells as well as B cells. The leukocytes present in the infiltrate mediate beta-cell killing via direct cytotoxicity (using Fas and perforin/granzyme) and indirect mediators (proinflammatory cytokines and free radical production; reviewed in[12]). Several cell types have also been implicated in playing critical roles in the targeting and destruction of beta cells, including MΦs, DCs, T-cell subsets, and B cells. Therefore, the pathologic conditions demonstrated in the NOD in mice is similar to those observed in the human disease.

The immunologic characterization of T1D has been conflicting and challenging. Most human lymphocyte studies have used peripheral blood, whereas those using the NOD mouse have been more extensive and invasive. Antibodies specific for pancreatic islet antigens are present in both species, yet, the presence of autoantibodies in mouse seems to be far less predictive of the development of T1D in man. In some cases, beta-cell autoantibodies are observed in several mouse strains that do not develop T1D.[13,14] Although antibodies likely do not play a role in T1D development in the NOD mouse, complement-fixing antibodies are present in patients with T1D and are cytolytic to human beta cells.[15] Work in the NOD mouse that demonstrates a lack of antibodies in T1D pathogenesis as well as adoptive transfer studies that demonstrate the important role of T cells in murine T1D have been major contributing factors to the belief that T cells are the main effectors of beta-cell destruction in T1D. Patients and NOD mice exhibit autoreactivity of CD4[+] and CD8[+] T-cell subsets as well as altered function of regulatory T cells. However, as there is little evidence to support the specific mechanism of destruction or the cell types that participate in beta-cell death during progression of human T1D, data collected from studies with the NOD mouse remain the basis for much of the current dogma.

Genetically modified and transgenic NOD mice have provided models to establish the role of different cell types in the pathogenesis of T1D. Innate immune cells, including DCs and MΦs, are critical for initiating the process of beta-cell death during T1D. DCs and MΦs are found in early insulitic infiltrates and are implicated in driving

Table 2
Insulin-dependent diabetes loci mapped in mouse models of T1D

Idd	Chr	Position (Base Pairs)	Outcross Partner	T1D Incidence of Congenic (%)	Year of Latest Publication	Gene Candidate	Homologous Human Locus	Gene Candidate
Idd1	17	34,132,973-35,404,440	NON.C57BL/10, C57BL/6	0[50]	2005[107]	MHC	IDDM1	HLA
Idd1.1	17					H2-Ab1		
Idd1.2	17					H2-Ea		
Idd2	9	99,810,752-99,810,847	NON	ND	1998[108]	Znf202	IDDM3	
Idd3	3	60,270,627-60,270,801	B10.H2g7, B6.PL-Thy1a	15[106]	2009[109]	Il2, Il21		
Idd4	11	74,677,336-74,677,434	C57BL/6, C57BL/ B10.H2g7		2007[110]			
Idd5	1	40.0 cM[a]	B10.H2g7	50[111]	2009[112]		IDDM6, IDDM7	
Idd5.1	1	60,883,084-62,840,206		50[43,106]	2009[68]	Ctla4, Icos, Als2cr19, Nrp2	IDDM12	CTLA4
Idd5.2	1	73,984,129-75,465,013		90[43]	2009[113]	Slc1a1, Il8rb	IDDM13	SLC11A1, IGFBP-2.5
Idd6	6	73.0 cM[a]	NON.H2g7	10[114,115]	2008[116]	HIF1β		
Idd6.1	6	146,377,508-149,517,037	C3H		2006[114]			
Idd6.2	6	137,388,269-146,377,508	C3H		2008[116]			
Idd6.3	6	146,261,958-147,388,045	C3H		2006[114]			

Idd7	7	19,998,822–19,998,946	NON.H2g7, B10.H2g7	ND	2008[117]		
Idd8	14	21,656,627–21,656,804	B10.H2g7		1993[118]		
Idd9	4	124,439,115–124,439,213	B10.H2g7, B6.PL-Thy1a, NON.H2g7	5[59,119]	2007[110]		
Idd9.1	4	128,365,830–131,179,223			2010[120]		
Idd9.2	4	144,968,503–149,098,840		30[121]	2010[121]		
Idd9.3	4	149,300,308–150,522,796		60[121]	2010[121]		
Idd10	3	48.5 cM[a]	B10.H2g7, B6.PL-Thy1a, NON.H2g7		2005[122]	CD101	
Idd11	4	64.6 cM[a]	C57BL/6	17–27[123]	2006[124]	Slc9a1	IDDM16
Idd12	14	35,170,432–35,170,533	C57BL/6		1994[125]		
Idd13	2	71.0 cM[a]	NOR	0[126]	2007[110]		
Idd13.1	2		C57BL/6			B2m	
Idd13.2	2		C57BL/6			Mertk	
Idd14	13	41,008,627–41,008,790	NON.H2g7, C57BL/ 6- susceptible allele	+33[127, b]	2007[110]		IDDM15

(continued on next page)

Table 2
(continued)

Idd	Chr	Position (Base Pairs)	Outcross Partner	T1D Incidence of Congenic (%)	Year of Latest Publication	Gene Candidate	Homologous Human Locus	Gene Candidate
Idd15	5	8,797,672–8,797,875	NON.H2g7	ND	1995[48]			
Idd16	17	33,737,692–33,737,814	CT5, C57BL/6, R209, ALR		2004[128]	*Tnf*		
Idd16.1	17	18.0 cM[a]	C57BL/6, R209		2005[59]	*H2K*		
Idd16.a	17	19.0 cM[a]	ALR		2005[59]	*H2-Ddx*		
Idd16.b	17	17.0 cM[a]	ALR		2005[59]			
Idd17	3	79,484,163–87,105,657	NON.H2g7, C57BL/6J		2004[129]			
Idd18	3	53.3 cM[a]	NON.H2g7, C57BL/6J		2009[112]			
Idd19	6	117,439,553–128,469,043	PWK	No change[130]	2006[130]	*Tnfrsf7, Tnfrsf1a, Hrh1*		
Idd20	6	83,595,701–91,990,027	C3H/H3J		2006[130]			
Idd21	18	24.5 cM[a]	ABH Biozzi	35[131]	2003[131]			
Idd21.a	18	74,588,921–84,295,862			2005[132]			
Idd21.b	18	61,299,030–74,588,997			2005[132]			
Idd21.c	18	6,108,402–21,671,921			2005[132]			

Idd22	8	90,626,802–90,626,908	ALR	ND	2008[67]	Nod2, Klf2, Ndufa13	
Idd23	17	8 cM[a]	C57BL/6		2004[128]		
Idd24	17	35,340,111–41,438,922	C57BL/6				
Idd25	4	133,341,830–133,341,946	NOR		2005[133]		
Idd26	1	19,802,051–40,319,403	NOR		2005[133]		
Idd27	7	86,521,272–127,029,671	CBcNO6/Lt		2005[134]		
mt-Nd2	mt	4738	ALR	ND	2008[66]	mt-Nd2	mt-ND2
Susp	3		ALR	ND	2008[66]		
Rthyd1	7	60.0 cM[a]	B10.Br/SgSnJxNOD-H2<k>		2004[135]		
Rthyd4	14	27.5 cM[a]	B10.Br/SgSnJxNOD-H2<k>		2004[135]		
Rthyd5	15	22.0 cM[a]	B10.Br/SgSnJxNOD-H2<k>		2004[135]		
Ssial3	7	58.7 cM[a]			2002[136]		

a centiMorgan (cM) position used when base pair interval is not defined.
b B6 susceptibility allele increases incidence in NOD.

early autoreactive immune responses.[16,17] Depletion of MΦs protects NOD mice from T1D and insulitis.[18] T cells from a MΦ-deficient environment lack diabetogenic potential, yet islet reactivity is restored when MΦs are replenished.[19] Antigen-presenting cells (APCs) play an essential role in CTL activation.[20] DCs are also critical in the initiation of T-cell responses or induction of tolerance, depending on the DC subset and T-cell requirement.[21–23] These data demonstrate the importance of innate immune cells to activate adaptive immunity, promoting pathogenic or tolerogenic responses, and these cells are therefore potential targets for therapies aimed at preventing T1D. It has been proposed that T1D develops in mice and humans because of a break in or lack of tolerance resulting from poor APC function; clinical trials are currently underway to investigate the safety and potential of DC therapy to promote tolerance or enhanced regulation of self-reactive T cells in human cohorts.[24]

Adaptive immune cells, specifically T lymphocytes, are implicated as the final effectors that drive beta-cell death, resulting in overt diabetes, based on work in human samples and NOD mice. Autoreactive responses of CD4+ and CD8+ T cells to islet antigens have been implicated in the pathogenesis of diabetes in humans and NOD mice (see **Table 1**). Using the NOD model, adoptive transfer experiments using CD4+ and CD8+ T cells demonstrated the necessity of both T-cell subsets for T1D induction.[25] T cells recognize specific peptide antigens when presented in the context of MHC molecules, also known as human leukocyte antigens (HLAs). This recognition is mediated by the T-cell receptor (TCR). During the maturation of T cells in the thymus, TCR, MHC, and antigen play essential roles. Defects in T-cell development are proposed to provide significant contributions to T1D susceptibility and pathogenesis. Likewise, polymorphisms in MHC are strongly associated with susceptibility in human and murine autoimmunity, and because MHC molecules are important for T-cell development and activation, these molecules greatly influence selection as well as tolerance in the periphery.

The recognition of autoantigens in the context of MHC is fundamental to initiating an autoimmune response in diabetes in humans and NOD mice. There are striking similarities in the autoantigens that are responded to in both species. T-cell responses and levels of circulating antibodies to more than 15 different antigens have been measured in T1D patients and at-risk individuals, whereas immune responses against 8 antigens have been measured in the NOD mouse (listed in **Table 1**). Of those autoantigens found in the NOD mice, dystrophia myotonica–protein kinase and chromogranin A have not yet been identified as autoantigens in humans, and many of the antigens in humans have not yet been tested for in NOD mice, demonstrating a need to further characterize potential autoreactive targets in mice and humans. Therefore, the T1D-prone mouse has lost tolerance to many of the same antigens against which T1D patients exhibit autoantigenic responses. In conclusion, diabetes in NOD mice has histologic and immune similarities with the human disease and, as described in the following section, these mice have similar genetic susceptibilities as humans.

GENETICS

T1D is a polygenic disease. To date, more than 50 genetic linkages have been associated with this autoimmune disease. However, the linkage to HLA class II (termed insulin-dependent diabetes mellitus 1 [IDDM1]) is by far the dominant susceptibility locus.[26] DQB alleles with serine (Ser), alanine (Ala), or valine (Val) at amino acid residue 57 are associated with T1D susceptibility, whereas those alleles containing an aspartic acid (Asp) residue are considered protective. The non-Asp-containing alleles cause a local rearrangement within the peptide-binding site, which alters the peptide-binding specificity,[27] resulting in altered T-cell recognition and thymic selection.[28] Likewise, susceptibility has also been linked to specific HLA-A and HLA-B class I alleles[29]; however, little is known about the role of the disease-associated variants in T1D. It should, however, be noted that when HLA-B*39 is combined with an HLA haplotype with DRB1*0404-DQB1*0302, patients are at significantly higher risk.[30] This event is a demonstration of gene-gene interaction or epistasis, controlling T1D onset.

Although HLA is by far the most highly associated *IDDM* locus, several non-HLA linkages have been identified. Of the more than 50 other linkages mapped in genome-wide association studies (GWASs), *INS* (*IDDM2*), *PTPN22* (*IDDM5*), and CTL antigen 4 (*CTLA-4, IDDM12*) have repeatedly been associated with T1D.[26] The insulin gene contains a variable number of tandem repeats (VNTRs) in the 5' flanking region. The VNTR class I alleles with 26 to 63 repeats are associated with recessive susceptibility, whereas the dominantly protective class III alleles have significantly more repeats (140 to >200 repeats). The allelic effects on insulin gene transcription can be measured in vitro and in vivo. Specifically, the class III alleles are believed to induce higher thymic expression and potentially enhanced deletion of insulin-reactive T cells.[31] At present, it is unknown how the risk alleles of *PTPN22* and *CTLA-4* contribute to T1D in humans; however, as discussed later, efforts using the NOD mouse are making progress in identifying mechanisms.

Although the aforementioned linkages, and many others, have been identified using population-based genome-wide scans or association studies, candidate gene testing has continued for the past 20 years. Most candidate testing projects have not been successful.[32–37] Polymorphisms of von Willebrand factor A domain containing 2 (*VWA2* or AMACO [*IDDM17*]) have been associated with dominant protection against T1D.[38] Even so, a potential mechanism for the protection provided by AMACO has yet to be published. These studies have provided details on linkages that have potentially profound significance to human T1D. A promoter polymorphism in *SLC11A1* (*NRAMP1* [natural resistance-associated macrophage protein 1]) (*IDDM7*) was identified and later confirmed as contributing to T1D.[39,40] NRAMP1 regulates the activation of MΦs and therefore the proliferation of intracellular pathogens. The T1D-resistance allele of *SCL11A1* is associated with lower levels of expression.[41] Another gene that was identified is *mt-ND2* (NADH dehydrogenase subunit 2), a mitochondrially encoded subunit of complex I of the electron transport chain.[42] These latter 2 genes have also been identified as contributing to T1D in mouse models.[43,44] Therefore, genetic studies have identified regions that predispose to and protect against T1D, and there is overlap in the regions or genes when comparing humans to mice.

In the late 1980s, the first genome-wide screens of the NOD mouse strain were executed with the goal to identify disease susceptibility/resistance loci or *Idd* (insulin-dependent diabetes).[45,46] In the mouse, more than 30 linkages have been mapped (see **Table 2**); however, only a few of the genes responsible have been identified. Similar to the human condition, the most significant associations are with the MHC alleles.[45–48] The NOD MHC class II molecule, I-Ag7 (*H2-Aa^{g7}*), as well as absence of H2-Ea expression are critical for T1D development.[49,50] The H2^{g7} MHC haplotype of NOD allele shares homology with the human T1D susceptibility HLA-DQB1 locus. DQB alleles with Ser, Ala, or Val at position 57 are associated with T1D susceptibility, and the NOD I-Ag7 also contains a nonaspartic residue at position 57.[51–53] Congenic mice have been a major asset for determining the genes and loci in T1D. Congenic mice are those that have been bred to be genotypically different at a particular locus. NOD mice that are congenic for MHC have been used to investigate the diabetogenic potential of the MHC haplotypes associated with T1D susceptibility or resistance. Congenic replacement of the NOD MHC haplotype H2^{g7} with MHC haplotype from strains that do not spontaneously develop T1D, for example, the

$H2^b$ of C57BL/6 (B6), prevents NOD insulitis and overt diabetes development.[50] These data demonstrate that alleles encoded within the $H2^{g7}$ haplotype are critical for T1D. However, introduction of $H2^{g7}$ on a B6 background does not induce T1D. Therefore, MHC alone is not sufficient to cause disease.[50] The situation is the same in humans; only a few individuals with risk-associated HLA alleles develop diabetes. Transgenic mice have also been instrumental in demonstrating the diabetogenic potential of human HLA genes.[54] NOD mice transgenically expressing human risk HLA alleles, such as HLA-DR3 or DQ8, develop T1D. Susceptibility, however, was modulated with the coexpression of HLA-DR4 or DQ6 protective alleles, correlating with human epidemiologic data[55,56] and confirming the effect of HLA alleles on T1D susceptibility. Work to understand the diabetogenic role of HLA class I has also used the NOD mouse. NOD mice expressing HLA-A*0201 and a deletion of the murine MHC class I genes (NOD.HHD) have been produced and have an accelerated form of T1D.[57,58] These studies highlight the importance of the NOD mice in defining the role of MHC in T1D.

Similarly, class I alleles have also been associated with T1D in the mouse. A polymorphism found in the ALR strain as well as the diabetes-resistant cataract Shionogi strain creates a unique allele, $H2-D^{dx}$. Introducing this allele to the NOD background significantly reduces T1D.[59] Likewise, introduction of the MHC class I allele $H2-K^{wm7}$ to the NOD background confers protection (see **Table 2**).[60] Analysis of the $H2-K^{wm7}$ MHC molecule defined a single peptide specificity.[61] This finding suggests that protection is afforded based on the lack of beta-cell antigen presented over other nondiabetogenic antigens, with a higher affinity for a particular MHC allele. Similarly, in the HLA linkage analysis, certain alleles provided either susceptibility or protection. Conversely, not all genes providing genetic risk are shared between the species. For example, on mouse Chromosome 1, a linkage was mapped to the gene β_2-microglobulin (B2m) and later confirmed using transgenic rescue[62]; however, B2M has not been identified as a candidate gene in humans. B2m is a component of MHC class I molecules. It has been conclusively demonstrated that the NOD allele provides dominant susceptibility.[62] However, as B2m is an important component of the HLA/MHC, this nonorthologous linkage demonstrates that even when exact synteny, or colocalization of loci, is not achieved, T1D-associated genes mapped in the NOD mice may point to important pathways that are affected in patients with T1D. Therefore, the study of homologous murine alleles along with human alleles expressed in transgenic mice affords researchers the model to evaluate and define autoantigen versus nondiabetogenic antigen expression.

In situations in which a mutation associated with or even proved to play a role in T1D is shared between mice and humans, the NOD systems can be used to better understand the function of the mutation and the role it plays in T1D onset. The class II HLA/MHC is one example of a shared mutation; another is the single-nucleotide polymorphism in mt-ND2 and mt-Nd2. In the human and mouse, there is a cytosine to adenine nucleotide substitution, resulting in a leucine to methionine amino acid substitution.[42,63] To determine how this mutation modifies mitochondrial function, the mouse was used to ensure genetic homogeneity at all loci save mt-Nd2; therefore, the genetic element was isolated. Ensuing studies were able to determine that the protective allele suppressed mitochondrial reactive oxygen species (ROS) production.[64,65] This reduction in mitochondrial ROS has been highly correlated with an enhanced protection against beta-cell apoptosis.[66,67] The use of mice enabled these studies to be performed in a clean genetic environment at a much faster rate than if using only human samples. A second example would be that of Nramp1. Although the polymorphism in the mouse is not identical to that in the human, the result of the sequence variation is the same: reduced expression and function of the enzyme. Using NOD models, including a novel RNA interference (RNAi) transgenic NOD for Nramp1, it was demonstrated that knockdown of Nramp1 was protective from T1D[43] and that the role of this enzyme in T1D was altered processing and presentation of pancreatic islet antigens.[68]

With the technology to genetically manipulate mouse models and the development of humanized models, the role of T1D-linked genes can be isolated and tested. Increased thymic expression of insulin mRNA was linked with individuals with INS-protective alleles.[69,70] Using genetically manipulated NOD mice, insulin expression in the thymus has been increased or deleted, resulting in altered T-cell insulin autoreactivity, demonstrating that the natural levels of thymic insulin expression are important for T1D and deletion of insulin-specific autoreactive T cells.[71–73] Specific knockout of insulin expression in the thymus induced diabetes in the NOD background as early as 3 weeks of age, demonstrating a critical loss of tolerance resulting from a lack of negative selection.[74] PTPN22, a negative regulator of T-cell activation,[75,76] is associated with T1D,[77,78] as well as other autoimmune diseases.[78,79] Studies using NOD congenics for PTPN22 ortholog, Ptpn8, showed modified incidence of T1D, demonstrating a role for PTPN22 in human and murine T1D.[80] Through further examination of NOD congenic and murine models, the role of lymphoid tyrosine phosphatase and pathways involved in T1D susceptibility can be examined and applied to human disease.

GWASs are another tool that has provided additional information on regions of the genome where T1D susceptibility is linked. Depending on the initial analysis, the genetic region containing the responsible gene may be large. In these cases, a sub-phenotype may be used to more quickly identify genes that may contribute to the gross phenotype of T1D. For example, Ctla4, a candidate gene for T1D (see **Table 2**), is involved in controlling the function of regulatory T cells.[81,82] By evaluating the subphenotype, a genetic region can be identified. Databases can then be used to identify a small number of candidate genes associated with this subphenotype and T1D. This process may also speed up the discovery of the gene in the interval. The process of subphenotypic analysis in many cases is preferable to positional cloning because creating a congenic mouse to identify only a single gene is a demanding, protracted, and therefore a costly process. Subphenotypic analysis has been successfully performed to determine whether Slc11a1 (Nramp1) was a contributing gene for T1D in the NOD mouse[43] and to confirm the T1D-associated polymorphisms in patients with T1D.[40]

This process can also be beneficial to identify the role of a single locus or multiple loci with epistatic interactions. When the Idd5 locus was initially detailed, it became apparent that there were at least 4 genes within this region contributing to T1D. However, the effect for each of these 4 regions is different, with the NOD allele at Idd5.1 demonstrating the most susceptibility. Congenic mice harboring this segment had a markedly reduced risk for T1D (50% compared with 85% in NOD mice).[83] However, the NOD-Idd5.2 had exactly the same T1D incidence as NOD mice. An epistatic interaction between these 2 regions was realized in NOD mice with both regions [NOD.Idd5.1/5.2]. These NOD-Idd5.1/5.2 mice had a T1D incidence of about 10%, demonstrating that, when combined, the protective genes in these 2 regions (likely Ctla4 and Slc11a1) synergized for T1D protection. Moving forward, the transgenic expression or knockin of human T1D susceptibility alleles into the NOD mouse will allow for rigorous testing of epistasis for resistance or susceptibility to T1D.

Technological advances, including sequencing of the mouse genome, genome-wide maps, and databases that allow targeted searches of these data assist researchers in defining and studying susceptibility and resistant loci. Databases are integral components in research of genetic diseases and in defining *Idd* loci. National Center for Biotechnology Information and Mouse Genome Informatics are databases for genetic and mapping data from various mouse strains, providing information on the sequence of the NOD genome, microsatellite markers, single-nucleotide polymorphisms, and known and predicted genes. T1Dbase provides a catalog of human *IDDM* and murine *Idd* loci and genes. These major advances in technology continue to provide information that should speed up the discovery of mechanisms influencing T1D onset.

The development of humanized mice is another advance that is expected to help researchers bridge the gap in translation from mouse to man. Humanized mice are those that are engrafted with human cells or that express human transgenes, allowing researchers to study human cells in vivo in the context of an autoimmune animal. Immunodeficient NOD mice were found to support engraftment of human hematopoietic cells[84] and hematolymphoid tissues.[85] Through the introduction of a targeted mutation in the interleukin-2 receptor common gamma chain, mice with severe defects in innate and adaptive immune cells can be used to study and characterize human hematopoietic stem cells and the function of the multiple lineages produced.[86] The ability to transplant xenogeneic islet grafts to immunodeficient mice provides researchers the ability to study human beta-cell function and response to killing. However, there are still problems in these models, including level of engraftment, the need for chemically induced hyperglycemia, and islet stem cell progenitor sensitivity. Current work is underway to eliminate the need for diabetes induction, thus optimizing and stabilizing engraftment to provide models to study human islets as well as the diabetogenic potential of human immune system (reviewed in[87]). These latest models should accelerate discovery by allowing more invasive studies to be performed on the genetics and immunopathology of diabetes using human effectors cells, such as human beta cells, in the context of human susceptibility/resistance genes.

PRECLINICAL TRIALS

Insulin treatment is needed for T1D to maintain euglycemia, but it is not a cure. Patients are still at risk for serious complications. The primary goals of ongoing research of T1D in the NOD mouse are to determine factors that contribute to and drive autoimmune pathogenesis, develop ways to intervene and/or reverse the course of beta-cell loss, and ultimately apply these therapeutics to cure and prevent human T1D. Therapies to modulate tolerance to autoantigens, such as insulin, have been tested in NOD mice[88–90] and human patients.[91] Treatments to modulate the immune response through administration of anti-CD3 in mouse[92–95] and humans[96] as well as antithymocyte globulin[97] have also been investigated. Although such treatments are effective in the mouse, responses in human patients have been underwhelming, demonstrating the need to better bridge the gap in the understanding of how to apply and translate dosing and timing requirements as well as evaluation of subgroups to determine which regimens are the most successfully stratified by biologic markers and disease state.

Using the genetic information of homologous NOD and human T1D susceptibility (see **Table 2**) to determine potential therapeutic targets is an important starting point. As previously discussed, NOD and human T1D susceptibility has strong correlation to MHC/HLA haplotypes, which can be used to screen for risk. Of other non-MHC–linked alleles, an important linkage, CTLA-4, has been described in NOD and humans. CTLA-4 is expressed on activated T cells and has been functionally characterized as a negative regulator of T-cell activity.[98] Binding of CTLA-4 to B7 molecules signals inhibition of effector T cells.[99] Genetic analysis linked a splice variant of CTLA-4 (liCTLA4) with

T1D in the NOD mouse. It has been shown that liCTLA4 inhibits T-cell reactivity and is more highly expressed in T cells from T1D-resistant NOD congenics.[100] NOD mice treated with CTLA-4 immunoglobulin or anti–B7-2 were protected from T1D onset. However, treatment was only protective when given early, before disease onset, and did not reduce insulitis.[101] Blocking CTLA-4 in NOD transgenic mice[102,103] and partial reduction of expression in lentivirus-transduced RNAi mice[104] accelerated disease onset. Also, beta cells expressing a single-chain anti–CTLA-4 in transgenic NOD mice were protected from T-cell–mediated destruction.[105] These data highlight an essential role for CTLA-4 in modulating peripheral tolerance in early diabetes progression. CTLA-4 is also proposed as the candidate gene for *Idd5.1*[106] and *IDDM12* (see **Table 2**). Therefore, CTLA-4 is a potential target for immune modulation and protection from T-cell–mediated beta-cell destruction. At present, a phase 2 clinical trial administering CTLA-4 immunoglobulin to patients with new-onset T1D is in progress. Continued use of the NOD mouse to determine the roles of *Idd/IDDM* in T1D will help determine the multitherapeutic approaches needed to significantly intervene in autoreactivity and beta-cell death.

Much of the work in the NOD mouse demonstrates that diabetes is a multigenic, multifaceted disease, and there are most likely many genetic and immunologic dysfunctions that, when combined with environmental factors, influence disease pathogenesis. Investigation of T-cell activation demonstrates that many conditions can affect activation status. Cytokine production and mechanisms of killing involve multiple pathways with overlap and redundancy, suggesting that therapeutics targeting these products will require multidrug approaches. There are dozens of therapies that can prevent and a few that can reverse T1D in the NOD mouse (reviewed in[49,91]). This fact has led some investigators to criticize the usefulness of the NOD mouse. However, these failures in translation may prove useful in exposing the similarities and differences between diabetes in mouse and in human. These observations also reinforce the need to standardize disease state, assessment of biologic targets, and outcome of therapies in the NOD mouse. Timing and dosing thresholds for effective prevention or reversal are critical. Similarly, standardized definitions of biomarker positivity, such as autoantibody titer, C-peptide, and markers of immune modulation, during the course of treatment are needed to assist researchers in comparing successes and failures within and between laboratories and to assist in the translation of these data to human T1D trials.

SUMMARY

The use of NOD mice has significantly enabled the understanding of the histology, pathology, and genetics associated with autoimmunity. The speed of disease onset and the relative ease of disease prevention and reversal in this animal model emphasize the lack of complete translatability to human T1D. As such, disease mechanisms clarified in the NOD mouse should be translated to human T1D with considerable caution. Despite its limitations, the NOD mouse may play a critical role in furthering the development of therapies for T1D. Humanized NOD mice models likely represent the next major technological advancement in murine models designed to study the pathophysiology of human T1D and evaluate potential therapeutic targets for immune modulation and enhanced beta-cell survival.

REFERENCES

1. Like AA, Butler L, Williams RM, et al. Spontaneous autoimmune diabetes mellitus in the BB rat. Diabetes 1982;31:7–13.

2. Like AA, Kislauskis E, Williams RR, et al. Neonatal thymectomy prevents spontaneous diabetes mellitus in the BB/W rat. Science 1982;216:644–6.
3. Makino S, Kunimoto K, Muraoka Y, et al. Breeding of a non-obese, diabetic strain of mice. Jikken Dobutsu 1980;29:1–13.
4. Atkinson MA, Leiter EH. The NOD mouse model of type 1 diabetes: as good as it gets? Nat Med 1999;5:601–4.
5. Roep BO, Atkinson M. Animal models have little to teach us about type 1 diabetes: 1. In support of this proposal. Diabetologia 2004;47:1650–6.
6. Roep BO, Atkinson M, von Herrath M. Satisfaction (not) guaranteed: re-evaluating the use of animal models of type 1 diabetes. Nat Rev Immunol 2004;4:989–97.
7. Willcox A, Richardson SJ, Bone AJ, et al. Analysis of islet inflammation in human type 1 diabetes. Clin Exp Immunol 2009;155:173–81.
8. Foulis AK, Liddle CN, Farquharson MA, et al. The histopathology of the pancreas in type 1 (insulin-dependent) diabetes mellitus: a 25-year review of deaths in patients under 20 years of age in the United Kingdom. Diabetologia 1986;29:267–74.
9. Hanafusa T, Imagawa A. Insulitis in human type 1 diabetes. Ann N Y Acad Sci 2008;1150:297–9.
10. Bouma G, Coppens JM, Mourits S, et al. Evidence for an enhanced adhesion of DC to fibronectin and a role of CCL19 and CCL21 in the accumulation of DC around the pre-diabetic islets in NOD mice. Eur J Immunol 2005;35:2386–96.
11. Delovitch TL, Singh B. The nonobese diabetic mouse as a model of autoimmune diabetes: immune dysregulation gets the NOD. Immunity 1997;7:727–38.
12. Pirot P, Cardozo AK, Eizirik DL. Mediators and mechanisms of pancreatic β-cell death in type 1 diabetes. Arq Bras Endocrinol Metabol 2008;52:156–65.
13. Abiru N, Yu L, Miao D, et al. Transient insulin autoantibody expression independent of development of diabetes: comparison of NOD and NOR strains. J Autoimmun 2001;17:1–6.
14. Robles DT, Eisenbarth GS, Dailey NJ, et al. Insulin autoantibodies are associated with islet inflammation but not always related to diabetes progression in NOD congenic mice. Diabetes 2003;52:882–6.
15. Radillo O, Nocera A, Leprini A, et al. Complement-fixing islet cell antibodies in type-1 diabetes can trigger the assembly of the terminal complement complex on human islet cells and are potentially cytotoxic. Clin Immunol Immunopathol 1996;79:217–23.
16. Jansen A, Homo-Delarche F, Hooijkaas H, et al. Immunohistochemical characterization of monocytes-macrophages and dendritic cells involved in the initiation of the insulitis and β-cell destruction in NOD mice. Diabetes 1994;43:667–75.
17. Kolb H, Kantwerk G, Treichel U. Prospective analysis of islet lesions in BB rats. Diabetologia 1986;29:A559.
18. Lee KU, Amano K, Yoon JW. Evidence for initial involvement of macrophage in development of insulitis in NOD mice. Diabetes 1988;37:989–91.
19. Jun HS, Yoon CS, Zbytnuik L, et al. The role of macrophages in T cell-mediated autoimmune diabetes in nonobese diabetic mice. J Exp Med 1999;189:347–58.
20. de Jersey J, Snelgrove SL, Palmer SE, et al. B cells cannot directly prime diabetogenic CD8 T cells in nonobese diabetic mice. Proc Natl Acad Sci U S A 2007;104:1295–300.
21. Clare-Salzler MJ, Brooks J, Chai A, et al. Prevention of diabetes in nonobese diabetic mice by dendritic cell transfer. J Clin Invest 1992;90:741–8.

22. Lo J, Clare-Salzler MJ. Dendritic cell subsets and type I diabetes: focus upon DC-based therapy. Autoimmun Rev 2006;5:419–23.

23. Papaccio G, Nicoletti F, Pisanti FA, et al. Prevention of spontaneous autoimmune diabetes in NOD mice by transferring in vitro antigen-pulsed syngeneic dendritic cells. Endocrinology 2000;141:1500–5.

24. Pasquali L, Giannoukakis N, Trucco M. Induction of immune tolerance to facilitate β cell regeneration in type 1 diabetes. Adv Drug Deliv Rev 2008;60:106–13.

25. Christianson SW, Shultz LD, Leiter EH. Adoptive transfer of diabetes into immunodeficient NOD-scid/scid mice. Relative contributions of CD4+ and CD8+ T-cells from diabetic versus prediabetic NOD.NON-Thy-1a donors. Diabetes 1993;42:44–55.

26. Barrett JC, Clayton DG, Concannon P, et al. Genome-wide association study and meta-analysis find that over 40 loci affect risk of type 1 diabetes. Nat Genet 2009;41:703–7.

27. Sato AK, Sturniolo T, Sinigaglia F, et al. Substitution of aspartic acid at β57 with alanine alters MHC class II peptide binding activity but not protein stability: HLA-DQ (alpha1*0201, β1*0302) and (alpha1*0201, β1*0303). Hum Immunol 1999;60:1227–36.

28. Antoniou AN, Elliott J, Rosmarakis E, et al. MHC class II Ab diabetogenic residue 57 Asp/non-Asp dimorphism influences T-cell recognition and selection. Immunogenetics 1998;47:218–25.

29. Howson JM, Walker NM, Clayton D, et al. Confirmation of HLA class II independent type 1 diabetes associations in the major histocompatibility complex including HLA-B and HLA-A. Diabetes Obes Metab 2009;11(Suppl 1):31–45.

30. Nejentsev S, Reijonen H, Adojaan B, et al. The effect of HLA-B allele on the IDDM risk defined by DRB1*04 subtypes and DQB1*0302. Diabetes 1997;46:1888–92.

31. Bennett ST, Wilson AJ, Esposito L, et al. Insulin VNTR allele-specific effect in type 1 diabetes depends on identity of untransmitted paternal allele. The IMDIAB Group. Nat Genet 1997;17:350–2.

32. Asano K, Ikegami H, Fujisawa T, et al. The gene for human IL-21 and genetic susceptibility to type 1 diabetes in the Japanese. Ann N Y Acad Sci 2006; 1079:47–50.

33. Bergholdt R, Brorsson C, Boehm B, et al. No association of the IRS1 and PAX4 genes with type I diabetes. Genes Immun 2009;10(Suppl 1):S49–53.

34. Ghandil P, Chelala C, Dubois-Laforgue D, et al. Crohn's disease associated CARD15 (NOD2) variants are not involved in the susceptibility to type 1 diabetes. Mol Genet Metab 2005;86:379–83.

35. Howson JM, Walker NM, Smyth DJ, et al. Analysis of 19 genes for association with type I diabetes in the Type I Diabetes Genetics Consortium families. Genes Immun 2009;10(Suppl 1):S74–84.

36. Smyth DJ, Howson JM, Payne F, et al. Analysis of polymorphisms in 16 genes in type 1 diabetes that have been associated with other immune-mediated diseases. BMC Med Genet 2006;7:20.

37. Zhang Y, Xiao X, Liu Y, et al. The association of the PAX4 gene with type 1 diabetes in Han Chinese. Diabetes Res Clin Pract 2008;81:365–9.

38. Eller E, Vardi P, Daly MJ, et al. IDDM17: polymorphisms in the AMACO gene are associated with dominant protection against type 1A diabetes in a Bedouin Arab family. Ann N Y Acad Sci 2004;1037:145–9.

39. Bassuny WM, Ihara K, Matsuura N, et al. Association study of the NRAMP1 gene promoter polymorphism and early-onset type 1 diabetes. Immunogenetics 2002;54:282–5.

40. Takahashi K, Satoh J, Kojima Y, et al. Promoter polymorphism of SLC11A1 (formerly NRAMP1) confers susceptibility to autoimmune type 1 diabetes mellitus in Japanese. Tissue Antigens 2004;63:231–6.

41. Sanjeevi C, Miller E, Dabadghao P, et al. Polymorphism at NRAMP1 and D2S1471 loci associated with juvenile rheumatoid arthritis. Clin Sci 2001;43: 1397–404.

42. Uchigata Y, Okada T, Gong JS, et al. A mitochondrial genotype associated with the development of autoimmune-related type 1 diabetes. Diabetes Care 2002; 25:2106.

43. Kissler S, Stern P, Takahashi K, et al. In vivo RNA interference demonstrates a role for Nramp1 in modifying susceptibility to type 1 diabetes. Nat Genet 2006;38:479–83.

44. Mathews CE, Suarez-Pinzon WL, Baust JJ, et al. Mechanisms underlying resistance of pancreatic islets from ALR/Lt mice to cytokine-induced destruction. J Immunol 2005;175:1248–56.

45. Prochazka M, Leiter EH, Serreze DV, et al. Three recessive loci required for insulin-dependent diabetes in nonobese diabetic mice. Science 1987;237: 286–9.

46. Wicker LS, Miller BJ, Coker LZ, et al. Genetic control of diabetes and insulitis in the nonobese diabetic (NOD) mouse. J Exp Med 1987;165:1639–54.

47. Mathews CE, Graser RT, Bagley RJ, et al. Genetic analysis of resistance to type-1 diabetes in ALR/Lt mice, a NOD-related strain with defenses against autoimmune-mediated diabetogenic stress. Immunogenetics 2003;55:491–6.

48. McAleer MA, Reifsnyder P, Palmer SM, et al. Crosses of NOD mice with the related NON strain. A polygenic model for IDDM. Diabetes 1995;44:1186–95.

49. von Herrath M, Nepom GT. Animal models of human type 1 diabetes. Nat Immunol 2009;10:129–32.

50. Yui MA, Muralidharan K, Moreno-Altamirano B, et al. Production of congenic mouse strains carrying NOD-derived diabetogenic genetic intervals: an approach for the genetic dissection of complex traits. Mamm Genome 1996; 7:331–4.

51. Acha-Orbea H, McDevitt HO. The first external domain of the nonobese diabetic mouse class II I-A β chain is unique. Proc Natl Acad Sci U S A 1987;84:2435–9.

52. Ridgway WM, Fasso M, Fathman CG. A new look at MHC and autoimmune disease. Science 1999;284:749 751.

53. Tisch R, McDevitt H. Insulin-dependent diabetes mellitus. Cell 1996;85:291–7.

54. Wong FS, Wen L. What can the HLA transgenic mouse tell us about autoimmune diabetes? Diabetologia 2004;47:1476–87.

55. Rajagopalan G, Kudva YC, Chen L, et al. Autoimmune diabetes in HLA-DR3/DQ8 transgenic mice expressing the co-stimulatory molecule B7-1 in the β cells of islets of Langerhans. Int Immunol 2003;15:1035–44.

56. Wen L, Wong FS, Tang J, et al. In vivo evidence for the contribution of human histocompatibility leukocyte antigen (HLA)-DQ molecules to the development of diabetes. J Exp Med 2000;191:97–104.

57. Jarchum I, Baker JC, Yamada T, et al. In vivo cytotoxicity of insulin-specific CD8+ T-cells in HLA-A*0201 transgenic NOD mice. Diabetes 2007;56: 2551–60.

58. Marron MP, Graser RT, Chapman HD, et al. Functional evidence for the mediation of diabetogenic T cell responses by HLA-A2.1 MHC class I molecules through transgenic expression in NOD mice. Proc Natl Acad Sci U S A 2002; 99:13753–8.

59. Pomerleau DP, Bagley RJ, Serreze DV, et al. Major histocompatibility complex-linked diabetes susceptibility in NOD/Lt mice: subcongenic analysis localizes a component of Idd16 at the H2-D end of the diabetogenic H2(g7) complex. Diabetes 2005;54:1603–6.
60. Hattori M, Yamato E, Itoh N, et al. Cutting edge: homologous recombination of the MHC class I K region defines new MHC-linked diabetogenic susceptibility gene(s) in nonobese diabetic mice. J Immunol 1999;163:1721–4.
61. Brims DR, Qian J, Jarchum I, et al. Predominant occupation of the class I MHC molecule H-2Kwm7 with a single self-peptide suggests a mechanism for its diabetes-protective effect. Int Immunol 2010;22:191–203.
62. Hamilton-Williams EE, Serreze DV, Charlton B, et al. Transgenic rescue implicates β2-microglobulin as a diabetes susceptibility gene in nonobese diabetic (NOD) mice. Proc Natl Acad Sci U S A 2001;98:11533–8.
63. Mathews CE, Leiter EH, Spirina O, et al. mt-Nd2 Allele of the ALR/Lt mouse confers resistance against both chemically induced and autoimmune diabetes. Diabetologia 2005;48:261–7.
64. Gusdon AM, Votyakova TV, Mathews CE. mt-Nd2a suppresses reactive oxygen species production by mitochondrial complexes I and III. J Biol Chem 2008;283: 10690–7.
65. Gusdon AM, Votyakova TV, Reynolds IJ, et al. Nuclear and mitochondrial interaction involving mt-Nd2 leads to increased mitochondrial reactive oxygen species production. J Biol Chem 2007;282:5171–9.
66. Chen J, Gusdon AM, Thayer TC, et al. Role of increased ROS dissipation in prevention of T1D. Ann N Y Acad Sci 2008;1150:157–66.
67. Chen J, Lu Y, Lee CH, et al. Commonalities of genetic resistance to spontaneous autoimmune and free radical–mediated diabetes. Free Radic Biol Med 2008;45: 1263–70.
68. Araki M, Chung D, Liu S, et al. Genetic evidence that the differential expression of the ligand-independent isoform of CTLA-4 is the molecular basis of the Idd5.1 type 1 diabetes region in nonobese diabetic mice. J Immunol 2009;183: 5146–57.
69. Vafiadis P, Bennett ST, Todd JA, et al. Insulin expression in human thymus is modulated by INS VNTR alleles at the IDDM2 locus. Nat Genet 1997;15:289–92.
70. Geenen V. Thymus-dependent T cell tolerance of neuroendocrine functions: principles, reflections, and implications for tolerogenic/negative self-vaccination. Ann N Y Acad Sci 2006;1088:284–96.
71. Chentoufi AA, Polychronakos C. Insulin expression levels in the thymus modulate insulin-specific autoreactive T-cell tolerance: the mechanism by which the IDDM2 locus may predispose to diabetes. Diabetes 2002;51:1383–90.
72. Nakayama M, Abiru N, Moriyama H, et al. Prime role for an insulin epitope in the development of type 1 diabetes in NOD mice. Nature 2005;435:220–3.
73. Tait KF, Collins JE, Heward JM, et al. Evidence for a type 1 diabetes-specific mechanism for the insulin gene-associated IDDM2 locus rather than a general influence on autoimmunity. Diabet Med 2004;21:267–70.
74. Fan Y, Rudert WA, Grupillo M, et al. Thymus-specific deletion of insulin induces autoimmune diabetes. EMBO J 2009;28:2812–24.
75. Cloutier JF, Veillette A. Cooperative inhibition of T-cell antigen receptor signaling by a complex between a kinase and a phosphatase. J Exp Med 1999;189: 111–21.
76. Hasegawa K, Martin F, Huang G, et al. PEST domain-enriched tyrosine phosphatase (PEP) regulation of effector/memory T cells. Science 2004;303:685–9.

77. Bottini N, Musumeci L, Alonso A, et al. A functional variant of lymphoid tyrosine phosphatase is associated with type I diabetes. Nat Genet 2004;36:337–8.

78. Dultz G, Matheis N, Dittmar M, et al. The protein tyrosine phosphatase non-receptor type 22 C1858T polymorphism is a joint susceptibility locus for immun-thyroiditis and autoimmune diabetes. Thyroid 2009;19:143–8.

79. Smyth D, Cooper JD, Collins JE, et al. Replication of an association between the lymphoid tyrosine phosphatase locus (LYP/PTPN22) with type 1 diabetes, and evidence for its role as a general autoimmunity locus. Diabetes 2004;53:3020–3.

80. Wicker LS, Clark J, Fraser HI, et al. Type 1 diabetes genes and pathways shared by humans and NOD mice. J Autoimmun 2005;25(Suppl):29–33.

81. Friedline RH, Brown DS, Nguyen H, et al. CD4+ regulatory T cells require CTLA-4 for the maintenance of systemic tolerance. J Exp Med 2009;206:421–34.

82. Ueda H, Howson JM, Esposito L, et al. Association of the T-cell regulatory gene CTLA4 with susceptibility to autoimmune disease. Nature 2003;423:506–11.

83. Wicker LS, Chamberlain G, Hunter K, et al. Fine mapping, gene content, comparative sequencing, and expression analyses support Ctla4 and Nramp1 as candidates for Idd5.1 and Idd5.2 in the nonobese diabetic mouse. J Immunol 2004;173:164–73.

84. Mosier DE, Gulizia RJ, Baird SM, et al. Transfer of a functional human immune system to mice with severe combined immunodeficiency. Nature 1988;335:256–9.

85. Greiner D. Use of NOD/LtSz-scid/scid mice in biomedical research. In: Letier E, Atkinson M, editors. NOD mice and related strains: research applications in diabetes, AIDS, cancer, and other diseases. Austin (TX): RG Landes; 1998. p. 173–204.

86. Shultz LD, Ishikawa F, Greiner DL. Humanized mice in translational biomedical research. Nat Rev Immunol 2007;7:118–30.

87. King M, Pearson T, Rossini AA, et al. Humanized mice for the study of type 1 diabetes and β cell function. Ann N Y Acad Sci 2008;1150:46–53.

88. Atkinson MA, Maclaren NK, Luchetta R. Insulitis and diabetes in NOD mice reduced by prophylactic insulin therapy. Diabetes 1990;39:933–7.

89. Zhang ZJ, Davidson L, Eisenbarth G, et al. Suppression of diabetes in nonobese diabetic mice by oral administration of porcine insulin. Proc Natl Acad Sci U S A 1991;88:10252–6.

90. Harrison LC, Dempsey-Collier M, Kramer DR, et al. Aerosol insulin induces regulatory CD8 gamma delta T cells that prevent murine insulin-dependent diabetes. J Exp Med 1996;184:2167–74.

91. Shoda LK, Young DL, Ramanujan S, et al. A comprehensive review of interventions in the NOD mouse and implications for translation. Immunity 2005;23: 115–26.

92. Hayward AR, Shreiber M. Neonatal injection of CD3 antibody into nonobese diabetic mice reduces the incidence of insulitis and diabetes. J Immunol 1989;143: 1555–9.

93. Chatenoud L, Thervet E, Primo J, et al. [Remission of established disease in diabetic NOD mice induced by anti-CD3 monoclonal antibody]. C R Acad Sci III 1992;315:225–8 [in French].

94. Chatenoud L, Thervet E, Primo J, et al. Anti-CD3 antibody induces long-term remission of overt autoimmunity in nonobese diabetic mice. Proc Natl Acad Sci U S A 1994;91:123–7.

95. Mottram PL, Murray-Segal LJ, Han W, et al. Remission and pancreas isograft survival in recent onset diabetic NOD mice after treatment with low-dose anti-CD3 monoclonal antibodies. Transpl Immunol 2002;10:63–72.

96. Keymeulen B, Vandemeulebroucke E, Ziegler AG, et al. Insulin needs after CD3-antibody therapy in new-onset type 1 diabetes. N Engl J Med 2005;352:2598–608.

97. Parker MJ, Xue S, Alexander JJ, et al. Immune depletion with cellular mobilization imparts immunoregulation and reverses autoimmune diabetes in nonobese diabetic mice. Diabetes 2009;58:2277–84.

98. Walunas TL, Lenschow DJ, Bakker CY, et al. CTLA-4 can function as a negative regulator of T cell activation. Immunity 1994;1:405–13.

99. Krummel MF, Allison JP. CD28 and CTLA-4 have opposing effects on the response of T cells to stimulation. J Exp Med 1995;182:459–65.

100. Vijayakrishnan L, Slavik JM, Illes Z, et al. An autoimmune disease-associated CTLA-4 splice variant lacking the B7 binding domain signals negatively in T cells. Immunity 2004;20:563–75.

101. Lenschow DJ, Ho SC, Sattar H, et al. Differential effects of anti-B7-1 and anti-B7-2 monoclonal antibody treatment on the development of diabetes in the nonobese diabetic mouse. J Exp Med 1995;181:1145–55.

102. Luhder F, Chambers C, Allison JP, et al. Pinpointing when T cell costimulatory receptor CTLA-4 must be engaged to dampen diabetogenic T cells. Proc Natl Acad Sci U S A 2000;97:12204–9.

103. Luhder F, Hoglund P, Allison JP, et al. Cytotoxic T lymphocyte-associated antigen 4 (CTLA-4) regulates the unfolding of autoimmune diabetes. J Exp Med 1998;187:427–32.

104. Chen Z, Stockton J, Mathis D, et al. Modeling CTLA4-linked autoimmunity with RNA interference in mice. Proc Natl Acad Sci U S A 2006;103:16400–5.

105. Shieh SJ, Chou FC, Yu PN, et al. Transgenic expression of single-chain anti-CTLA-4 Fv on β cells protects nonobese diabetic mice from autoimmune diabetes. J Immunol 2009;183:2277–85.

106. Hunter K, Rainbow D, Plagnol V, et al. Interactions between Idd5.1/Ctla4 and other type 1 diabetes genes. J Immunol 2007;179:8341–9.

107. Ivakine EA, Fox CJ, Paterson AD, et al. Sex-specific effect of insulin-dependent diabetes 4 on regulation of diabetes pathogenesis in the nonobese diabetic mouse. J Immunol 2005;174:7129–40.

108. Fox CJ, Danska JS. Independent genetic regulation of T-cell and antigen-presenting cell participation in autoimmune islet inflammation. Diabetes 1998;47:331–8.

109. McGuire HM, Vogelzang A, Hill N, et al. Loss of parity between IL-2 and IL-21 in the NOD Idd3 locus. Proc Natl Acad Sci U S A 2009;106:19438–43.

110. Takenaka K, Prasolava TK, Wang JC, et al. Polymorphism in Sirpa modulates engraftment of human hematopoietic stem cells. Nat Immunol 2007;8:1313–23.

111. Hill NJ, Lyons PA, Armitage N, et al. NOD Idd5 locus controls insulitis and diabetes and overlaps the orthologous CTLA4/IDDM12 and NRAMP1 loci in humans. Diabetes 2000;49:1744–7.

112. Mangada J, Pearson T, Brehm MA, et al. Idd loci synergize to prolong islet allograft survival induced by costimulation blockade in NOD mice. Diabetes 2009;58:165–73.

113. Dai YD, Marrero IG, Gros P, et al. Slc11a1 enhances the autoimmune diabetogenic T-cell response by altering processing and presentation of pancreatic islet antigens. Diabetes 2009;58:156–64.

114. Hung MS, Avner P, Rogner UC. Identification of the transcription factor ARNTL2 as a candidate gene for the type 1 diabetes locus Idd6. Hum Mol Genet 2006;15:2732–42.

115. Vallois D, Grimm CH, Avner P, et al. The type 1 diabetes locus Idd6 controls TLR1 expression. J Immunol 2007;179:3896–903.
116. Vallois D, Gagnerault MC, Avner P, et al. Influence of a non-NK complex region of chromosome 6 on CD4+ invariant NK T cell homeostasis. J Immunol 2008;181:1753–9.
117. Serreze DV, Choisy-Rossi CM, Grier AE, et al. Through regulation of TCR expression levels, an Idd7 region gene(s) interactively contributes to the impaired thymic deletion of autoreactive diabetogenic CD8+ T cells in nonobese diabetic mice. J Immunol 2008;180:3250–9.
118. Ghosh S, Palmer SM, Rodrigues NR, et al. Polygenic control of autoimmune diabetes in nonobese diabetic mice. Nat Genet 1993;4:404–9.
119. Lyons PA, Hancock WW, Denny P, et al. The NOD Idd9 genetic interval influences the pathogenicity of insulitis and contains molecular variants of Cd30, Tnfr2, and Cd137. Immunity 2000;13:107–15.
120. Yamanouchi J, Puertas MC, Verdaguer J, et al. Idd9.1 locus controls the suppressive activity of FoxP3+CD4+CD25+ regulatory T-cells. Diabetes 2010;59:272–81.
121. Hamilton-Williams EE, Wong SB, Martinez X, et al. Idd9.2 and Idd9.3 protective alleles function in CD4+T-cells and non-lymphoid cells to prevent expansion of pathogenic islet specific CD8+T-cells. Diabetes 2010;59:1478–86.
122. Yamaji K, Ikegami H, Fujisawa T, et al. Evidence for Cd101 but not Fcgr1 as candidate for type 1 diabetes locus, Idd10. Biochem Biophys Res Commun 2005;331:536–42.
123. Brodnicki TC, Fletcher AL, Pellicci DG, et al. Localization of Idd11 is not associated with thymus and nkt cell abnormalities in NOD mice. Diabetes 2005;54:3453–7.
124. Benavides F, Perez C, Blando J, et al. The radiation-induced nackt (nkt) allele is a loss-of-function mutation of the mouse cathepsin L gene. J Immunol 2006;176:702–3.
125. Morahan G, McClive P, Huang D, et al. Genetic and physiological association of diabetes susceptibility with raised Na+/H+ exchange activity. Proc Natl Acad Sci U S A 1994;91:5898–902.
126. Serreze DV, Bridgett M, Chapman HD, et al. Subcongenic analysis of the Idd13 locus in NOD/Lt mice: evidence for several susceptibility genes including a possible diabetogenic role for β 2-microglobulin. J Immunol 1998;160:1472–8.
127. Brodnicki TC, Quirk F, Morahan G. A susceptibility allele from a non-diabetes-prone mouse strain accelerates diabetes in NOD congenic mice. Diabetes 2003;52:218–22.
128. Deruytter N, Boulard O, Garchon HJ. Mapping non-class II H2-linked loci for type 1 diabetes in nonobese diabetic mice. Diabetes 2004;53:3323–7.
129. Koarada S, Wu Y, Fertig N, et al. Genetic control of autoimmunity: protection from diabetes, but spontaneous autoimmune biliary disease in a nonobese diabetic congenic strain. J Immunol 2004;173:2315–23.
130. Morin J, Boitard C, Vallois D, et al. Mapping of the murine type 1 diabetes locus Idd20 by genetic interaction. Mamm Genome 2006;17:1105–12.
131. Hall RJ, Hollis-Moffatt JE, Merriman ME, et al. An autoimmune diabetes locus (Idd21) on mouse chromosome 18. Mamm Genome 2003;14:335–9.
132. Hollis-Moffatt JE, Hook SM, Merriman TR. Colocalization of mouse autoimmune diabetes loci Idd21.1 and Idd21.2 with IDDM6 (human) and Iddm3 (rat). Diabetes 2005;54:2820–5.
133. Reifsnyder PC, Li R, Silveira PA, et al. Conditioning the genome identifies additional diabetes resistance loci in type I diabetes resistant NOR/Lt mice. Genes Immun 2005;6:528–38.

134. Chen J, Reifsnyder PC, Scheuplein F, et al. "Agouti NOD": identification of a CBA-derived Idd locus on Chromosome 7 and its use for chimera production with NOD embryonic stem cells. Mamm Genome 2005;16:775–83.
135. Liston A, Lesage S, Gray DH, et al. Generalized resistance to thymic deletion in the NOD mouse; a polygenic trait characterized by defective induction of Bim. Immunity 2004;21:817–30.
136. Boulard O, Fluteau G, Eloy L, et al. Genetic analysis of autoimmune sialadenitis in nonobese diabetic mice: a major susceptibility region on chromosome 1. J Immunol 2002;168:4192–201.

The Intestinal Microbiome: Relationship to Type 1 Diabetes

Josef Neu, MD[a],*, Graciela Lorca, PhD[b], Sandra D.K. Kingma, MD[c],
Eric W. Triplett, PhD[b]

KEYWORDS

• Type 1 diabetes • Microbiome • Microbes

Environmental influences that have not yet been identified appear to play a major role in the pathogenesis of type 1 diabetes (T1D).[1] It is clear that autoimmune pancreatic beta cell destruction with resultant life-threatening metabolic aberrations that lead to organ failure comprises the final end result. Emerging evidence, however, implicates interplay between the developing intestinal microbial environment with the intestinal mucosal immune system[2] as an early and potentially manageable component in the pathogenesis. The concept of a core microbiome whose alteration may result in major shifts in the intestinal mucosal inflammatory and immune responses is likely to play a significant role in the pathogenesis of many forms of autoimmune and metabolic diseases, including T1D.[3]

Novel and rapidly emerging high-throughput nonculture-based technologies dependent on microbial DNA analysis are opening exciting new opportunities to explore the relationship of previously uncharacterized microbes and their ecologic niches with various diseases. With the recent advent of the Human Microbiome Project,[4] further taxonomic information coupled to known data about functionality of newly characterized microbes may provide clues to the relationship of the resident microbes (or lack of resident microbes) to the disease. Additional information in the form of how these microbes interact with mucosal surfaces, their metabolic product, and their interaction with the immune system will need to be garnered to clarify the relationships in autoimmunity and TID.

This article discusses recent evidence that associates the developing intestinal microbiome to the pathogenesis of autoimmune T1D. It attempts to identify avenues

[a] Department of Pediatrics, University of Florida, Gainesville, FL 326101, USA
[b] Department of Microbiology and Cell Science, University of Florida, Gainesville, FL, USA
[c] VU University Medical Center, Amsterdam, The Netherlands
* Corresponding author.
E-mail address: neuj@peds.ufl.edu

Endocrinol Metab Clin N Am 39 (2010) 563–571
doi:10.1016/j.ecl.2010.05.008
0889-8529/10/$ – see front matter © 2010 Elsevier Inc. All rights reserved.

that should be pursued that relate this new evidence to interventions that eventually could result in prevention.

THE HUMAN SUPERORGANISM

Only a fraction of the microbiota that associate closely with people has been genetically characterized and identified. With the advent of new technologies that enable characterization of previously noncultivatable microbes, it is becoming clear that a vastly larger number of microbial species than previously thought shares a common environment with the human host.[4] People are born with a genome that is almost exclusively human, but in the first years after birth, it evolves into a superorganism with a combined genome (the metagenome) that is 90% bacterial working both in parallel and in concert with the indigenous human genome.[5] This developmental shift is one that cannot be ignored when discussing disease pathogenesis, especially entities involving immunity.

The vast number of microbes residing in the human gastrointestinal (GI) tract interacts closely with the intestinal mucosal immune system, especially in the first years of life. Aberrations in this relationship may have life-long effects, since these microbes are actively participating in the shaping of the innate and adaptive immune networks of the host during critical windows of development.[6,7]

The presence of a commensal intestinal microbiota in infancy is critical for numerous physiologic processes (**Fig. 1**), including growth, angiogenesis, optimization of nutrition, and stimulation of various arms of the innate and adaptive immune systems.[8,9] This microbiota metabolize otherwise indigestible compounds such as carbohydrate fibers to form various energy substrates and bioactive small molecules such as acetate and butyrate (a bioreactor role); they also modulate immune

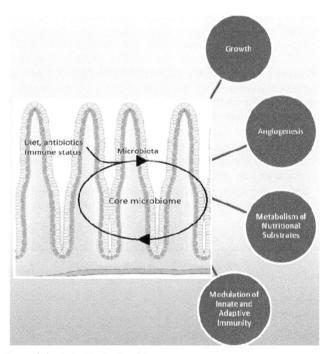

Fig. 1. Functions of the intestinal microbiome.

responses against both commensal and invasive pathogens.[10] The epithelial cells of the intestine, which comprise the largest surface area of the body, are the primary interface between the vast number of microbes in the lumen, and these cells contain signaling pathways that operate via epithelial receptors that selectively relay information to the submucosa using various transduction pathways.

During the life of the individual person, it has been found that the intestinal microbiota are in a constant state of flux, depending on diet, immune status of the host, and use of antibiotics. More recent information suggests that despite this constant change, there is a constant subset of genes, the core microbiome that is present in most healthy individuals, but if some of the core genes are lacking, various metabolic conditions may result, including obesity[11] and autoimmune diseases.[3]

INTESTINAL MUCOSAL IMMUNOLOGY IN RELATION TO T1D

In addition to comprising the largest surface area of the body, the intestinal mucosa is constantly exposed to a vast array of microbes, food antigens, and toxins. The intestinal epithelium must discriminate between pathogenic and nonpathogenic organisms, as well as food antigens. It must tolerate the commensal flora that maintain mucosal homeostasis by controlling inflammatory responses and sensing danger signals of potentially harmful pathogens. It is becoming increasingly clear that the nexus of intestinal microbiota composition, the intestinal barrier, and the mucosal immune system plays pivotal roles in the development of various allergic and autoimmune diseases.[3]

In T1D, evidence for a synergism between aberrant intestinal microbiota (autoimmune microbiomes), a leaky intestinal mucosal barrier, and altered mucosal immunity contributing to the disorder's pathogenesis has begun to evolve (**Fig. 2**).[2,12,13] If the proposed facets do indeed form integral components in the pathogenesis of T1D,[14] they also offer potential targets for intervention that would include maintenance of

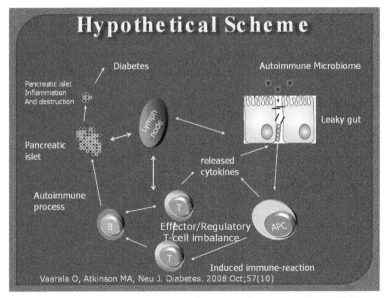

Fig. 2. Hypothetical scheme showing synergy between the intestinal microbiota, a permeability barrier and the immune system. (*Adapted from* Vaarala O, Atkinson MA, Neu J. The perfect storm for type 1 diabetes: the complex interplay between intestinal microbiota, gut permeability, and mucosal immunity. Diabetes 2008;57(10):2555–62; with permission.)

nondiabetogenic microbiota, tightening of interepithelial junctions, and prevention of propagation of inflammation and autoimmunity by nutritional or pharmacologic means.

ALTERED INTESTINAL MICROBIOTA IN T1D

With the knowledge that environment influences the development of T1D and that the GI tract provides the greatest surface area for interaction of the environment, this is an area that begs further investigation. Among the most promising molecular techniques that have recently been developed to fill this void are those that enable detection of uncultivatable species and are amenable to statistical microecologic analyses.[14–18] Some of these methods target 16Ss RNA gene sequences, as they contain signatures of phylogenetic groups and sometimes even species. Other techniques apply polymerase chain reaction (PCR) with denaturing or temperature gradient gel electrophoresis, fluorescent in situ hybridization and shotgun sequencing DNA, and whole metagenomic approaches. These techniques offer promise for future efforts seeking to establish a causal link between the intestinal microbiota and T1D, as well as to the identification of aberrant microbiota that could be targeted for disease prevention strategies.

Obtaining data on the intestinal microecologic conditions before the onset of TID offers significant challenges. Stool samples obtained over time in individuals at risk for the development of diabetes present an opportunity to compare the microecology of those who seroconvert to a diabetic phenotype or who actually develop the disease with those who do not. Animal models such as the biobreeding diabetes-prone (BBDP) rat or nonobese diabetic (NOD) mouse are also available. In a recent set of experiments, bacteria associated with the onset of TID in a rat model system were identified. Stool samples were collected at three time points after birth from BBDP and biobreeding diabetes-resistant (BBDR) rats.[19] DNA was isolated from these samples, and the 16S rRNA gene was amplified using universal primer sets. In the first experiment, bands specific to BBDP and BBDR genotypes were identified by automated ribosomal intergenic spacer analysis[18] at the time of diabetes onset in BBDP. *Lactobacillus* and *Bacteroides* strains were identified in the BBDR- and BBDP-specific bands, respectively. Sanger sequencing showed that the BBDP and BBDR bacterial communities differed significantly. but too few reads were available to identify significant differences at the genus or species levels. A second experiment confirmed these results using higher throughput pyrosequencing and quantitative PCR of 16S rRNA with more rats per genotype. An average of 4541 and 3381 16S rRNA bacterial reads were obtained from each of the 10 BBDR and 10 BBDP samples collected at time of diabetes onset. Nine genera were more abundant in BBDP, whereas another nine genera were more abundant in BBDR. Thirteen and eleven species were more abundant in BBDP and BBDR, respectively. An average of 23% and 10% of all reads could be classified at the genus and species levels, respectively. Quantitative PCR verified the higher abundance of *Lactobacillus* and *Bifidobacterium* in the BBDR samples[19] (**Fig. 3**). Whether these changes are caused by diabetes or are involved in the development remains to be determined, but the fact that the microbial ecology differed before onset of the disease supports an etiologic role.

INTESTINAL MUCOSAL BARRIER—MICROBIAL INTERACTION

The incidence of TID has increased steadily over the past several decades in developed countries, suggesting an environmental component to disease induction.[1,20] Germane to the microbial pathology is the fact that diabetes development in the NOD mouse model is increased when mice are reared in a germ-free environment. Whether this response is signaled through toll-like receptors (TLRs), receptors that

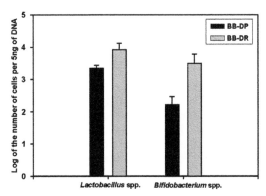

Fig. 3. Log of the number of *Lactobacillus* and *Bifidobacterium* cells per 5 ng of DNA from bio-breeding diabetes resistant (BBDR) and bio-breeding diabetes-prone (BBDP) stool samples. (*From* Roesch LF, Lorca GL, Casella G, et al. Culture-independent identification of gut bacteria correlated with the onset of diabetes in a rat model. ISME J 2009;3(5): 536–48; with permission.)

are known to recognize bacteria, was evaluated in a recent study designed to understand how microbial sensing impacted the progression of T1D. In this study, NOD mice were crossed with specific pathogen-free mice, lacking Myd88 protein (adaptor for multiple innate immune receptors that recognize microbial stimuli instead of Myd88-deficient animals), and disease was monitored.[21] Wild-type NOD mice developed diabetes as early as 10 weeks, but MyD88-deficient animals were completely devoid of autoimmunity, suggesting that microbial signals initiate disease. When these animals were rederived in a germ-free environment, the incidence of disease dramatically increased, suggesting that the presence of the microbiota is protective even in the absence of signaling by TLRs. Thus, bacterial sensing by TLRs enhances the development of TID, while mechanisms that do not require TLRs induce protective responses.

The link between an abnormally permeable intestine and T1D has been demonstrated in animal models of autoimmune diabetes, in which the immune-mediated destruction of insulin-producing β-cells develops spontaneously, and in human T1D. In BBDP rats as well as in BBDR rats, structural changes in the intestinal morphology together with increased permeability have been reported.[13,22] The expression of tight junction proteins claudin-1 and occludin was decreased BBDP and BBDR rats when compared with control Wistar rats.[13] In BBDP rats, the number of mucus-secreting goblet cells was higher than in BBDR rats, which could be a marker of inflammation.[13] The increased gut permeability was demonstrated transiently at early life both in BBDP and BBDR rats, whereas morphologic changes and signs of inflammation were seen in only BBDP rats.[13] Collectively, these data support the authors' hypothesis that an unhealthy collection of bacteria in the intestine (an autoimmune microbiome) leads to leaks in the epithelial layer of the gut which, in turn, causes a large increase in specific immune responses that eventually destroy the insulin-producing pancreatic islets. More extensive studies in people from cohorts such as The Environmental Determinants of Diabetes in the Young (TEDDY) are needed to further test this hypothesis.

The small intestinal mucosa of children with T1D shows increased expression of inflammatory cytokines, human leukocyte antigen (HLA)-class 2 molecules, and lymphocyte adhesion molecules.[23] Inflammatory mediators, such as interleukin (IL)-4 and interferon (IFN)-g, can increase the gut permeability.[24,25] A more recent study[26] in individuals at risk of T1D suggests that increased intestinal permeability may actually precede clinical onset of T1D. Out of 18 at-risk individuals with β-cell autoantibodies, all showed increased urinary lactulose mannitol ratio, suggestive of increased paracellular permeability, which is consistent with the previous studies in BBDP rats.

Intestinal microbes and infections are known modifiers of the intestinal barrier. Pattern recognition receptors expressed on the surface and cytoplasm of intestinal epithelial cells that recognize various microbial components play a significant role in controlling the epithelial barrier. Ligands of TLRs, for example actively mediate intestinal inflammation. TLR-2, as an example, controls mucosal inflammation via regulation of the epithelial barrier function.[27] Thus, changes in the normal flora could be of importance in the development of autoimmune diabetes by affecting intestinal permeability. Furthermore, manipulations such as antibiotic treatment, administration of prebiotics and probiotics also could alter the composition of microbes and therefore the mucosal barrier function.[28]

The composition of the intestinal microbiota may not only affect permeability but may also directly have immune-modulating effects via other cell types such as dendritic cells, which mediate the differentiation of T cells into effector or regulatory cells. The latter can control tolerance[29] via elaboration of anti-inflammatory agents such as IL-10 and transforming growth factor (TGF)-β.[29] The tolerogenic effect of the commensal microbes and the mechanisms of action on how development of both innate and adaptive immunity are affected are active areas of current investigation.[30]

PROBIOTICS AND T1D

There is a possibility that modulation of gut-associated lymphoid tissue may provide a means to affect the pathogenesis of T1D. In a study of NOD mice, VSL#3, a probiotic, was administered to determine whether it could prevent diabetes.[31] Probiotic-treated mice showed reduced insulitis and a decreased rate of beta cell destruction. Prevention was associated with an increased production of IL-10 from Peyer patches and the spleen and with increased IL-10 expression in the pancreas, where IL-10-positive islet-infiltrating mononuclear cells were detected.

MICROBIAL INTERACTION WITH NUTRIENTS, IMMUNITY AND PATHOGENESIS OF T1D

The role of colonic microbes as bioreactors in the fermentation of complex carbohydrates has been suggested as playing a role in the pathogenesis of T1D.[32] Breakdown of these complex carbohydrates into short chain fatty acids such as acetate, propionate, and butyrate may function as energy substrates to colonocytes, but in addition, may it also be involved in intestinal differentiation and other critical intestinal functions.[33] For example, butyrate has been found to be a powerful inducer of tight junction formation in intestinal epithelium.[34] The role of this in the pathogenesis of T1D is yet to be explored.

Vitamin D deficiency and gene polymorphism involved in vitamin D metabolism have been suggested as risk factors of T1D.[35,36] In a recent study,[36] the role of vitamin D in maintenance of mucosal integrity was supported by demonstrating its role controlling gut permeability. 1,25-(OH)2D3-enhanced tight junctions formed by Caco-2 monolayers by increasing tight-junction proteins, such as ZO-1, claudin-1, claudin-2 and E-cadherin and concurrently increased transepithelial electric resistance (TER) in these cells.

Microbial imbalance also may disable vitamin D receptor gene expression, and in turn cause the active metabolite to rise to excessively high levels where it could inhibit expression by the bulk of the body's other nuclear receptors.[3] Thus, the dual role of microbes as they relate to vitamin D and the pathogenesis of T1D remains unclear but is a fertile area for future investigation.

SUMMARY

The microbial ecology of the developing GI tract is clearly becoming a target for future strategies aimed at prevention of various autoimmune diseases including T1D. With emerging techniques that not only help characterize the various microbial taxa in the GI tract, but also aid in the understanding of the interaction of these microbes with the developing immune system and their metabolic roles, one can be confident that new interventions will be discovered that will prevent this devastating disease.

REFERENCES

1. Knip M, Veijola R, Virtanen SM, et al. Environmental triggers and determinants of type 1 diabetes. Diabetes 2005;54(Suppl 2):S125–36.
2. Vaarala O, Atkinson MA, Neu J. The perfect storm for type 1 diabetes: the complex interplay between intestinal microbiota, gut permeability, and mucosal immunity. Diabetes 2008;57(10):2555–62.
3. Proal AD, Albert PJ, Marshall T. Autoimmune disease in the era of the metagenome. Autoimmun Rev 2009;8(8):677–81.
4. Turnbaugh PJ, Ley R, Hamad YM, et al. The human microbiome project. Nature 2007;449(164):804–10.
5. Goodacre R. Metabolomics of a superorganism. J Nutr 2007;137(Suppl 1): 259S–66S.
6. Bailey M, Haverson K, Inman C, et al. The development of the mucosal immune system pre- and postweaning: balancing regulatory and effector function. Proc Nutr Soc 2005;64(4):451–7.
7. Björkstén B. Disease outcomes as a consequence of environmental influences on the development of the immune system. Curr Opin Allergy Clin Immunol 2009; 9(3):185–9.
8. Hooper LV. Bacterial contributions to mammalian gut development. Trends Microbiol 2004;12(3):129–34.
9. Stappenbeck TS, Hooper LV, Gordon JI. Developmental regulation of intestinal angiogenesis by indigenous microbes via Paneth cells. Proc Natl Acad Sci U S A 2002;99(24):15451–5.
10. Neish AS. Microbes in gastrointestinal health and disease. Gastroenterology 2009;136(1):65–80.
11. Turnbaugh P, Gordon JI. The core gut microbiome, energy balance and obesity. J Physiol 2009;587(Pt 17):4153–8.
12. Meddings JB, Jarand J, Urbanski SJ, et al. Increased gastrointestinal permeability is an early lesion in the spontaneously diabetic BB rat. Am J Physiol 1999;276:G951–7.
13. Neu J, Reverte CM, Mackey AD, et al. Changes in intestinal morphology and permeability in the biobreeding rat before the onset of type 1 diabetes. J Pediatr Gastroenterol Nutr 2005;40(5):589–95.
14. Vael CA, Desager KB. The importance of the development of the intestinal microbiota in infancy 2009;21(6):794–800.

15. Huson DH, Richter DC, Mitra S, et al. Methods for comparative metagenomics. BMC Bioinformatics 2009;10(Suppl 1):S12.
16. Raes J, Foerstner KU, Bork P. Get the most out of your metagenome: computational analysis of environmental sequence data. Curr Opin Microbiol 2007; 10(5):490–8.
17. Relman DA. New technologies, human–microbe interactions, and the search for previously unrecognized pathogens. J Infect Dis 2002;186(Suppl 2):S254–8.
18. Fisher MM, Triplett EW. Automated approach for ribosomal intergenic spacer analysis of microbial diversity and its application to freshwater bacterial communities. Appl Environ Microbiol 1999;65(10):4630–6.
19. Roesch LF, Lorca GL, Casella G, et al. Culture-independent identification of gut bacteria correlated with the onset of diabetes in a rat model. ISME J 2009;3(5):536–48.
20. Patterson CC, Dahlquist G, Soltesz G, et al. Is childhood-onset type I diabetes a wealth-related disease? An ecological analysis of European incidence rates. Diabetologia 2001;44(Suppl 3):B9–16.
21. Wen L, Ley RE, Volchkov PY, et al. Innate immunity and intestinal microbiota in the development of type 1 diabetes. Nature 2008;455:1109–13.
22. Graham S, Courtois P, Malaisse WJ, et al. Enteropathy precedes type 1 diabetes in the BB rat. Gut 2004;53(10):1437–44.
23. Westerholm-Ormio M, Vaarala O, Pihkala P, et al. Immunologic activity in the small intestinal mucosa of pediatric patients with type 1 diabetes. Diabetes 2003;52(9):2287–95.
24. Colgan SP, Resnick MB, Parkos CA, et al. IL-4 directly modulates function of a model human intestinal epithelium. J Immunol 1994;153(5):2122–9.
25. Bruewer M, Utech M, Ivanov AI, et al. Interferon-gamma induces internalization of epithelial tight junction proteins via a macropinocytosis-like process. FASEB J 2005;19(8):923–33.
26. Bosi E, Molteni L, Radaelli MG, et al. Increased intestinal permeability precedes clinical onset of type 1 diabetes. Diabetologia 2006;49(12):2824–7.
27. Cario E, Gerken G, Podolsky DK. For whom the bell tolls!—innate defense mechanisms and survival strategies of the intestinal epithelium against lumenal pathogens. Z Gastroenterol 2002;40(12):983–90.
28. Brugman S, Klatter FA, Visser JT, et al. Antibiotic treatment partially protects against type 1 diabetes in the bio-breeding diabetes-prone rat. Is the gut flora involved in the development of type 1 diabetes? Diabetologia 2006;49(9):2105–8.
29. Coombes JL, Powrie F. Dendritic cells in intestinal immune regulation. Nat Rev Immunol 2008;8(6):435–46.
30. Round JL, O'Connell RM, Mazmanian SK. Coordination of tolerogenic immune responses by the commensal microbiota. J Autoimmun 2009;34(3):J220–5.
31. Calcinaro FDS, Marinaro M, Candeloro P, et al. Oral probiotic administration induces interleukin-10 production and prevents spontaneous autoimmune diabetes in the non-obese diabetic mouse. Diabetologia 2005;48(8):1565–75.
32. Samuelsson U, Ludvigsson J. The concentrations of short-chain fatty acids and other microflora-associated characteristics in faeces from children with newly diagnosed type 1 diabetes and control children and their family members. Diabet Med 2004;21(1):64–7.
33. Roy CC, Kien CL, Bouthillier L, et al. Short-chain fatty acids: ready for prime time? Nutr Clin Pract 2006;21(4):351–66.
34. Peng L, Li ZR, Green RS, et al. Butyrate enhances the intestinal barrier by facilitating tight junction assembly via activation of AMP-activated protein kinase in Caco-2 cell monolayers. J Nutr 2009;139(9):1619–25.

35. Zipitis CS, Akobeng AK. Vitamin D supplementation in early childhood and risk of type 1 diabetes: a systematic review and meta-analysis. Arch Dis Child 2008; 93(6):512–7.
36. Kong J, Zhang Z, Musch MW, et al. Novel role of the vitamin D receptor in maintaining the integrity of the intestinal mucosal barrier. Am J Physiol Gastrointest Liver Physiol 2008;294(1):G208–16.

Contemporary Management of Patients with Type 1 Diabetes

Sanjeev N. Mehta, MD, MPH[a,b], Joseph I. Wolfsdorf, MB, BCh[a,c],*

KEYWORDS

• Diabetes • Management • Intensive therapy • Outcomes

HISTORICAL BACKGROUND

Successful management of type 1 diabetes (T1D) requires meticulously balancing insulin replacement with diet and exercise. Scientific and technological advances, of which arguably the most important are the ability to self-monitor blood glucose (BG) and measure glycated hemoglobin (HbA1c), introduced into routine clinical care in the late 1970s,[1,2] have led to a gradual evolution of treatment strategies. In 1993, the Diabetes Control and Complications Trial (DCCT) showed that a system of intensive diabetes management aimed at near-normal glycemic control dramatically reduces the risk of microvascular complications and favorably affects the risk of macrovascular complications.[3–5] However, the treatment regimens used by subjects randomized to the intensive treatment arm of the DCCT also significantly increased their risk of severe hypoglycemia and led to more weight gain.[6,7]

The principal goals of contemporary diabetes management are outlined below. In the post-DCCT era, clinicians are challenged to implement intensive diabetes management in routine clinical care, but most do not have the resources available to the DCCT investigators.[8] Since the publication of the DCCT results more than 15 years ago, a variety of insulin analogues, better and more sophisticated insulin pumps, and faster and more accurate glucose meters have become widely used in the

This work was supported by a National Institutes of Health Training Grant in Pediatric Endocrinology (K12 DK639605).

[a] Harvard Medical School, 25 Shattuck Street, Boston, MA 02115, USA
[b] Pediatric, Adolescent and Young Adult Section and Genetics and Epidemiology Section, Joslin Diabetes Center, 1 Joslin Place, Boston, MA 02215, USA
[c] Division of Endocrinology, Children's Hospital Boston, 300 Longwood Avenue, Boston, MA 02115, USA
* Corresponding author. Division of Endocrinology, Children's Hospital Boston, 300 Longwood Avenue, Boston, MA 02115.
E-mail address: Joseph.Wolfsdorf@childrens.harvard.edu

treatment of T1D. This brief overview of contemporary diabetes management focuses on the assimilation of these advances into routine clinical care, with an emphasis on health outcomes in the post-DCCT era.

Goals of Contemporary Diabetes Management

- Utilize intensive therapy aimed at near-normal BG and hemoglobin A1c levels
- Prevent diabetic ketoacidosis and severe hypoglycemia
- Achieve the highest quality of life compatible with the daily demands of diabetes management
- In children, achieve normal growth and physical development and psychological maturation
- Establish realistic goals adapted to each individual's circumstances.

MULTIDISCIPLINARY DIABETES TEAM

Optimal management of T1D is time-consuming and requires considerable personnel resources. The provision of health care to individuals with T1D, ideally, involves a collaboration between a primary care clinician and a diabetes care team.[9] Intensive diabetes case management provided by a diabetes team is an efficient and effective means of health care delivery.[10,11] The team should consist of a diabetes specialist, diabetes educator, dietitian, and mental health professional, who collaborate to assess, educate, and treat the individual with T1D.[12] The roles of team members are well defined, but frequently overlap; good communication among team members is essential to ensure that the patient receives accurate and consistent information. The patient or a family member should be able to contact a member of the care team at any time for advice on urgent matters, for example, sick-day management. To be successful, the multidisciplinary team must recognize and adapt to the patient's priorities, diabetes knowledge, and readiness to implement the treatment plan. The patient, therefore, must be the central member of the team.

Intensive case management is an ongoing process that begins at the time of diagnosis. If the patient is clinically stable (eg, absence of diabetic ketoacidosis [DKA] or severe dehydration), the initial assessment, management, and education may be accomplished in either an inpatient or outpatient setting, depending on local resources and practice patterns.[13] In addition to providing emotional support, the diabetes team must provide the basic skills required to safely administer insulin, make appropriate dietary choices, monitor BG levels, and manage hypoglycemia. During the first few months after diagnosis, the patient will require more frequent contact with members of the diabetes team. Thereafter, routine diabetes care should be delivered at least quarterly; follow-up consultations with a dietitian and mental health specialist are recommended at least annually. The adoption of new technologies (eg, commencing insulin pump therapy or continuous glucose monitoring [CGM]) or the need to address a significant deterioration in glycemic control requires more frequent encounters. Periodic physical examinations, laboratory assessments, and subspecialty referral (eg, ophthalmologist) are required for assessment and management of diabetes-related complications and comorbidities. Recommendations are summarized in **Tables 1** and **2**.[14–21]

INSULIN ANALOGUES

Intensive diabetes therapy aims to mimic physiologic insulin replacement.[22,23] Normal insulin production has two principal components: basal insulin secretion that suppresses lipolysis and balances hepatic glucose production with glucose use by obligate glucose consumers (eg, brain and erythrocytes) and prandial insulin release that inhibits hepatic glucose production and stimulates glucose uptake after eating. The ability to simulate endogenous insulin production via subcutaneous administration is limited by two factors: (1) delivery of insulin into the systemic circulation as opposed to the portal system, and (2) the inability in clinical practice to reproduce the two distinct phases of prandial insulin release.[23]

In the 1980s, human regular (soluble) insulin produced by recombinant DNA technology became available and rapidly replaced animal source insulins. Regular insulin is a short-acting prandial insulin that also imparts a significant basal component. Neutral protamine Hagedorn (NPH), an intermediate-acting insulin that has been widely used to provide the basal component of insulin regimens, has a broad peak action that imparts a substantial prandial component. Over the past 15 years, several insulin analogues have been developed as alternatives to regular and NPH insulin with pharmacodynamic profiles that more closely mimic prandial (insulins lispro, aspart, and glulisine) and basal (insulins glargine and detemir) insulin profiles, respectively.[23,24] Pharmacodynamic profiles of available insulins and insulin preparations are summarized in **Table 3**.

Rapid-Acting Insulins

Compared with regular insulin, these analogues have a faster onset and shorter duration of action. Unlike regular insulin, their time to peak action is independent of the dose, and their pharmacologic properties are unaffected by renal or hepatic dysfunction.[26,27] Intra- and interindividual absorption of rapid-acting analogues are less variable than regular insulin.[28] For all these reasons they are considered first-line prandial or bolus insulins. Rapid-acting analogues should be administered 10 to 15 minutes before meals to match glucose absorption and achieve a prandial peak effect that limits postprandial glucose excursions.[29,30] This is a major practical advantage as compared with regular insulin, which must be administered at least 30 minutes before a meal.[31,32] In special circumstances, rapid-acting analogues may be administered after eating to safely manage unpredictable food intake (eg, very young children, sick-day management).[29,33]

The use of these analogues has been associated with significantly less postprandial hyperglycemia and postabsorptive hypoglycemia when compared with regular insulin.[23,24] However, several meta-analyses have concluded that in adults with T1D, use of rapid-acting analogues as compared with regular insulin is associated with a clinically insignificant 0.1% reduction in HbA1c (**Table 4**). In children, no significant impact on HbA1c has been demonstrated using rapid-acting analogues (**Table 5**).[24,35,38] Their use in insulin pumps, however, is associated with a modest 0.2% reduction in HbA1c.[37]

When compared with regular insulin, the effect of rapid-acting analogues on hypoglycemia is inconsistent (see **Tables 4** and **5**). Rapid-acting analogues are associated with a significant reduction in severe hypoglycemia in adults, but not children.[24,34,36–38] Rapid-acting analogues reduce the frequency of nocturnal hypoglycemia in adults and adolescents, but not in prepubertal children, and their use in pump therapy is associated with decreased nocturnal hypoglycemia.[38] These analogues are associated with modest reductions in overall frequency of hypoglycemia in children, but not adults.[39] When compared head-to-head, insulin lispro and aspart have equivalent effects on HbA1c and risk of both overall and nocturnal hypoglycemia (see **Tables 4** and **5**).[40] There are insufficient data to comment on the relative effectiveness of insulin glulisine.

Table 1
Summary of recommendations for routine health maintenance of individuals with type 1 diabetes

	ADA[14]	AACE[15]	NICE[16,17]	CDA[18]	ISPAD[19,20]	APEG[21]
Hemoglobin A1c	2–4 times per year		2–6 times per year	4 times per year	3–6 times per year	2–4 times per year
Growth (height, weight)	4 times per year		Every visit		4 times per year	4 times per year
Nutritionist	Diagnosis, then every year				Diagnosis, then every year	Diagnosis, then every year
Lipid profile	Adult: at diagnosis, then every 1–2 y; Child (low-risk): age ≥10 y; then every 1–5 y; Child (high-risk): after age 2 y, then every 1–5 y		Adult: every year; Child: not indicated	Adult: at diagnosis, then every 1–3 y; Child (low-risk): ages 12 and 17 y; Child (high-risk): age <12 y	Child (low-risk): every 5 y after age 12 y; Child (high-risk): every 5 y after age 2 y	Prepubertal child: within 6–12 mo, then every 5 y; Pubertal child: within 6–12 mo, then every 2 y
Blood pressure	Every physical examination		Every year after age 12 y	Adult: every physical examination; Child: 2 times per year	Every year	Every year
Nephropathy	Albumin/creatinine ratio; Every year once diabetes duration >5 y and age >10 y; Serum creatinine: every year (adults only)	Albumin/creatinine ratio; Every year after 5 y duration; Serum creatinine: every year after 5 y duration	Albumin/creatinine ratio; Every year from age 12 y; Serum creatinine: every year from age 12 y	Albumin/creatinine ratio; Every year after 5 y duration; Serum creatinine: every year after 5 y duration	Albumin/creatinine ratio; Every year from age 11 y (after 2 y duration) or from age 9 y (after 5 y duration)	Albumin/creatinine ratio; Prepubertal child: every year after 5 y duration; Pubertal child: every year after 2 y duration

Retinopathy	Adult: within 5 y of diagnosis, then every year Child: 10 y of age and 3–5 y duration, then every year	Every year after 5 y duration	Every year from age 12 y	15 y of age and 5 y duration, then every year	After diagnosis, then every year from age 11 y (after 2 y duration) or age 9 y (after 5 y duration)	Prepubertal child: every year after 5 y duration Pubertal child: every year after 2 y duration
Neuropathy	Distal symmetric polyneuropathy: every year; autonomic neuropathy: after 5 y duration	Every year after 5 y duration	Adult: every year Child: not indicated	Every year after 5 y postpubertal duration	Every year after 5 y duration	Every year if poor glycemic control
Foot examination	Every year	Every year	Every year	Every year	Every year	
Thyroid disease	TSH; TPO and TG Abs After metabolic control achieved, then every 1–2 y; antibodies at diagnosis		TSH At diagnosis, then every year	TSH; TPO and TG Abs At diagnosis, then every 1–2 y; antibodies at diagnosis	TSH Adults: every year Children: at diagnosis, then every 1–2 y	TSH; TPO and TG Abs Every 1–2 y
Celiac disease	TTG or EMA IgA and serum IgA After diagnosis, then periodically		EMA IgA and serum IgA At diagnosis, then every 3 y	EMA IgA and serum IgA As clinically indicated	TTG IgA and serum IgA Every 2 y	EMA IgA and serum IgA At diagnosis, then every 2–3 y
Dental examination	Every 2 y					Every 6 mo

Abbreviations: AACE, American Association of Clinical Endocrinologists; Abs, antibodies; ADA, American Diabetes Association; APEG, Australasian Paediatric Endocrine Group; CDA, Canadian Diabetes Association; EMA, endomysial antibody; IgA, immunoglobulin A; ISPAD, International Society for Pediatric and Adolescent Diabetes; NICE, National Institute for Health and Clinical Excellence; TG, thyroglobulin; TPO, thyroid peroxidase; TSH, thyroid-stimulating hormone; TTG, tissue transglutaminase.

Table 2
Summary of target ranges for glycemic control and cardiovascular risk factors for individuals with type 1 diabetes

	ADA[14]	AACE[15]	NICE[16,17]	CDA[18]	ISPAD[19,20]	APEG[21]
Hemoglobin A1c	<6 y: <8.5% 6–12 y: <8.0% 13–19 y: <7.5% Adults: <7.0%	≤6.5%	<7.5%	<6 yr: <8.5% 6–12 yr: <8.0% 13–18 yr: ≤7.0% Adults: ≤7.0%	<7.5%	<7.5%
Nutrition (% TEI)	Carb+MUFA: 60%–70% Protein: 15%–20% PUFA: 10% Sat fat: <7%	Carb: 45%–65% Protein: 15%–20% Total fat: <30% Sat fat: <10%	Carb: >50% Protein: 10%–15% Total fat: 30%–35% Sat fat: <10%	Carb: 45%–60% Protein: 15%–20% Total fat: <35% Sat fat: <7%	Carb: 50%–55% Protein: 10%–15% Total fat: 30%–35% Sat+trans fat: <10%	Carb: 50%–55% Protein: 15%–20% Total fat: 25%–40% Sat fat: <10%
Lipid profile	LDL: <100 mg/dL HDL: >50 mg/dL TG: <150 mg/dL	LDL: <100 mg/dL HDL: >40 mg/dL (males); >50 mg/dL (females) TG: <150 mg/dL		LDL: ≤2.0 mmol/L TC/HDL: <4.0 mmol/L TG: <4.5 mmol/L	LDL: <2.6 mmol/L HDL: >1.1 mmol/L TG: <1.7 mmol/L	
Blood pressure (mm Hg)	Adult: SBP <130, DBP <80 Child: SBP, DBP <90% for age, gender, height	SBP <130 DBP <80	SBP <135 DBP <85	SBP <130 DBP <80	SBP, DBP <95 for age, gender, height	SBP, DBP <95% for age, gender, height
Urine ACR	Normal: <30 Micro: 30–299 Macro: ≥300 (μg/mg Cr)	Normal: <30 Micro: 30–299 Macro: ≥300 (μg/mg Cr)	Males: ≤2.5 Females: ≤3.5 (mg/mmol Cr)	Males: normal <2 Micro: 2–20 Macro: >20 Females: normal <2.8 Micro: 2–28 Macro: >28 (mg/mmol Cr)	Males: 2.5–25 Females: 3.5–25 (mg/mmol Cr)	Normal: <30 Micro: 30–299 Macro: ≥300 (μg/mg Cr)

Conversions: To convert albumin to creatinine ratio from mg/mmol to μg/mg, multiply by 8.84. To convert total, HDL, and LDL cholesterol from mmol/L to mg/dL, multiply by 38.67. To convert triglycerides from mmol/L to mg/dL, multiply by 88.57.

Abbreviations: AACE, American Association of Clinical Endocrinologists; ACR, albumin/creatinine ratio; ADA, American Diabetes Association; APEG, Australasian Paediatric Endocrine Group; carb, carbohydrate; CDA, Canadian Diabetes Association; DBP, diastolic blood pressure; HDL, high-density lipoprotein cholesterol; ISPAD, International Society for Pediatric and Adolescent Diabetes; LDL, low-density lipoprotein cholesterol; Macro, macroalbuminuria; Micro, microalbuminuria; MUFA, monounsaturated fat; NICE, National Institute for Health and Clinical Excellence; PUFA, polyunsaturated fat; sat, saturated; SBP, systolic blood pressure; TEI, total energy intake; TG, triglycerides.

Table 3
Pharmacodynamic profiles of available insulins and insulin preparations

	Onset	Peak Action	Effective Duration
Rapid acting			
Insulin lispro (analogue)[a]	5–15 min	30–90 min	3–5 h
Insulin aspart (analogue)[a]	5–15 min	30–90 min	3–5 h
Insulin glulisine (analogue)	5–15 min	30–90 min	3–5 h
Short acting			
Regular (soluble)	30–60 min	2–3 h	5–8 h
Intermediate acting			
NPH (isophane)	2–4 h	4–10 h	10–16 h
Long acting			
Insulin glargine (analogue)	2–4 h	Peakless	20–24 h
Insulin detemir (analogue)	2–4 h	6–14 h	16–20 h
Combinations			
70% NPH, 30% regular	30–60 min	Dual	10–16 h
70% NPA, 30% aspart	5–15 min	Dual	10–16 h
75% NPL, 25% lispro	5–15 min	Dual	10–16 h
50% NPH, 50% regular	30–60 min	Dual	10–16 h

[a] Per manufacturers' data; other data indicate equivalent pharmacodynamic effect.[25]
Data from Wolfsdorf JI, editor. Intensive diabetes management. 4th edition. Alexandria (VA): American Diabetes Association; 2009.

In open-label studies, rapid-acting analogues have been associated with modest, but statistically significant, improvements in quality of life (QOL) attributable to the convenience of more flexible regimens and the shorter interval between insulin administration and food consumption.[24,36,39] A double-blind randomized controlled trial, however, did not demonstrate a significant improvement in QOL with rapid-acting analogues.[41] Regular insulin and rapid-acting analogues have similar frequencies and types of other adverse events, including DKA.[36,37] There are insufficient data regarding their impact on long-term complications and death.[39]

Long-Acting Insulins

NPH insulin is a suspension-based formulation with inconsistent absorption and action resulting in highly variable pharmacodynamic effects.[42] In contrast, the long-acting analogues are relatively peakless and have significantly less dose-to-dose variability resulting in more reproducible action profiles. Their duration of action is longer, and they can often be administered once daily to achieve 24-hour basal coverage. Insulin detemir, however, may require 2 injections daily to provide stable 24-hour basal coverage. The doses should be administered at approximately the same time ($\pm$2 hours) of the day and should not be mixed with prandial insulins.

Several meta-analyses show that use of long-acting analogues is associated with modest (~0.1%) to no reduction in HbA1c when compared with NPH and ultralente insulins.[24,36,38] These findings are consistent in both adults and children with T1D (see **Tables 4** and **5**). Long-acting analogues are associated with significantly less severe hypoglycemia and nocturnal hypoglycemia in adults with T1D.[24] The reduction in hypoglycemia is primarily attributed to their peakless and more consistent pharmacologic profiles;

Table 4
Summary of meta-analyses examining the impact of insulin analogues on health outcomes of adults with T1D

Study	A1c	Frequency of Hypoglycemia			Quality of Life
		Severe	Nocturnal	Overall	
Rapid-acting analogues					
Brunelle et al (1998)[34]	No difference[a,b]	Decreased[a,b]			
Siebenhofer et al (2004)[35]	0.08%–0.19% reduction	Decreased[a,b]		No difference[a,b]	
Plank et al (2005)[36]	0.12% reduction[a,b]			No difference[a,b]	Inconsistent; some improvement
Siebenhofer et al (2006)[37]	0.1% reduction[a,b]	Decreased[a,b]	Decreased[a,b]	No difference[a,b]	Inconsistent; some improvement
Singh et al (2009)[38]	0.09%[a]–0.13%[b] reduction	No difference,[b] decreased[a]	Decreased[a,b]	No difference[a,b]	Improvement[a,b]
Basal analogues					
Singh et al (2009)[38]	No difference,[d] 0.11% reduction[c]	No difference,[c] decreased[d]	No difference,[c] decreased[d]	No difference[c,d]	No difference[c,d]

a Insulin lispro.
b Insulin aspart.
c Insulin glargine.
d Insulin detemir.

Table 5
Summary of meta-analyses examining the impact of insulin analogues on health outcomes of children with T1D

| | Study | A1C | Frequency of Hypoglycemia | | | Quality of Life |
			Severe	Nocturnal	Overall	
Rapid-acting analogues	Plank et al (2005)[36]	No difference			No difference to decreased[a,b]	
	Siebenhofer et al (2006)[37]	No difference	No difference[a,b]	No difference to decreased[a,b]	No difference to decreased[a,b]	
	Singh et al (2009)[38]	No difference[a,b]	No difference[a,b]	No difference,[b] decreased[a]	Decreased[a,b]	No data
Basal analogues	Singh et al (2009)[38]	No difference[c,d]	No difference,[c] decreased[d]	Decreased[d]	Decreased[d]	No data

[a] Insulin lispro.
[b] Insulin aspart.
[c] Insulin glargine.
[d] Insulin detemir.

however, Singh and colleagues[38] found no difference in any type of hypoglycemia in studies using the same prandial insulin (see **Table 4**). In children, long-acting analogues reduce the risk of severe hypoglycemia and are associated with modest reductions in the occurrence of overall and nocturnal hypoglycemia (see **Table 5**).[24,38]

In adults with T1D, long-acting analogues are associated with significant improvements in QOL, including reduced fear of hypoglycemia; QOL data for children are lacking. Compared with NPH-based regimens, long-acting analogues are not associated with changes in daily insulin requirement. Insulin detemir, but not insulin glargine, has been associated with favorable effects on weight.[43–45] Insulin glargine may cause an uncomfortable sensation of stinging or pain at the injection site. Recent observational studies have raised concerns about the mitogenic and carcinogenic potential of insulin glargine; however, careful analyses of the epidemiologic data have concluded that insulin glargine is safe.[46]

INSULIN REGIMENS

In the DCCT, the intensively treated cohort used various insulin regimens. At a minimum, subjects were required to administer at least 3 insulin injections daily or use an insulin pump.[47] Intensive insulin regimens can be classified as modified fixed dose (sliding scale) or flexible (basal-bolus).

A modified fixed-dose insulin regimen refers to the use of prandial and NPH insulin in the morning before breakfast, prandial insulin before dinner, and intermediate- or long-acting insulin at bedtime. The prandial doses of rapid-acting insulin typically are adjusted using a sliding scale based on the preprandial BG level. In a modified fixed-dose regimen, the peak action of the morning dose of NPH may obviate the need for a lunchtime insulin dose. This regimen requires consistent timing and quantity of meals and snacks to be effective. Some flexibility in meal quantity is possible by including insulin-to-carbohydrate ratios for breakfast, dinner, and additional snacks.

Flexible insulin regimens can be delivered using either multiple daily injections (MDI) or an insulin pump. These regimens separate the basal and prandial components of insulin replacement. Doses of rapid-acting insulin are based on the current BG level (using an insulin sensitivity or correction factor) and the anticipated amount of carbohydrate in the meal or snack (using an insulin-to-carbohydrate ratio); additional adjustments are made for recent or planned exercise. Basal insulin is provided using once or twice daily doses of a long-acting analogue for injection-based therapy or continuous infusion of rapid-acting insulin (using basal rates) for insulin pump therapy.

Insulin regimens based on 1 or 2 daily injections (referred to as conventional therapy) cannot achieve optimal glycemic control in patients with severe insulin deficiency. For a limited period of time after the diagnosis of T1D, however, patients with persistent endogenous insulin production in partial or complete remission (the "honeymoon period") can maintain tight glycemic control using once or twice daily insulin regimens.[48] In general, the use of these regimens, including the use of premixed (combination) insulins, should be reserved for patients in whom there are insurmountable barriers that preclude the use of intensive insulin therapy.[49]

The SEARCH for Diabetes in Youth study recently reported epidemiologic data on the use of insulin regimens in 2743 youths with T1D in the United States.[50] Four insulin regimens were used with nearly equal frequency: insulin pump (22%), injection-based flexible (24%), modified fixed dose (27%), and conventional (26%). Use of an insulin pump was associated with lower HbA1c levels; however, socioeconomic status may have confounded this finding. Modified fixed-dose insulin regimens were associated with lowest body mass index (BMI) Z-scores, but the worst overall glycemic control and, when compared with insulin pump use, more frequent hospitalizations. Conventional regimens were more commonly used by patients with shorter diabetes duration or higher fasting C-peptide levels, suggesting persistent endogenous insulin production. Neither the risk of hypoglycemia nor the frequency of emergency room visits was associated with insulin regimen.

In the SEARCH study, more than 70% of the cohort had HbA1c levels greater than 7.5%,[50] and 5 years after the DCCT, the Hvidore Study Group reported no significant association between insulin regimen and HbA1c over a 3-year period; more than 70% of subjects had HbA1c levels greater than 8%.[51] This study preceded the widespread use of insulin analogues and flexible insulin regimens, and only 1% of subjects used an insulin pump. However, subsequent studies by the Hvidore Study Group have shown that despite increased use of insulin analogues, flexible insulin regimens, and pumps, it has been difficult to demonstrate significant improvements in metabolic outcomes in adolescents 11 to 18 years old.[51–53]

In the DCCT, the mean HbA1c level in the intensive treatment group was 7.2% compared with 9.1% in the conventional treatment group. It is noteworthy that after completion of the DCCT when subjects were returned to diabetes care supervised by their own clinicians, the mean values of HbA1c during the first 7-year period of follow-up in the Epidemiology of Diabetes Interventions and Complications (EDIC) study increased to 8.1% in the group that had received intensive treatment during the DCCT and decreased to 8.3% in the group that had received conventional treatment.[54] The adolescent cohort assigned to either the intensive or conventional arms of the DCCT failed to achieve the same level of glycemic control (their mean HbA1c levels were 8.06% and 9.76%, respectively) as their adult counterparts. And, during follow-up in the EDIC study, mean HbA1c levels were similar, 8.38% and 8.45%, in the former adolescents treated intensively and conventionally, respectively.[55]

It has been suggested that flexible regimens are the "gold standard" for intensive insulin therapy.[56] Whereas these regimens have the potential to most closely simulate physiologic insulin production, the requirements for their successful implementation limit their effectiveness for many individuals with T1D. In clinical practice, the prescription of a more flexible insulin regimen does not per se guarantee improved glycemic control. Patients with T1D should be informed about the requirements, risks, and benefits of intensive insulin regimens and encouraged to choose the regimen to which they will most likely be able to consistently adhere.

INSULIN PUMP THERAPY

Continuous subcutaneous insulin infusion, commonly referred to as insulin pump therapy, was introduced in the late 1970s,[57,58] and use of pump therapy increased dramatically following publication of the DCCT results. Over the last 30 years, technological advancements have led to smaller and safer insulin pumps with numerous "user-friendly" technical features that facilitate calculation of insulin doses and enable insulin boluses to be delivered in a variety of formats appropriate to various types of meals (**Table 6**).[56,59,60]

The clinical effectiveness of pump therapy has been evaluated in adults with T1D; however, many studies are limited by small sample sizes, lack of control groups, observational or retrospective analyses, as well as significant temporal trends in diabetes care (eg, adoption of rapid-acting analogues), all of which may confound results.[35,56,61] Pump therapy is safe and effective in children and adolescents.[62,63]

In a meta-analysis performed by Weissberg-Benchell and colleagues,[64] adults using insulin pump therapy showed a significant 0.95% reduction in HbA1c when

Table 6 Technological features of insulin pumps[a]	
Insulin delivery	Small bolus increments: 0.05–0.10 units
	Extended boluses for delayed digestion or grazing
	Multiple insulin-to-carbohydrate ratios, sensitivity factors, BG targets
	Bolus calculators (based on BG level and carbohydrate quantity)
	Low basal rates: 0.025–0.05 units/h
	Multiple basal rates
	Temporary basal rates and suspension mode
Safety features	Alarms for occlusion and low insulin reservoir
	Active insulin to prevent insulin stacking
	Keypad lock
	Waterproof or watertight
Miscellaneous	Electronic logbook software (insulin doses, BG levels, carbohydrates)
	Integrated food databases with customization
	Reminder alarms for BG checks, bolus doses
	Wireless communication with remote glucose meter
	Integration with continuous glucose monitoring technology

[a] Available features will vary by insulin pump make and model.

compared with MDI; however, most studies included in this meta-analysis predated the DCCT. Comparison studies of longer duration (more than 6–12 months) and with higher baseline HbA1c levels are associated with larger HbA1c reductions in pump users.[64–68] More recent meta-analyses have reported 0.2% to 0.5% lower HbA1c levels with pump use compared with MDI.[65,69,70] Adolescents, but not prepubertal children, using pump therapy had significant reductions in HbA1c when compared with those using MDI.[62,65]

Retrospective and uncontrolled studies of pump therapy demonstrate significant reductions in hypoglycemia, including severe hypoglycemia, in children and adults with T1D.[67,71–75] Recurrent hypoglycemia is considered to be a specific indication for pump therapy; however, meta-analyses of randomized controlled trials using paired or crossover study designs have failed to show significant reductions in overall or severe hypoglycemia when pump use is compared with MDI.[64–66,70] Insulin pump use may reduce the risk of nocturnal hypoglycemia.[38]

Compared with MDI regimens, pump therapy is associated with significantly lower daily insulin requirements, but no effect on weight or BMI.[64–66,68,69] Overall, it appears that insulin pump therapy offers the opportunity to significantly improve glycemic control without increasing severe hypoglycemia or untoward weight gain.

The QOL of pump users appears to be the same or better than those using MDI.[62,64] In children, the most dramatic improvement in QOL follows transition from conventional insulin regimens to pump therapy as opposed to transition from flexible, injection-based regimens.[76] Indeed, many studies describing the impact of insulin regimen on QOL predate the widespread use of flexible injection-based regimens with long-acting analogues. It is not surprising, therefore, that improvements in QOL are primarily related to increased flexibility around mealtimes.

The absence of an subcutaneous insulin depot increases the risk of DKA with pump therapy; however, increased experience with their use and technological improvements in pump design have significantly reduced the rates of major adverse events.[66,77,78] At present, the risk of DKA is marginally higher with pump therapy, highlighting the need to emphasize DKA prevention strategies for individuals who use a pump.[61] Missed mealtime boluses, especially among adolescents, is common, and Burdick and colleagues[79] showed that youth who miss 2 meal boluses per week (the average rate in this study) have a 0.5% increase in HbA1c; a linear increase in HbA1c occurred with more frequent missed boluses.[61,79] Skin infection at the site of cannula insertion is a common adverse event.[80] At present, about 60% to 80% of individuals who initiate pump therapy do not revert to injection-based regimens.[64,81,82]

Patients considering pump use must be motivated, informed of the risks and benefits, technically capable of managing the device, and willing to perform frequent BG monitoring.[83] The ability to accurately count carbohydrates is required for the successful implementation of any intensive insulin regimen. Older children and adolescents should express a desire to use a pump and not merely the desire to appease their parents or health care provider. Because young children are unable to participate in the decision, attention to the child's physical and emotional well-being should inform the decision to continue pump therapy.[84,85]

Some individuals who use injection-based regimens experience recurrent hypoglycemia, unpredictable glycemic fluctuations, or persistent elevations in HbA1c despite concerted efforts to optimize their glycemic control. Such individuals may be able to improve their control with pump therapy.[86,87] Others may simply want to improve their QOL by avoiding MDI or taking advantage of the flexibility afforded by pump therapy. It is the authors' practice to offer pump therapy to any individual who is informed, motivated, and demonstrates the ability to adhere to the minimum diabetes self-care requirements necessary to use a pump safely. Successful implementation requires the support of a diabetes team experienced in the use of pump therapy.

MEDICAL NUTRITION THERAPY

Medical nutrition therapy (MNT) emphasizes the important role of nutrition in normal growth and physical development and optimizing glycemic control, lipid profiles, and blood pressure in individuals with T1D.[88,89] Successful diabetes management requires daily attention to nutrition principles, especially diet quality and accurate estimation of the carbohydrate content of food. Numerous individual and dietary factors, many of which cannot be readily quantified, affect postprandial glycemic responses; consequently, it can be difficult for both patients and the diabetes team to assess the unique impact of diet on daily BG fluctuations and HbA1c values.

A registered dietitian (RD) experienced in T1D management is an essential member of the diabetes team.[90] All individuals with T1D should meet with an RD at the time of diagnosis, undergo a comprehensive nutrition assessment, and receive counseling. Thereafter, patients should meet with an RD at least once per year. Individuals who are in the process of becoming more independent in their care, transitioning to more flexible regimens, or struggling to achieve desired health outcomes may benefit from more frequent consultations.

Carbohydrates are the principal determinant of postprandial BG excursions.[91,92] Regardless of insulin regimen, individuals with T1D must learn to balance insulin doses with anticipated carbohydrate consumption to optimize glycemic control.[89] In the DCCT, several meal-planning strategies were used according to center preference and the participants' ability to successfully implement variably complex approaches.[93] Carbohydrate counting has become the most widely implemented meal-planning strategy in intensive diabetes management. Limitations include not addressing carbohydrate quality, diet composition, or total caloric intake. These nutrition principles must be learned and applied in conjunction with carbohydrate counting to optimize overall nutrition. Carbohydrate counting may be too difficult for some individuals who will require more basic and structured meal-planning strategies that emphasize consistent timing and amount of food consumption.[94]

MNT also provides basic nutrition education that includes the components of a healthful diet, understanding macronutrients, and determining individual caloric requirements. Carbohydrate restriction is not recommended. Patients should be encouraged to consume whole foods such as fruits, vegetables, and whole grains to maximize the fiber, vitamin, and mineral content of their diet. Low glycemic index diets are associated with lower HbA1c levels.[95] Protein should comprise 15% to 20% of total caloric intake; high-protein diets (to avoid carbohydrate consumption or facilitate weight loss) are not recommended. Total fat should be limited to about 30% and *trans* fat should be avoided completely (see **Table 2**).

The effectiveness of MNT has been evaluated during the DCCT and short-term dietary interventions, and in cross-sectional analyses.[93,96,97] Dietary adherence is associated with improved glycemic control, including lower HbA1c values and reduced postprandial glycemic excursions.[94,96,98] Recent studies have demonstrated that carbohydrate counting is related to lower HbA1c levels, supporting its use in intensive diabetes management.[99–101] In North America, Europe, and Asia, diet quality in individuals with T1D has consistently been found to be suboptimal.[102–104] Excessive saturated fat and low fiber intake with inadequate fruit and vegetable consumption are common. The epidemic of obesity has not spared children with T1D; a recent SEARCH study publication showed a higher prevalence of overweight in youth with T1D when compared with similarly aged youth without diabetes (22.1% vs 16.1%, $P<.05$).[105] In addition to secular dietary trends, a singular focus on carbohydrate quantity may be partially responsible for these dietary trends.[106] Therefore, MNT must address both dietary quality and health outcomes while remaining sensitive to the patient's lifestyle, taste preferences, and QOL.

BLOOD GLUCOSE MONITORING

Frequent self-monitoring of BG (SMBG) is a fundamental component of T1D management, providing immediate feedback on the effects of insulin doses, food choices, exercise, and physiologic stress on BG values. Individuals with T1D should measure their BG level at least 4 times daily, typically before meals and at bedtime, with periodic assessments overnight. Patients and care providers should be taught to use written logbooks or electronically downloaded SMBG data to identify glycemic patterns that guide adjustment of the diabetes treatment plan to optimize glycemic control. Systematic recording of insulin doses, dietary information, and exercise are essential for interpreting SMBG data. SMBG rapidly confirms symptomatic hypoglycemia allowing for timely treatment, and patients with impaired hypoglycemia awareness should check BG values more frequently. Likewise, more frequent SMBG can facilitate therapy adjustments during exercise, illness, and situations associated with increased risk such as driving, swimming, and alcohol consumption. More frequent SMBG has consistently been reported to be a significant and independent predictor of lower HbA1c levels.[107–112]

BG meters have become smaller, faster, and more accurate. Current meters require only 0.3 to 1.5 μL of blood and provide accurate BG values within 5 seconds. These meters can store hundreds of BG values, and some include event markers to tag meals, exercise, and insulin doses, which enhance interpretation of downloaded data. Alternative site testing, identification of test solution results, larger or backlit displays, and stability in extreme temperatures are additional features of current devices. CGM, reviewed by Aye and colleagues elsewhere in this issue, is a potentially valuable adjunct to daily SMBG.

SUMMARY

In 1993, the DCCT showed that any sustained reduction in HbA1c level lowers the risk of diabetic complications, and intensive diabetes management aimed at near-normal glycemia has become the standard of care for patients with T1D. Intensive insulin regimens, frequent SMBG, MNT, and the guidance and support of a diabetes team are well-established components of contemporary diabetes management. Therapeutic innovations allowing for more physiologic and flexible insulin regimens together with more frequent BG monitoring and CGM, use of carbohydrate counting, and patient empowerment have made it possible to achieve previously unattainable levels of glycemic control and reduced risk of severe hypoglycemia. Sustained improvement in glycemic control should prevent or, at least, delay the appearance of the chronic complications of diabetes. The prospects for patients with T1D are far better than they were in the past.[113,114]

In most individuals with T1D, however, the goal of near-normalization of HbA1c remains elusive. Several large, multicenter studies demonstrate a persistent gap between attained and target HbA1c levels. Successful implementation of intensive diabetes management in routine clinical practice continues to be a major challenge. The unremitting daily task of controlling BG while avoiding hypoglycemia is arduous and often frustrating. Recent meta-analyses show that the use of insulin analogues and pump therapy, when compared with conventional insulins and injection-based regimens, respectively, have had only a modest impact on glycemic control and rates of adverse events. Reliance on available technology is insufficient to achieve optimal health outcomes. Patients also require considerable psychosocial support, ongoing education, and guidance from a cohesive diabetes team that works with each patient to set and achieve individualized treatment goals. Major scientific advances, such as successful β-cell replacement or the development of closed-loop systems, will be required to reduce the burden of care and improve health outcomes for patients with T1D.

REFERENCES

1. Skyler JS, Lasky IA, Skyler DL, et al. Home blood glucose monitoring as an aid in diabetes management. Diabetes Care 1978;1:150–7.
2. Sonksen PH, Judd SL, Lowy C. Home monitoring of blood-glucose. Method for improving diabetic control. Lancet 1978;1:729–32.
3. The DCCT Research Group. The effect of intensive treatment of diabetes on the development and progression of long-term complications in insulin-dependent diabetes mellitus. N Engl J Med 1993;329:977–86.
4. Nathan DM, Cleary PA, Backlund JY, et al. Intensive diabetes treatment and cardiovascular disease in patients with type 1 diabetes. N Engl J Med 2005; 353:2643–53.
5. Lachin JM, Genuth S, Nathan DM, et al. Effect of glycemic exposure on the risk of microvascular complications in the Diabetes Control and Complications Trial—revisited. Diabetes 2008;57:995–1001.
6. The Diabetes Control and Complications Trial Research Group. Adverse events and their association with treatment regimens in the Diabetes Control and Complications Trial. Diabetes Care 1995;18:1415–27.
7. Hypoglycemia in the Diabetes Control and Complications Trial. The Diabetes Control and Complications Trial Research Group. Diabetes 1997;46:271–86.

8. The Diabetes Control and Complications Trial Research Group Resource utilization and costs of care in the Diabetes Control and Complications Trial. Diabetes Care 1995;18:1468–78.
9. Wegner SE, Lathren CR, Humble CG, et al. A medical home for children with insulin-dependent diabetes: comanagement by primary and subspecialty physicians—convergence and divergence of opinions. Pediatrics 2008;122:e383–7.
10. The Diabetes Control and Complications Research Group. Lifetime benefits and costs of intensive therapy as practiced in the Diabetes Control and Complications Trial. JAMA 1996;276:1409–15.
11. Herman WH, Dasbach EJ, Songer TJ, et al. The cost-effectiveness of intensive therapy for diabetes mellitus. Endocrinol Metab Clin North Am 1997;26:679–95.
12. The team approach. In: Wolfsdorf JI, editor. Intensive diabetes management. 4th edition. Alexandria (VA): American Diabetes Association; 2009. p. 15–28.
13. Clar C, Waugh N, Thomas S. Routine hospital admission versus out-patient or home care in children at diagnosis of type 1 diabetes mellitus. Cochrane Database Syst Rev 2007;2:CD004099.
14. American Diabetes Association. Standards of medical care in diabetes—2010. Diabetes Care 2010;33(Suppl 1):S11–62.
15. Rodbard HW, Blonde L, Braithwaite SS, et al. American Association of Clinical Endocrinologists medical guidelines for clinical practice for the management of diabetes mellitus. Endocr Pract 2007;13(Suppl 1):1–68.
16. National Collaborating Centre for Chronic Conditions. Type 1 diabetes in adults: National clinical guideline for diagnosis and management in primary and secondary care. Royal College of Physicians Press. Available at: http://www.nice.org.uk/CG15. Updated September 10, 2004. Accessed January 20, 2010.
17. National Collaborating Centre for Women's and Children's Health. Type 1 diabetes: diagnosis and management of type 1 diabetes in children and young people. Royal College of Physicians Press. Available at: http://www.nice.org.uk/CG15. Updated June 2009. Accessed January 20, 2010.
18. Canadian Diabetes Association Clinical Practice Guidelines Expert Committee. Canadian Diabetes Association 2008 clinical practice guidelines for the prevention and management of diabetes in Canada. Can J Diabetes 2008;32:S1–201.
19. Pihoker C, Forsander G, Wolfsdorf J, et al. The delivery of ambulatory diabetes care to children and adolescents with diabetes. Pediatr Diabetes 2009;10(Suppl 12):58–70.
20. Smart C, Aslander-van Vliet E, Waldron S. Nutritional management in children and adolescents with diabetes. Pediatr Diabetes 2009;10(Suppl 12):100–17.
21. Australasian Paediatric Endocrine Group. Clinical practice guidelines: Type 1 diabetes in children and adolescents. National Health and Medical Research Council. Available at: http://www.nhmrc.gov.au/publications/synopses/cp102syn.htm. Updated March 9, 2005. Accessed January 20, 2010.
22. Schade DS, Santiago JV, Skyler J, et al. Insulin secretion in non-diabetic and insulin-dependent subjects. Intensive insulin therapy. Princeton (NJ): Excerpta Medica; 1983. p. 23–35.
23. Hirsch IB. Insulin analogues. N Engl J Med 2005;352:174–83.
24. Rachmiel M, Perlman K, Daneman D. Insulin analogues in children and teens with type 1 diabetes: advantages and caveats. Pediatr Clin North Am 2005;52:1651–75.
25. Plank J, Wutte A, Brunner G, et al. A direct comparison of insulin aspart and insulin lispro in patients with type 1 diabetes. Diabetes Care 2002;25:2053–7.
26. Holleman F, Hoekstra JB. Insulin lispro. N Engl J Med 1997;337:176–83.

27. Holmes G, Galitz L, Hu P, et al. Pharmacokinetics of insulin aspart in obesity, renal impairment, or hepatic impairment. Br J Clin Pharmacol 2005;60:469–76.
28. Howey DC, Bowsher RR, Brunelle RL, et al. [Lys(B28), Pro(B29)]-human insulin. A rapidly absorbed analogue of human insulin. Diabetes 1994;43:396–402.
29. Danne T, Aman J, Schober E, et al. A comparison of postprandial and preprandial administration of insulin aspart in children and adolescents with type 1 diabetes. Diabetes Care 2003;26:2359–64.
30. Swan KL, Weinzimer SA, Dziura JD, et al. Effect of puberty on the pharmacodynamic and pharmacokinetic properties of insulin pump therapy in youth with type 1 diabetes. Diabetes Care 2008;31:44–6.
31. Dimitriadis GD, Gerich JE. Importance of timing of preprandial subcutaneous insulin administration in the management of diabetes mellitus. Diabetes Care 1983;6:374–7.
32. Lean ME, Ng LL, Tennison BR. Interval between insulin injection and eating in relation to blood glucose control in adult diabetics. Br Med J (Clin Res Ed) 1985;290:105–8.
33. Deeb LC, Holcombe JH, Brunelle R, et al. Insulin lispro lowers postprandial glucose in prepubertal children with diabetes. Pediatrics 2001;108:1175–9.
34. Brunelle BL, Llewelyn J, Anderson JH Jr, et al. Meta-analysis of the effect of insulin lispro on severe hypoglycemia in patients with type 1 diabetes. Diabetes Care 1998;21:1726–31.
35. Siebenhofer A, Plank J, Berghold A, et al. Meta-analysis of short-acting insulin analogues in adult patients with type 1 diabetes: continuous subcutaneous insulin infusion versus injection therapy. Diabetologia 2004;47:1895–905.
36. Plank J, Siebenhofer A, Berghold A, et al. Systematic review and meta-analysis of short-acting insulin analogues in patients with diabetes mellitus. Arch Intern Med 2005;165:1337–44.
37. Siebenhofer A, Plank J, Berghold A, et al. Short acting insulin analogues versus regular human insulin in patients with diabetes mellitus. Cochrane Database Syst Rev 2006;2:CD003287.
38. Singh SR, Ahmad F, Lal A, et al. Efficacy and safety of insulin analogues for the management of diabetes mellitus: a meta-analysis. CMAJ 2009;180:385–97.
39. Siebenhofer A, Jeitler K, Berghold A, et al. Severe hypoglycaemia and glycaemic control in type 1 diabetes: meta-analysis of multiple daily insulin injections compared with continuous subcutaneous insulin infusion. Diabet Med 2009; 26:311–2.
40. Bode B, Weinstein R, Bell D, et al. Comparison of insulin aspart with buffered regular insulin and insulin lispro in continuous subcutaneous insulin infusion: a randomized study in type 1 diabetes. Diabetes Care 2002;25:439–44.
41. Gale EA. A randomized, controlled trial comparing insulin lispro with human soluble insulin in patients with type 1 diabetes on intensified insulin therapy. The UK Trial Group. Diabet Med 2000;17:209–14.
42. Binder C, Lauritzen T, Faber O, et al. Insulin pharmacokinetics. Diabetes Care 1984;7:188–99.
43. Vague P, Selam JL, Skeie S, et al. Insulin detemir is associated with more predictable glycemic control and reduced risk of hypoglycemia than NPH insulin in patients with type 1 diabetes on a basal-bolus regimen with premeal insulin aspart. Diabetes Care 2003;26:590–6.
44. Standl E, Lang H, Roberts A. The 12-month efficacy and safety of insulin detemir and NPH insulin in basal-bolus therapy for the treatment of type 1 diabetes. Diabetes Technol Ther 2004;6:579–88.

45. De Leeuw I, Vague P, Selam JL, et al. Insulin detemir used in basal-bolus therapy in people with type 1 diabetes is associated with a lower risk of nocturnal hypoglycaemia and less weight gain over 12 months in comparison to NPH insulin. Diabetes Obes Metab 2005;7:73–82.

46. Garg SK, Hirsch IB, Skyler JS. Insulin glargine and cancer—an unsubstantiated allegation. Diabetes Technol Ther 2009;11:473–6.

47. The DCCT Research Group. Implementation of treatment protocols in the Diabetes Control and Complications Trial. Diabetes Care 1995;18:361–76.

48. Kobayashi T, Nakanishi K, Murase T, et al. Small doses of subcutaneous insulin as a strategy for preventing slowly progressive beta-cell failure in islet cell antibody-positive patients with clinical features of NIDDM. Diabetes 1996;45: 622–6.

49. Hirsch IB. Intensive treatment of type 1 diabetes. Med Clin North Am 1998;82: 689–719.

50. Paris CA, Imperatore G, Klingensmith G, et al. Predictors of insulin regimens and impact on outcomes in youth with type 1 diabetes: the SEARCH for Diabetes in Youth study. J Pediatr 2009;155:183–9.

51. Holl RW, Swift PG, Mortensen HB, et al. Insulin injection regimens and metabolic control in an international survey of adolescents with type 1 diabetes over 3 years: results from the Hvidore study group. Eur J Pediatr 2003; 162:22–9.

52. Danne T, Mortensen HB, Hougaard P, et al. Persistent differences among centers over 3 years in glycemic control and hypoglycemia in a study of 3,805 children and adolescents with type 1 diabetes from the Hvidore Study Group. Diabetes Care 2001;24:1342–7.

53. de Beaufort CE, Swift PG, Skinner CT, et al. Continuing stability of center differences in pediatric diabetes care: do advances in diabetes treatment improve outcome? The Hvidore Study Group on Childhood Diabetes. Diabetes Care 2007;30:2245–50.

54. Writing Team for the Diabetes Control and Complications Trial/Epidemiology of Diabetes Interventions and Complications Research Group. Effect of intensive therapy on the microvascular complications of type 1 diabetes mellitus. JAMA 2002;287:2563–9.

55. White NH, Cleary PA, Dahms W, et al. Beneficial effects of intensive therapy of diabetes during adolescence: outcomes after the conclusion of the Diabetes Control and Complications Trial (DCCT). J Pediatr 2001;139:804–12.

56. Weinzimer SA, Sikes KA, Steffen AT, et al. Insulin pump treatment of childhood type 1 diabetes. Pediatr Clin North Am 2005;52:1677–88.

57. Pickup JC, Keen H, Parsons JA, et al. Continuous subcutaneous insulin infusion: an approach to achieving normoglycaemia. Br Med J 1978;1:204–7.

58. Tamborlane WV, Sherwin RS, Genel M, et al. Reduction to normal of plasma glucose in juvenile diabetes by subcutaneous administration of insulin with a portable infusion pump. N Engl J Med 1979;300:573–8.

59. Boland EA, Grey M, Oesterle A, et al. Continuous subcutaneous insulin infusion. A new way to lower risk of severe hypoglycemia, improve metabolic control, and enhance coping in adolescents with type 1 diabetes. Diabetes Care 1999;22: 1779–84.

60. Wood JR, Laffel LMB. Technology and intensive management in youth with type 1 diabetes: State of the art. Curr Diab Rep 2007;7:104–13.

61. Danne T, Lange K, Kordonouri O. New developments in the treatment of type 1 diabetes in children. Arch Dis Child 2007;92:1015–9.

62. Eugster EA, Francis G. Position statement: continuous subcutaneous insulin infusion in very young children with type 1 diabetes. Pediatrics 2006;118:e1244–9.

63. Phillip M, Battelino T, Rodriguez H, et al. Use of insulin pump therapy in the pediatric age-group: consensus statement from the European Society for Paediatric Endocrinology, the Lawson Wilkins Pediatric Endocrine Society, and the International Society for Pediatric and Adolescent Diabetes, endorsed by the American Diabetes Association and the European Association for the Study of Diabetes. Diabetes Care 2007;30:1653–62.

64. Weissberg-Benchell J, Antisdel-Lomaglio J, Seshadri R. Insulin pump therapy: a meta-analysis. Diabetes Care 2003;26:1079–87.

65. Jeitler K, Horvath K, Berghold A, et al. Continuous subcutaneous insulin infusion versus multiple daily insulin injections in patients with diabetes mellitus: systematic review and meta-analysis. Diabetologia 2008;51:941–51.

66. Retnakaran R, Hochman J, DeVries JH, et al. Continuous subcutaneous insulin infusion versus multiple daily injections: the impact of baseline A1c. Diabetes Care 2004;27:2590–6.

67. Nimri R, Weintrob N, Benzaquen H, et al. Insulin pump therapy in youth with type 1 diabetes: a retrospective paired study. Pediatrics 2006;117:2126–31.

68. Pickup J, Mattock M, Kerry S. Glycaemic control with continuous subcutaneous insulin infusion compared with intensive insulin injections in patients with type 1 diabetes: meta-analysis of randomised controlled trials. BMJ 2002;324:705.

69. Colquitt JL, Green C, Sidhu MK, et al. Clinical and cost-effectiveness of continuous subcutaneous insulin infusion for diabetes. Health Technol Assess 2004;8: iii–xii, 1–171.

70. Fatourechi MM, Kudva YC, Murad MH, et al. Clinical review: hypoglycemia with intensive insulin therapy: a systematic review and meta-analyses of randomized trials of continuous subcutaneous insulin infusion versus multiple daily injections. J Clin Endocrinol Metab 2009;94:729–40.

71. Bode BW, Steed RD, Davidson PC. Reduction in severe hypoglycemia with long-term continuous subcutaneous insulin infusion in type I diabetes. Diabetes Care 1996;19:324–7.

72. Plotnick LP, Clark LM, Brancati FL, et al. Safety and effectiveness of insulin pump therapy in children and adolescents with type 1 diabetes. Diabetes Care 2003;26:1142–6.

73. Willi SM, Planton J, Egede L, et al. Benefits of continuous subcutaneous insulin infusion in children with type 1 diabetes. J Pediatr 2003;143:796–801.

74. Springer D, Dziura J, Tamborlane WV, et al. Optimal control of type 1 diabetes mellitus in youth receiving intensive treatment. J Pediatr 2006;149:227–32.

75. Pickup JC, Sutton AJ. Severe hypoglycaemia and glycaemic control in type 1 diabetes: meta-analysis of multiple daily insulin injections compared with continuous subcutaneous insulin infusion. Diabet Med 2008;25:765–74.

76. Cogen FR, Henderson C, Hansen JA, et al. Pediatric quality of life in transitioning to the insulin pump: does prior regimen make a difference? Clin Pediatr (Phila) 2007;46:777–9.

77. Guerci B, Meyer L, Salle A, et al. Comparison of metabolic deterioration between insulin analog and regular insulin after a 5-hour interruption of a continuous subcutaneous insulin infusion in type 1 diabetic patients. J Clin Endocrinol Metab 1999;84:2673–8.

78. Egger M, Davey SG, Stettler C, et al. Risk of adverse effects of intensified treatment in insulin-dependent diabetes mellitus: a meta-analysis. Diabet Med 1997; 14:919–28.

79. Burdick J, Chase HP, Slover RH, et al. Missed insulin meal boluses and elevated hemoglobin A1c levels in children receiving insulin pump therapy. Pediatrics 2004;113:e221–4.

80. Conwell LS, Pope E, Artiles AM, et al. Dermatological complications of continuous subcutaneous insulin infusion in children and adolescents. J Pediatr 2008;152:622–8.

81. Schifferdecker E, Schmidt K, Boehm BO, et al. Long-term compliance of intensified insulin therapy. Diabetes Res Clin Pract 1994;23:17–23.

82. Wood JR, Moreland EC, Volkening LK, et al. Durability of insulin pump use in pediatric patients with type 1 diabetes. Diabetes Care 2006;29:2355–60.

83. Lenhard MJ, Reeves GD. Continuous subcutaneous insulin infusion: a comprehensive review of insulin pump therapy. Arch Intern Med 2001;161:2293–300.

84. Litton J, Rice A, Friedman N, et al. Insulin pump therapy in toddlers and preschool children with type 1 diabetes mellitus. J Pediatr 2002;141:490–5.

85. Kaufman FR, Halvorson M, Fisher L, et al. Insulin pump therapy in type 1 pediatric patients. J Pediatr Endocrinol Metab 1999;12(Suppl 3):759–64.

86. Pickup J, Keen H. Continuous subcutaneous insulin infusion in type 1 diabetes. BMJ 2001;322:1262–3.

87. Weinzimer SA, Ahern JH, Doyle EA, et al. Persistence of benefits of continuous subcutaneous insulin infusion in very young children with type 1 diabetes: a follow-up report. Pediatrics 2004;114:1601–5.

88. Gunther AL, Liese AD, Bell RA, et al. Association between the dietary approaches to hypertension diet and hypertension in youth with diabetes mellitus. Hypertension 2009;53:6–12.

89. Bantle JP, Wylie-Rosett J, Albright AL, et al. Nutrition recommendations and interventions for diabetes: a position statement of the American Diabetes Association. Diabetes Care 2008;31(Suppl 1):S61–78.

90. Khakpour D, Thomson L. The nutrition specialist on the diabetes management team. Clin Diabetes 1998;16:21–2.

91. Halfon P, Belkhadir J, Slama G. Correlation between amount of carbohydrate in mixed meals and insulin delivery by artificial pancreas in seven IDDM subjects. Diabetes Care 1989;12:427–9.

92. Wheeler ML, Pi-Sunyer FX. Carbohydrate issues: type and amount. J Am Diet Assoc 2008;108:S34–9.

93. Anderson EJ, Richardson M, Castle G, et al. Nutrition interventions for intensive therapy in the Diabetes Control and Complications Trial. The DCCT Research Group. J Am Diet Assoc 1993;93:768–72.

94. Wolever TM, Hamad S, Chiasson JL, et al. Day-to-day consistency in amount and source of carbohydrate associated with improved blood glucose control in type 1 diabetes. J Am Coll Nutr 1999;18:242–7.

95. Brand-Miller J, Hayne S, Petocz P, et al. Low-glycemic index diets in the management of diabetes: a meta-analysis of randomized controlled trials. Diabetes Care 2003;26:2261–7.

96. Delahanty LM. Clinical significance of medical nutrition therapy in achieving diabetes outcomes and the importance of the process. J Am Diet Assoc 1998;98: 28–30.

97. Pastors JG, Warshaw H, Daly A, et al. The evidence for the effectiveness of medical nutrition therapy in diabetes management. Diabetes Care 2002;25: 608–13.

98. Mehta SN, Volkening LK, Anderson BJ, et al. Dietary behaviors predict glycemic control in youth with type 1 diabetes. Diabetes Care 2008;31:1318–20.

99. Mehta SN, Quinn N, Volkening LK, et al. Impact of carbohydrate counting on glycemic control in children with type 1 diabetes. Diabetes Care 2009;32: 1014–6.
100. Smart CE, Ross K, Edge JA, et al. Children and adolescents on intensive insulin therapy maintain postprandial glycaemic control without precise carbohydrate counting. Diabet Med 2009;26:279–85.
101. Bishop FK, Maahs DM, Spiegel G, et al. The Carbohydrate Counting in Adolescents with Type 1 Diabetes (CCAT) study. Diabetes Spectr 2009;22:56–62.
102. Mayer-Davis EJ, Nichols M, Liese AD, et al. Dietary intake among youth with diabetes: the SEARCH for Diabetes in Youth Study. J Am Diet Assoc 2006; 106:689–97.
103. Overby NC, Flaaten V, Veierod MB, et al. Children and adolescents with type 1 diabetes eat a more atherosclerosis-prone diet than healthy control subjects. Diabetologia 2007;50:307–16.
104. Saito M, Kuratsune H, Nitta H, et al. Plasma lipid levels and nutritional intake in childhood- and adolescence-onset young type 1 diabetic patients in Japan. Diabetes Res Clin Pract 2006;73:29–34.
105. Liu LL, Lawrence JM, Davis C, et al. Prevalence of overweight and obesity in youth with diabetes in USA: the SEARCH for Diabetes in Youth Study. Pediatr Diabetes 2010;11(1):4–11.
106. Mehta SN, Haynie DL, Higgins LA, et al. Emphasis on carbohydrates may negatively influence dietary patterns in youth with type 1 diabetes. Diabetes Care 2009;32:2174–6.
107. Karter AJ, Ackerson LM, Darbinian JA, et al. Self-monitoring of blood glucose levels and glycemic control: the Northern California Kaiser Permanente Diabetes registry. Am J Med 2001;111:1–9.
108. Levine BS, Anderson BJ, Butler DA, et al. Predictors of glycemic control and short-term adverse outcomes in youth with type 1 diabetes. J Pediatr 2001; 139:197–203.
109. Nathan DM, McKitrick C, Larkin M, et al. Glycemic control in diabetes mellitus: have changes in therapy made a difference? Am J Med 1996;100:157–63.
110. Strowig SM, Raskin P. Improved glycemic control in intensively treated type 1 diabetic patients using blood glucose meters with storage capability and computer-assisted analyses. Diabetes Care 1998;21:1694–8.
111. Evans JM, Newton RW, Ruta DA, et al. Frequency of blood glucose monitoring in relation to glycaemic control: observational study with diabetes database. BMJ 1999;319:83–6.
112. Dorchy H, Roggemans MP, Willems D. Glycated hemoglobin and related factors in diabetic children and adolescents under 18 years of age: a Belgian experience. Diabetes Care 1997;20:2–6.
113. Nordwall M, Bojestig M, Arnqvist HJ, et al. Declining incidence of severe retinopathy and persisting decrease of nephropathy in an unselected population of type 1 diabetes—the Linkoping Diabetes Complications Study. Diabetologia 2004;47:1266–72.
114. Nathan DM, Zinman B, Cleary PA, et al. Modern-day clinical course of type 1 diabetes mellitus after 30 years' duration: the Diabetes Control and Complications Trial/Epidemiology of Diabetes Interventions and Complications and Pittsburgh Epidemiology of Diabetes Complications Experience (1983–2005). Arch Intern Med 2009;169:1307–16.

Inpatient Management of Adults and Children with Type 1 Diabetes

David M. Tridgell, MD[a],*, Angela H. Tridgell, MD[b],
Irl B. Hirsch, MD[c]

KEYWORDS

- Type 1 diabetes mellitus • Insulin • Management • Inpatient
- Adult • Children • Steroid-induced hyperglycemia

Type 1 diabetes is a chronic autoimmune condition caused by destruction of the insulin-producing pancreatic beta cells, with subsequent loss of endogenous insulin production. This condition results in a lifelong need for exogenous insulin to prevent hyperglycemia, diabetic ketoacidosis (DKA), and ultimately death. This absolute need for continuous exogenous insulin results in unique insulin management challenges for the inpatient provider. In addition, inpatient hyperglycemia is often associated with increased mortality, morbidity, and longer hospital stays, whereas hypoglycemia is also an independent risk factor for mortality.[1] Perhaps not surprisingly, recent clinical trials of tight glucose control (TGC) in critically ill patients have shown inconsistent results, possibly attributable to the increase in hypoglycemia.[1]

However, it would be an error to abandon attempts to control hyperglycemia and conclude that doing so provides no benefit or has too high a risk. Protocols aimed at controlling hyperglycemia that are started in the emergency department[2] and outside of the intensive care unit[3] have shown cost savings and shorter hospital stays. Consultation with endocrinology and diabetes control teams have also been shown to shorten hospitalization.[4] In comparison, use of traditional sliding scale–only approaches can give patients an inconsistent message as to the importance of

Conflicts of Interest: David and Angela Tridgell: none; Irl Hirsch is a consultant for Roche and Johnson & Johnson, and has received research grants from Novo Nordisk and Mannkindk.
[a] Division of Metabolism, Endocrinology and Nutrition, University of Washington, 1959 NE Pacific Street, Box 356426, Seattle, WA 98195, USA
[b] Division of Endocrinology and Diabetes, Seattle Children's Hospital, University of Washington, 4800 Sandpoint Way NE, Mailstop A5902, Seattle, WA 98105, USA
[c] Division of Metabolism, Endocrinology and Nutrition, University of Washington, 4225 Roosevelt Way NE, Suite 101, Seattle, WA 98105, USA
* Corresponding author.
E-mail address: tridge@uw.edu

Endocrinol Metab Clin N Am 39 (2010) 595–608
doi:10.1016/j.ecl.2010.05.014
0889-8529/10/$ – see front matter © 2010 Elsevier Inc. All rights reserved.

glycemic control and can result in increased rates of hyperglycemia, hypoglycemia, and DKA.[5–7] Patients accustomed to TGC may feel extremely frustrated with poor inpatient control, particularly if it is the result of providers having poor knowledge of the use of modern insulin regimens.[8] This article focuses on the "how to" of inpatient insulin management in noncritical, nonpregnant adults and pediatric patients with type 1 diabetes. These principles can also be applied to patients with steroid-induced hyperglycemia.

INSULIN PHARMACOKINETICS AND PHARMACODYNAMICS

Insulin is associated with a high rate of medical errors and is considered a high-alert medication.[9,10] The advent of insulin analogs has conceptually simplified diabetes management through allowing for more physiologic basal–bolus therapy, but the larger selection of insulins may lead to confusion for inexperienced providers. Therefore, inpatient providers must know the generic names, trade names, and pharmacokinetics of currently available insulins (**Table 1**). The astute reader will note the absence of premixed insulins from **Table 1**, because the authors do not recommend their use in any patient with type 1 diabetes, whether inpatient or outpatient.

Trade names of standard human insulin (regular and neutral protamine Hagedorn [NPH]) end with the suffix -lin, as in the trade names Humulin and Novolin. This suffix distinguishes these human insulin preparations from the newer rapid-acting insulin analogs whose trade name suffixes are -log (Humalog and Novolog), as in *analog*. Insulin lispro, insulin aspart, and insulin glulisine may be substituted for one another due to similar pharmacokinetics.

When given subcutaneously, rapid-acting analogs are absorbed more quickly and achieve higher peak serum concentrations than regular insulin (pharmacokinetics, **Fig. 1**A). However, the downstream effect on glucose disposal into the cell (pharmacodynamics) when administered subcutaneously is closer to regular insulin than

Table 1
Pharmacokinetics of various insulin preparations when administered subcutaneously

Generic Name	Trade Names	Onset of Action	Peak Action	Effective Duration
Standard				
Regular	Humulin R Novolin R	30–60 min	2–3 h	8–10 h
NPH	Humulin N Novolin N	2–4 h	4–10 h	12–18 h
Rapid-acting analogs				
Lispro	Humalog	5–15 min	30–90 min	4–6 h
Aspart	Novolog	5–15 min	30–90 min	4–6 h
Glulisine	Apidra	5–15 min	30–90 min	4–6 h
Long-acting analogs				
Glargine	Lantus	2–4 h	None	20–24 h
Detemir	Levemir		None	6–23 h[a]

Abbreviation: NPH, neutral protamine Hagedorn.
  [a] Assumes 0.1–0.2 U/kg per injection. Onset and duration may vary significantly by injection site.
  Data from Rodbard HW, Blonde L, Braithwaite SS, et al. American Association of Clinical Endocrinologists medical guidelines for clinical practice for the management of diabetes mellitus. Endocr Pract 2007;13(Suppl 1):17.

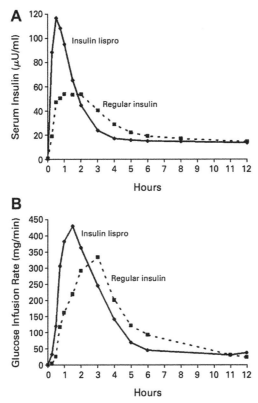

Fig. 1. Insulin pharmacokinetics and pharmacodynamics. Effects of subcutaneous administration of insulin lispro and regular insulin on serum insulin concentrations (*A*) and the rate of glucose infusion necessary to maintain normoglycemia (*B*) in 10 normal subjects. To convert values for insulin to picomoles per liter, multiply by 6.0; to convert values for the glucose infusion rate to millimoles per minute, multiply by 0.005551. (*From* Holleman F, Hoekstra JB. Insulin lispro. N Engl J Med 1997;337(3):178; with permission.)

would be predicted by pharmacokinetics alone (see **Fig. 1**B). When given intravenously, regular insulin and insulin lispro have identical pharmacokinetics and pharmacodynamic properties.[11] Although some of the rapid-acting analogs are approved by the US Food and Drug Administration for intravenous use, the authors only recommend regular insulin be used intravenously because of the identical pharmacokinetics/pharmacodynamics and lower cost compared with rapid-acting analogs.

FUNDAMENTALS OF INSULIN MANAGEMENT

In their clinical practice guidelines, the American Diabetes Association[12] (ADA) recommends the terminology *basal, prandial, nutritional,* and *correction* insulin be used when referring to the basic components of insulin therapy. *Basal insulin* is the background insulin that is needed constantly to prevent ketosis, unchecked hepatic gluconeogenesis, and subsequent hyperglycemia. *Prandial insulin* is required to prevent the postprandial rise in blood glucose caused by peripheral glucose disposal at the level of the muscle. The term *nutritional insulin* is used instead of *prandial insulin* when calories are provided by tube feeds, total parenteral nutrition (TPN), or intravenous dextrose.

Correction insulin (also referred to as *supplemental insulin*) refers to the additional insulin given to correct for hyperglycemia (**Fig. 2**).

The *insulin sensitivity factor* (ISF, also called *correction factor*) refers to how much one unit of insulin will usually lower plasma glucose. The insulin-to-carbohydrate (I:C) ratio refers to how many grams of carbohydrate one unit of insulin will cover to maintain plasma glucose. In a healthy, nonstressed individual with normal insulin sensitivity and oral intake, basal and prandial insulin each account for approximately 50% of the total daily dose. In a typical adult one unit of insulin will lower plasma glucose by approximately 50 mg/dL (an ISF of 1:50) and one unit of insulin will cover 15 g of carbohydrate (I:C ratio of 1:15). These ratios vary between individuals and are higher or lower depending on age, pubertal status, weight, and general level of activity.

METHODS OF SUBCUTANEOUS INSULIN ADMINISTRATION

Although definitions vary, *sliding scale* commonly refers to administration of regular insulin based only on the blood glucose either four times daily or every 6 hours, regardless of meals or activity level. Thus, sliding scale reacts to hyperglycemia rather than trying to prevent it. It is nonphysiologic and may result in higher rates of hyperglycemia, hypoglycemia, and DKA,[5–7] and therefore should no longer be used. Many patients and providers still use the term *sliding scale* to refer to correction dose insulin. However, the authors recommend both providers and patients adopt the newer terminology for improved standardization.

Conventional insulin therapy (CIT) usually refers to two injections of insulin daily, most commonly a mixture of regular and NPH insulin injected twice daily before breakfast and dinner. This technique is no longer standard of care given the advent of insulin analogs, and the authors recommend switching to a more physiologic regimen, as described later. However, recent epidemiologic data showed that 40% of children on CIT are from low-income households, and nearly 35% have no medical insurance.[13]

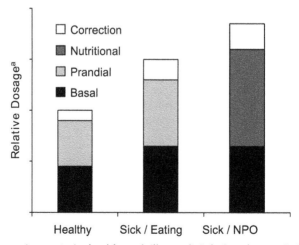

Fig. 2. Insulin requirements in health and illness. [a] Relative dosage is for illustrative purposes only, because actual insulin needs may vary widely. NPO, nothing by mouth. (*Adapted from* Clement S, Braithwaite SS, Magee MF, et al. Management of diabetes and hyperglycemia in hospitals. Diabetes Care 2004;27(2):565; with permission.)

Modern multiple daily injection (MDI) therapy combines a long-acting insulin analog (insulin glargine or insulin detemir) to provide basal insulin, with multiple injections of a rapid-acting analog to provide prandial and correction dose insulin. Regular insulin is occasionally used instead of rapid-acting analogs, such as in patients with gastroparesis with slower digestion. Occasionally MDI refers to multiple injections of regular insulin at meals, and NPH insulin in the morning and at bedtime. Insulin glargine is usually given once daily at approximately the same time (often at bed time, although this is not necessary), although it can be divided into two separate doses. Insulin detemir is generally given twice daily because of its shorter duration of action. Correction dose insulin should not be given any more frequently than every 4 to 6 hours to prevent "insulin stacking" and hypoglycemia. For an inpatient, correction dose insulin (rapid acting analog) should generally be given only at meal times or bedtime to prevent insulin stacking and hypoglycemia, or every 6 hours for patients receiving nothing by mouth (NPO; who should also receive basal insulin). Bedtime and overnight correction dose insulin is often reduced by 25% to 50% of daytime dosage to prevent nocturnal hypoglycemia.

Continuous subcutaneous insulin infusion (CSII) refers to an insulin pump that delivers insulin through plastic tubing to an infusion set (in most pumps). Infusion sets are small subcutaneous plastic catheters that must be replaced every 2 to 3 days. Pumps are programmed to deliver a rapid-acting analog (regular insulin, although no longer standard of care, can also be used) in small, incremental doses to provide basal insulin, thus taking the place of a long-acting analog.

Larger doses, known as a *bolus*, provide for prandial or correction dose insulin. Hyperglycemia and DKA can develop quickly if insulin administration is interrupted or discontinued, because of the lack of a long-acting subcutaneous basal insulin depot. Unexplained hyperglycemia without ketosis in a patient using CSII who has not disconnected the pump is more often caused by infusion set problems (such as local inflammation, lipohypertrophy, or kinked tubing) than the pump itself, and should prompt immediate replacement of the infusion set. Patients using CSII during their hospitalization must come prepared with extra infusion sets and pump supplies, because these are not provided by the hospital given the wide variety of supplies.

The I:C, ISF, and blood sugar targets are programmed into modern insulin pumps. Patients enter in the estimated carbohydrate amount and blood glucose. The pump calculates the recommended insulin dose, subtracting any insulin "on board" from the calculation to prevent insulin stacking. The user may override the recommended amount, giving more or less insulin than recommended. Pump keypads can be locked to prevent small children from dosing without supervision.

INPATIENT GLYCEMIC GOALS

Hyperglycemia has been associated with increased mortality and morbidity (ie, increased infection rates) in hospitalized patients, and hypoglycemia also has been recognized as a risk factor for mortality.[1] Randomized controlled trails in critically ill adults with hyperglycemia (most without a history of diabetes) have shown both increased and decreased mortality with intensive insulin management. The possibility exists that any benefits of intensive insulin management in this patient population may be offset by adverse events resulting from higher rates of hypoglycemia in these trials. Thus, recommended glucose targets for critically ill patients were relaxed to 140 to 180 mg/dL in a recent consensus statement. This administration should be performed with a validated insulin infusion protocol with frequent glucose monitoring, demonstrated safety, and low rates of hypoglycemia (**Table 2**).[1] For patients who are not

Table 2		
Recommended inpatient target glucose values for adults		
	Plasma Blood Glucose Range (mg/dL)	
Critically ill	140–180	
	Before meals	Random
Non–critically ill	<140	<180

Consider modifying regimen if sugar drops below 100 mg/dL, and modify regimen if less than 70 mg/dL unless the event is easily explained (such as a missed meal).

critically ill, the premeal glucose should generally be less than 140 mg/dL, with random measurements of less than 180 mg/dL (see **Table 2**). More stringent targets may be appropriate for patients with previous TGC, whereas less-stringent targets may be appropriate for patients with comorbidities.[1] Because no randomized controlled trials have studied intensive insulin management outside of the intensive care unit setting, these targets were based on clinical experience and judgement.[1] Although the targets for non–critically ill adults are lower than for critically ill patients, critically ill patients may be less able to recognize hypoglycemia given comorbidities or sedation.

The only recommendations proposed for inpatient glycemic goals in children with type 1 diabetes are expert opinion, apply to surgical admissions, and differ slightly in their recommended targets.[14,15] No consensus exists for steroid-induced hyperglycemia in children. Numerous observational studies support the conclusion that hyperglycemia and hypoglycemia in children are associated with longer hospitalizations and increased inpatient morbidity.[16–20] Only two randomized controlled trials have studied glucose management in pediatric critical illness.[21,22] The glucose targets were lower than currently recommended for adult critical illness, and both trials had high rates of hypoglycemia. One study was stopped early because of potential harm.[22]

Children may be less able to communicate hypoglycemic symptoms, resulting in increased susceptibility to hypoglycemia and risk of possible long-term neurologic sequelae. Therefore, the authors recommend using the current adult critical illness glycemic goals (140–180 mg/dL) in pediatric critical illness, and extend this recommendation for intraoperative use with an insulin drip (**Table 3**).

For non–critically ill children with type 1 diabetes or steroid-induced hyperglycemia, the authors have modified the ADA outpatient age-based blood glucose targets for inpatient use to reduce the risk of hypoglycemia. The ADA outpatient targets were designed to reduce the risk for long-term complications, and have not been studied

Table 3		
Recommended inpatient target glucose values for children		
	Plasma Blood Glucose Range (mg/dL)	
Critically ill	140–180	
	Before meals	Bedtime/overnight
Toddlers and preschoolers (age, 0–6 years)	<180	150–200
School-aged (age, 6–12 years)	<180	150–200
Adolescents and young adults (age, 13–19 years)	<140	150–200

Pediatric recommendations modified from the ADA outpatient age-based guidelines. Consider modifying regimen if sugar drops below 100 mg/dL, and modify regimen if less than 70 mg/dL unless the event is easily explained (such as a missed meal).

Data from Silverstein J, Klingensmith G, Copeland K, et al. Care of children and adolescents with type 1 diabetes: a statement of the American Diabetes Association. Diabetes Care 2005;28:186–212.

for use in the hospital.[23] Additionally, because bedtime glucose levels correlate with overnight hypoglycemia risk,[24,25] the authors recommend a higher bedtime glucose target of 150 to 200 mg/dL for all age groups, with a reduction of bedtime correction dose insulin by 25% to 50% of the normal daytime dosage (see **Table 3**). Additional studies are needed in this area to clarify optimal targets for both adults and children.

If the child is new to insulin, initial doses are based on pubertal status and weight. The total daily dose of insulin for prepubertal children is approximately 0.7 to 1.0 units/kg per day, whereas a pubertal child may need 1.0 to 2.0 units/kg per day. If the diagnosis of diabetes is recent, the dose may be closer to 0.5 units/kg per day because of remaining endogenous insulin secretion.

INSULIN SELF-MANAGEMENT

Insulin self-management allows appropriate patients to dose and administer their own insulin the way they would as an outpatient. This strategy acknowledges patient autonomy. Because many patients may understand their own diabetes better than their providers, control may be improved by insulin self-management.

Appropriate patients are lucid, have proficient outpatient skills (including performing self-monitoring of glucose at home, using MDI or CSII), are familiar with carbohydrate counting and sick-day management, demonstrate proper insulin administration technique, and have reasonable oral intake.[26] Patients with temporary or permanent physical disability who otherwise meet the above criteria may still be appropriate to dose their own insulin but may need nursing assistance for insulin administration.

Young children should not be allowed to attempt self-management. A family member who fulfills the above criteria and commits to staying in the hospital may be appropriate to perform this task. Teenagers may be allowed to co-manage their diabetes provided expectations are clear and there is good communication.

If the facility allows, patients may use their home glucose meters, provided an initial blood glucose result is within 15% of simultaneous laboratory measurement. Patients should be required to share subsequent glucose values and insulin doses (including basal rates for those on CSII) with nursing staff for documentation. Some patients may not be accustomed to the degree of hyperglycemia induced by their illness, and therefore providers still must assess glucose control and provide recommendations and teaching as needed. Insulin self-management is no longer appropriate when it results in uncontrolled hyperglycemia, hypoglycemia, or DKA.[26]

ADJUSTING THE INPATIENT REGIMEN

A hemoglobin A1c should be obtained at admission if a recent value is not available. The A1c may be inaccurate in the case of recent blood transfusions, anemia, erythrocytosis (including erythropoietin therapy), and hemoglobinopathy.

Factors contributing to inpatient hyperglycemia include infection, surgery, excess snacking, missed insulin doses, CSII device malfunction or infusion set problems, inactivity, mistiming of insulin administration, and mistiming of finger stick glucose measurements (ie, after the meal is started, rather than before).[27] The mistiming of insulin administration and glucose measurements can make control seem artificially worse, and can be avoided through proper coordination between dietary and nursing services.[27]

For patients on subcutaneous regimens, blood glucose should be monitored before meals and at bedtime in patients who are eating, and at minimum of every 6 hours for those who are NPO or on continuous tube feeds. Given the pharmacodynamics of insulin analogs, sufficient insulin lag time (the period between insulin injection and food intake) decreases postprandial hyperglycemia.[28] The authors recommend progressively longer lag times for rapid-acting prandial and correction dose insulin, depending on the degree of hyperglycemia (**Table 4**). Proper lag times may be best achieved by patients who are self-managing. For nauseated patients and children who are picky eaters, prandial insulin may be given during or immediately after a meal to prevent hypoglycemia. Prandial regular insulin is often indicated for patients with gastroparesis or cancer who may "graze," and should usually be given 30 minutes before the first bite of food. Clinical judgment is needed when patients are hypoglycemic at the start of a meal; insulin administration can be delayed for a brief time, and the insulin dose can be decreased or carbohydrate consumption increased.

Illness can dramatically increase insulin requirements in any hospitalized patient, and may fluctuate dramatically during and after hospitalization. Insulin regimens should be reassessed at least daily and after any changes in clinical or mental status, medications (ie, glucocorticoid dose), or nutritional status (ie, being made NPO for surgery).

ADJUSTING SUBCUTANEOUS INSULIN

Ideally, the basal insulin requirements should be evaluated first. If the bedtime blood glucose is in target range, little change between the bedtime glucose and the fasting morning glucose indicate the nocturnal basal dose is adequate, whereas dramatically rising or falling glucose values indicate the basal insulin dose is too low or too high, respectively. However, this presumes an ideal situation, characterized by a reasonable period between dinner and the bedtime glucose (ideally ≥4 hours), no snacking after dinner or overnight, no hypoglycemic episodes overnight, and no supplemental insulin at bedtime. All of these criteria rarely occur in the inpatient setting, and judgment is needed when confounding factors are present. If basal insulin is significantly greater than 50% of the total daily dose, major insulin adjustments likely will be required in the hospital to avoid hypoglycemia. The basal insulin can be adjusted by 10% to 20% every 1 to 2 days as needed,[27] or more rapidly for more critical hypo- or hyperglycemia. Adjustments of prandial and correction insulin doses for breakfast, lunch, and dinner are made based on the glucose response at lunch, dinner, and bedtime, respectively.

TPN, TUBE FEEDING, AND GLUCOCORTICOIDS

Components of insulin therapy for patients on TPN or tube feeds consist of basal, prandial, and correction dose insulin. Occasionally, patients will receive these nutritional modalities to supplement inadequate oral intake, in which case they may require both prandial insulin to cover their meals and nutritional insulin to cover tube feeds or TPN.

No controlled trials have evaluated optimal insulin administration for TPN. One approach is to titrate a separate insulin infusion (in addition to basal insulin for patients

Table 4	
Recommended lag times for preprandial (rapid-acting analog) insulin	
Preprandial Glucose (mg/dL)	**Lag Time (min)**
80–99	0
100–199	10–20
200–299	20–30
≥300	30–40

with type 1 diabetes) to estimate the required nutritional component, and then take 66% to 100% of the 24-hour requirement and add it to subsequent TPN bags.[26]

For patients on continuous tube feeds, nutritional insulin can be provided by regular insulin every 6 hours. Alternatively, basal and nutritional insulin can be provided by a combination of regular insulin and NPH insulin twice or three times daily. When the target rate for tube feeding has been met, the temptation may arise to cover basal and nutritional insulin needs with insulin glargine only. However, this approach risks hypoglycemia because of the frequency with which tube feeds are suddenly discontinued or rates are decreased. Alternatively, insulin detemir twice daily is used by some providers to provide both prandial and nutritional insulin. This approach offers greater flexibility than once-daily glargine, although given the relatively long duration of action, detemir still poses a high potential for hypoglycemia if tube feedings are suddenly discontinued. Blood glucose should be monitored every 4 to 6 hours during continuous tube feeds, and correction dose insulin should be provided through a rapid-acting analog. Blood glucose should be monitored every 1 to 2 hours when tube feed rates are unexpectedly decreased or discontinued, intravenous dextrose should be given as needed, and the insulin regimen should be promptly reevaluated and modified if necessary.[26]

A combination of regular and NPH insulin may be given before initiation of nocturnal tube feeds to provide nutritional insulin. Patients on bolus tube feeds can receive subcutaneous regular insulin or a rapid-acting analog before each tube feed bolus.[26] The most important pearl for success is to perform enough glucose testing to appreciate which insulin must be altered at any given time.

Glucocorticoids result in hyperglycemia and exert a greater effect on postprandial hyperglycemia than on fasting hyperglycemia. Accordingly, nutritional and correction insulin should be adjusted upward, or downward, as steroid doses increase or decrease. With prednisone doses in the range of 20 to 60 mg daily, the authors have found that adding NPH insulin in the morning (starting with 5–10 units), with otherwise minimal changes in the other components of the MDI regimen, works well. With higher doses of glucocorticoids, fasting hyperglycemia will result and basal insulin doses will also need to be increased. Intravenous insulin is indicated when subcutaneous insulin is inadequate, and may be preferable for short-term (2–3 days) pulses of high-dose steroids in which tapering will be rapid.[26]

INTRAVENOUS INSULIN

Intravenous insulin is indicated for patients with type 1 diabetes in moderate to severe DKA (pH <7.2 and bicarbonate <10). Mild DKA (pH 7.2–7.3 and bicarbonate 10–15) can be treated with either subcutaneous or intravenous insulin, depending on the clinical situation.[29] If subcutaneous insulin is used, a dosage increase of 5% to 10% of the total daily dose is necessary to counteract ketosis.[30] Intravenous insulin is indicated for critical illness, general anesthesia, myocardial infarction or cardiogenic shock, stroke, severe hyperglycemia secondary to high-dose glucocorticoid treatment, prolonged NPO status, and as a dose-finding strategy in anticipation of reinitiation of subcutaneous insulin therapy.[26] Numerous protocols for the administration of intravenous insulin have been published.[31,32] With proper protocols and staff training, intravenous insulin can be safely used outside of the intensive care unit, and the authors recommend implementing these protocols to prevent having to transfer patients to the intensive care unit just to receive an insulin drip. Occasionally, it may be appropriate to allow patients on an insulin drip to eat; this may occur when critical illness or DKA are resolving, during transition to subcutaneous insulin, or for patients on high-dose glucocorticoids. Eating will result in hyperglycemia. The use of subcutaneous prandial insulin in conjunction with the intravenous drip can mitigate much of this postprandial hyperglycemia.

PERIOPERATIVE INSULIN

Patients admitted for elective procedures will need outpatient instructions on insulin dosing before hospitalization. Reduction of long-acting basal insulin is unnecessary the night prior to or the morning of surgery for most patients with type 1 diabetes. However, patients receiving NPH insulin should reduce their morning dose by 50%. Patients on CSII should continue their basal insulin rates as usual. Nutritional insulin should not be given the morning of the procedure in any NPO patient. Correction dose insulin, if needed, should be reduced by 25% to 50% of the usual daytime dose.

Although some authors recommend that all patients with type 1 diabetes undergoing surgery be started on intravenous dextrose to prevent ketosis and hypoglycemia,[33] this article's authors believe there is room for some personal judgment, depending on the duration of NPO status. Young children may be susceptible to hypoglycemia when NPO, unlike adolescents and adults. Intravenous insulin and dextrose should be started for all major surgery or prolonged NPO status. All patients on insulin drips undergoing procedures should have hourly glucose measurements, although the optimal frequency has never been studied. For patients undergoing elective surgery not involving general anesthesia, intravenous insulin can be initiated when glucose exceeds the target range.

Patients using CSII should be placed on an insulin drip and discontinue their insulin pump whenever they will undergo general anesthesia, or any procedure that has the potential to last longer than 2 hours without the need for general anesthesia. The authors do not recommend CSII be used under general anesthesia because of the lack of familiarity of most operating room staff with CSII, coupled with the lack of flexibility and long lag time (relative to intravenous) of subcutaneous insulin.

TRANSITION FROM INTRAVENOUS TO SUBCUTANEOUS INSULIN

Several steps are necessary when transitioning from intravenous to subcutaneous insulin: determining the new total daily dose of subcutaneous insulin, apportioning the appropriate amount to basal and prandial/nutritional insulin, and the transition itself. Existing transition protocols have been studied in predominately a type 2 diabetes population.[34] The authors consider two subject groups: those with normal insulin sensitivity and those with insulin resistance. Patients undergoing elective procedures and some patients with DKA may have normal insulin sensitivity. For these patients, the home regimen may be continued, or modified as necessary when the home regimen was suboptimal or if the nutritional status of the patient will change (**Fig. 3**). Patients who still have a depot of long-acting subcutaneous basal insulin, such as those undergoing minor surgery or elective procedures, may not require any additional subcutaneous insulin when the intravenous insulin drip is discontinued. However, patients on CSII may need to reprime their infusion sets.

Increased insulin resistance may occur from illness or glucocorticoids. In these cases, the insulin drip rate can be used as a guide to estimate subcutaneous insulin needs, taking care to apportion the proper amount to basal and nutritional insulin, and then multiplied by a safety factor of 0.8 as shown in **Fig. 3**.[34] Patients who no longer have a depot of long-acting subcutaneous basal insulin must have an overlap of subcutaneous basal insulin with the intravenous insulin by approximately 2 hours. This strategy allows some absorption of subcutaneous insulin into the circulation and helps prevent hyperglycemia.

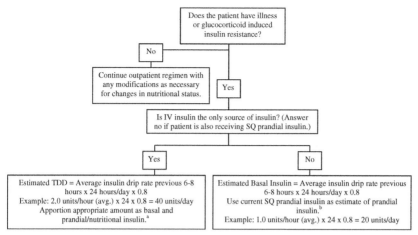

Fig. 3. Transitioning from intravenous to subcutaneous insulin. Please see text for examples of how the transition is done. [a] Note that glucocorticoids may result in prandial or nutritional insulin needs greater than 50% of TDD. [b] One way to estimate how accurately prandial insulin is dosed is to evaluate the postprandial glucose values and insulin drip change rates. Avg, average; IV, intravenous, TDD, total daily dose; SQ, subcutaneous.

Basal insulin should be given at the appropriate time of the day (ie, bedtime or morning) and not at an arbitrary time when intravenous insulin is discontinued (eg, at noon after the order has been written). Ideally, hospitals will have protocols that allow for intravenous insulin to be given outside of the intensive care unit to allow this transition. When this is not possible, a one-time dose of insulin of appropriate duration can be used as a bridge. For example, if a patient will transfer from the ICU at noon to a general medical floor, they can receive a one-time dose of NPH insulin as a bridge 2 to 3 hours before discontinuing the insulin drip, with initiation of insulin glargine or insulin detemir at bedtime. If the drip is going to be discontinued at dinner time, a one-time dose of a rapid-acting analog or regular insulin (estimated to provide for both short-term basal insulin and prandial or nutritional insulin, if appropriate) can be given 1 hour before discontinuing the drip, with initiation of the basal insulin at bedtime.

WRITING ORDERS

The authors encourage the use of standard order sets that address all three components of subcutaneous insulin therapy. Order sets should have nurse-driven protocols that do not rely on physician notification for treatment of hypoglycemia, but do notify the physician for hypoglycemia that is prolonged or results in adverse outcomes (eg, loss of consciousness, falls, seizures). These protocols should automatically check a 2 AM blood glucose after any incident of hypoglycemia. Checking a 2 AM blood glucose is also advisable whenever insulin dosing has changed, if blood sugars are unstable, or if the patient is NPO.[12]

Orders should specifically state when correction dose insulin should be given (ie, at meal times and bedtime only). Anecdotal cases exist of correction dose insulin administration with every blood glucose check (ie, every hour), resulting in insulin stacking and severe hypoglycemia or death. Correction dose insulin should generally not be given between meals. Order sets should include a prompt to reduce bedtime and overnight correction dose insulin by 25% to 50% of the daytime dose to prevent nocturnal hypoglycemia.

ADDITIONAL CONSIDERATIONS FOR CHILDREN

The authors advise that an endocrinologist be involved in the management of all hospitalized children with type 1 diabetes. The involvement may be as simple as evaluating the home insulin regimen that will be continued during the inpatient period, or as complete as full management of the diabetes by the endocrinology team. The different roles of the family members and nursing staff should be delineated, because family members often prefer to help manage the child's diabetes during hospitalization.

Some children require very small doses of insulin administered as diluted insulin, of which several common concentrations exist. The authors recommend diluted insulin be prepared by the inpatient pharmacy as 10 units per milliliter of commercial diluent (U10) to simplify dosing calculations. It is essential that unique labeling differentiate diluted insulin from standard insulin (U100).

DISCHARGE PLANNING

Hospital discharge provides an opportunity to reevaluate the previous outpatient regimen, modify or switch regimens in patients with previously poor control, and address any social or diabetes education needs of the patient or family. These considerations should be addressed several days before discharge to prevent delays in discharge. The hospitalization may provide an opportunity to switch patients previously on CIT to MDI. However, although not standard of care, some patients may be on CIT because of lack of financial resources. A social worker or patient representative may be invaluable when financial resources are lacking. Patients should always be cautioned about factors that are likely to cause changes in insulin needs. All patients should have appropriate plans for endocrinology follow-up after discharge.

SUMMARY

Inpatient TGC may lead to reduced morbidity, shorter hospital stays, and improved patient satisfaction, but must be balanced against the risks of hypoglycemia, as reflected in recent guidelines. Proper balance of TGC and safety requires familiarity with available insulin preparations, proper use of intravenous insulin, frequent testing, and MDI therapy that takes into account basal insulin, prandial or nutritional insulin, and correction insulin.

REFERENCES

1. Moghissi ES, Korytkowski MT, DiNardo M, et al. American Association of Clinical Endocrinologists and American Diabetes Association consensus statement on inpatient glycemic control. Diabetes Care 2009;32:1119–31.
2. Munoz C, Villanueva G, Fogg L, et al. Impact of a subcutaneous insulin protocol in the emergency department: RUSH Emergency Department Hyperglycemia Intervention (REDHI). J Emerg Med 2008. DOI:10.1016/j.jemermed.2008.03.017. [Epub ahead of print].
3. Olson L, Muchmore J, Lawrence CB. The benefits of inpatient diabetes care: improving quality of care and the bottom line. Endocr Pract 2006;12(Suppl 3):35–42.
4. Levetan CS, Salas JR, Wilets IF, et al. Impact of endocrine and diabetes team consultation on hospital length of stay for patients with diabetes. Am J Med 1995;99:22–8.
5. Queale WS, Seidler AJ, Brancati FL. Glycemic control and sliding scale insulin use in medical inpatients with diabetes mellitus. Arch Intern Med 1997;157:545–52.
6. Hirsch IB. Sliding scale insulin—time to stop sliding. JAMA 2009;301:213–4.

7. Umpierrez GE, Palacio A, Smiley D. Sliding scale insulin use: myth or insanity? Am J Med 2007;120:563–7.
8. Bhattacharyya A, Christodoulides C, Kaushal K, et al. In-patient management of diabetes mellitus and patient satisfaction. Diabet Med 2002;19:412–6.
9. Amori RE, Pittas AG, Siegel RD, et al. Inpatient medical errors involving glucose-lowering medications and their impact on patients: review of 2,598 incidents from a voluntary electronic error-reporting database. Endocr Pract 2008;14:535–42.
10. Cohen MR, Proulx SM, Crawford SY. Survey of hospital systems and common serious medication errors. J Healthc Risk Manag 1998;18:16–27.
11. Heinemann L, Woodworth J. Pharmacokinetics and glucodynamics of insulin lispro. Drugs Today 1998;34:24–36.
12. American Diabetes Association. Standards of medical care in diabetes–2009. Diabetes Care 2009;32(Suppl 1):S13–61.
13. Paris CA, Imperatore G, Klingensmith G, et al. Predictors of insulin regimens and impact on outcomes in youth with type 1 diabetes: the SEARCH for diabetes in youth study. J Pediatr 2009;155:183–9.
14. Betts P, Brink S, Silink M, et al. Management of children and adolescents with diabetes requiring surgery. Pediatr Diabetes 2009;10(Suppl 12):169–74.
15. Rhodes ET, Ferrari LR, Wolfsdorf JI. Perioperative management of pediatric surgical patients with diabetes mellitus. Anesth Analg 2005;101:986–99 table.
16. Verbruggen SC, Joosten KF, Castillo L, et al. Insulin therapy in the pediatric intensive care unit. Clin Nutr 2007;26:677–90.
17. Preissig CM, Rigby MR. Pediatric critical illness hyperglycemia: risk factors associated with development and severity of hyperglycemia in critically ill children. J Pediatr 2009;155:734–9.
18. Day KM, Haub N, Betts H, et al. Hyperglycemia is associated with morbidity in critically ill children with meningococcal sepsis. Pediatr Crit Care Med 2008;9:636–40.
19. Palacio A, Smiley D, Ceron M, et al. Prevalence and clinical outcome of inpatient hyperglycemia in a community pediatric hospital. J Hosp Med 2008;3:212–7.
20. Ulate KP, Lima Falcao GC, Bielefeld MR, et al. Strict glycemic targets need not be so strict: a more permissive glycemic range for critically ill children. Pediatrics 2008;122:e898–904.
21. Vlasselaers D, Milants I, Desmet L, et al. Intensive insulin therapy for patients in paediatric intensive care: a prospective, randomised controlled study. Lancet 2009;373:547–56.
22. Beardsall K, Vanhaesebrouck S, Ogilvy-Stuart AL, et al. Early insulin therapy in very-low-birth-weight infants. N Engl J Med 2008;359:1873–84.
23. Silverstein J, Klingensmith G, Copeland K, et al. Care of children and adolescents with type 1 diabetes: a statement of the American Diabetes Association. Diabetes Care 2005;28:186–212.
24. Kaufman FR, Austin J, Neinstein A, et al. Nocturnal hypoglycemia detected with the Continuous Glucose Monitoring System in pediatric patients with type 1 diabetes. J Pediatr 2002;141:625–30.
25. Woodward A, Weston P, Casson IF, et al. Nocturnal hypoglycaemia in type 1 diabetes–frequency and predictive factors. QJM 2009;102:603–7.
26. Clement S, Braithwaite SS, Magee MF, et al. Management of diabetes and hyperglycemia in hospitals. Diabetes Care 2004;27:553–91.
27. Inzucchi SE. Clinical practice. Management of hyperglycemia in the hospital setting. N Engl J Med 2006;355:1903–11.
28. Rassam AG, Zeise TM, Burge MR, et al. Optimal administration of lispro insulin in hyperglycemic type 1 diabetes. Diabetes Care 1999;22:133–6.

29. Wolfsdorf J, Glaser N, Sperling MA. Diabetic ketoacidosis in infants, children, and adolescents: a consensus statement from the American Diabetes Association. Diabetes Care 2006;29:1150–9.

30. Brink S, Laffel L, Likitmaskul S, et al. Sick day management in children and adolescents with diabetes. Pediatr Diabetes 2007;8:401–7.

31. Bode BW, Braithwaite SS, Steed RD, et al. Intravenous insulin infusion therapy: indications, methods, and transition to subcutaneous insulin therapy. Endocr Pract 2004;10(Suppl 2):71–80.

32. DeSantis AJ, Schmeltz LR, Schmidt K, et al. Inpatient management of hyperglycemia: the Northwestern experience. Endocr Pract 2006;12:491–505.

33. O'Malley CW, Emanuele M, Halasyamani L, et al. Bridge over troubled waters: safe and effective transitions of the inpatient with hyperglycemia. J Hosp Med 2008;3:55–65.

34. Schmeltz LR, DeSantis AJ, Schmidt K, et al. Conversion of intravenous insulin infusions to subcutaneously administered insulin glargine in patients with hyperglycemia. Endocr Pract 2006;12:641–50.

Toward Closing the Loop: An Update on Insulin Pumps and Continuous Glucose Monitoring Systems

Tandy Aye, MD, Jen Block, RN, CDE, Bruce Buckingham, MD*

KEYWORDS

- Insulin pumps • Continuous glucose monitoring
- Type 1 diabetes • Closed-loop therapy
- Artificial pancreas • Nocturnal hypoglycemia

Diabetes is a chronic disease that currently can only be controlled by constant vigilance. Chronic elevations, and likely fluctuations, of the blood glucose are associated with long-term complications (blindness, kidney failure, heart disease, and lower extremity amputations). Perversely, tight glucose control increases the risk of serious hypoglycemia. Despite insulin infusion pumps and programs that promote intensive diabetes management, the average A1c at major diabetes treatment centers remains higher than 8%,[1] well above the recommended goal of 7% for adults and for age-adjusted pediatric goals (**Table 1**).[2] Many factors contribute to this failure:

The difficulties in correctly estimating the amount of carbohydrates in a meal
Missed meal boluses
Anxiety about hypoglycemia resulting in under-treatment, especially overnight.

It has always been difficult to achieve compliance with complicated medical regimes, whether it is taking pills three or four times a day, or administration of insulin three or more times a day. As long as diabetes treatment demands constant direct

Dr Aye has no financial disclosures. Mrs Block has received honoraria and/or consulting fees from Medtronic MiniMed and Unomedical (Copenhagen, Denmark). Dr Buckingham receives research support from Medtronic MiniMed (Northridge, CA, USA), Abbott Diabetes Care (Alameda, CA, USA), and Dexcom (San Diego, CA, USA), and he is on medical advisory boards of Medtronic MiniMed, Unomedical, Biodel (Danbury, CT, USA), Animas (Chester, PA, USA), Novo-Nordisk (Princeton, NJ, USA), and Bayer (Tarrytown, NY, USA).
Department of Pediatrics, Stanford Medical Center, G-313, 300 Pasteur Drive, Stanford, CA 94305-5208, USA
* Corresponding author.
E-mail address: buckingham@stanford.edu

Table 1
Hemoglobin A1c goals by age

Age	Target Range[a]	HbA1c
0–5 years	80–200 mg/dL	7.5%–8.5%
6–11 years	70–180 mg/dL	<8%
12–20+ years	70–150 mg/dL	<7%

[a] American Diabetes Association. Standards of medical care in diabetes–2009. Diabetes Care 2009;32(Suppl 1):S13–61.

intervention, most people with diabetes will not meet treatment goals. By taking the patient out of the loop or closing the loop, an artificial pancreas would allow the person with diabetes to go about his or her daily activities without the need to constantly remember to check blood glucose, count carbohydrates, and take insulin multiple times each day.

An artificial pancreas consists of three components: an insulin infusion pump, a continuous glucose sensor, and an algorithm that translates data from the glucose sensor and determines insulin delivery. The most likely first closed-loop system would use a subcutaneous (SQ) sensor and insulin infusion pump. An implantable system, however, is also feasible. The main difficulties in optimizing a SQ system are

Accuracy of the SQ continuous glucose sensors
Lags in interstitial SQ glucose measurements when the glucose is changing rapidly
Delays in the onset of insulin action after an SQ injection
Prolonged insulin action of 4 to 6 hours following an SQ injection
Lack of algorithm models that exactly mimic islet physiology.

Thus, with current technology, a, SQ sensor–SQ insulin delivery system does not fully mimic normal beta cell function; however, initial studies indicate that excellent diabetes control can be achieved using such a system on a short-term basis.[3]

Before a functional artificial pancreas (AP) will receive US Food and Drug Administration (FDA) approval, clinical safety in an outpatient setting must be demonstrated. The most important safety issue in the short term will be the avoidance of severe hypoglycemic events. Fortunately, when subcutaneous glucose sensors fail, they generally indicate falsely low glucose readings. A falsely low glucose would cause underdelivery of insulin in a closed-loop system, resulting in hyperglycemia, not hypoglycemia. Hypoglycemia also can be avoided by aiming for a slightly higher glucose target. As an example, if the target is set to 120 mg/dL, and the sensor was inaccurate by 50%, glucose values would still be above 60 mg/dL. Current glucose sensors are more accurate above 70 mg/dL,[4–6] and because a closed loop generally would maintain glucose levels above this level, the system would be functioning in a glucose range where sensors have greater accuracy, which is another safety feature to prevent hypoglycemia. As algorithms improve, the amount of time spent above 200 mg/dL also can be progressively decreased. Currently, children with an average A1c of 6.9% spend an average of 6 hours with glucose readings above 200 mg/dL each day.[7] With a closed-loop system, it should be possible to significantly decrease the time spent in hyperglycemia without increasing hypoglycemia, and thereby decrease glycemic variability. Glycemic variability, independent of HbA1c levels, recently has been described as an independent risk factor for diabetic complications,[8,9] although this concept is controversial.[10]

SENSORS

Several devices and technologies have been proposed for continuous glucose monitoring, including the use of near-infrared and midinfrared spectroscopy, erythrocyte scattering, photoacoustic phenomenon, optical coherence tomography, thermo-optical techniques, Raman spectroscopy, and fluorescence measurements.[11] Currently commercially available continuous glucose sensors are based on measuring subcutaneous (interstitial) glucose levels. These are electrochemical sensors that use glucose oxidase and measure an electric current generated when glucose reacts with oxygen. They are coated with specialized membranes to make them biocompatible, generating almost no tissue reaction, and providing a barrier to potential cross-reactants such as acetaminophen. These sensors are relatively stable and generally provide a good glucose signal for 3 to 7 days.

There is a lag time between blood glucose readings and continuous glucose monitoring (CGM) readings. The lag time is due to three components:

1. A physiologic lag time between blood and interstitial glucose levels of about 3 to 8 minutes
2. Delays in the electrochemical sensor due to transit times for glucose to diffuse across the membranes coating the sensor of 1 to 2 minutes
3. Processing of the sensor signals, since these signals can be noisy and require digital filtering, which generally introduces an additional 3- to 12-minute delay in CGM readings.[12] As sensor technology improves, the sensor noise is reduced, which allows for less filtering and more rapid response times. A more rapid sensor response time is very important when using the sensor signals to drive a closed-loop system. In pigs, the temporal changes in interstitial blood glucose levels correlate better with changes in the central nervous system (CNS) glucose than to changes in the blood glucose.[13] Perhaps interstitial glucose levels would correlate better with CNS function than blood glucose levels, although this remains to be determined in people.

Although real-time CGM is not as accurate as discrete blood glucose monitoring, CGM values are generally within 15% of the discrete measurement. A discrete blood glucose has been compared with a snapshot, and real-time monitoring with a video, where there is less information in each frame, but the video provides the added dimension of glucose change over time that the snapshot cannot provide. There have been significant improvements in the accuracy of sensors over the last 6 to 10 years. In a study assessing the use of CGM in nondiabetic children in 2004, 20% of CGM readings were less than 60 mg/dL, and 54% of CGM values were greater than 150 mg/dL, whereas the range of reference glucose values was 60 to 140 mg/dL.[14] In a recent study conducted by the Juvenile Diabetes Research Foundation (JDRF) in nondiabetic children and adults using current CGM sensors, the sensor glucose concentrations were 71 to 120 mg/dL for 91% of the day, and sensor values were less than or equal to 60 or greater than 140 for only 0.2% and 0.4% of the day, respectively.[15] Glucose sensors also can be tuned to be more accurate in various glucose ranges. For example, the Medtronic Veo Glucose sensor (Northridge, CA, USA) uses the same sensor technology as the Medtronic Paradigm REAL-Time (Northridge, CA, USA), but the sensor calibration has been adjusted to be improve hypoglycemia sensitivity from 55% in the Paradigm REAL-Time to 82% in the Veo.[16]

There are other glucose sensing technologies other than the current glucose oxidase-based needle sensors that also can measure blood and subcutaneous glucose levels. One such technology uses a boronic acid matrix, which binds glucose and measures glucose levels by quenching of a fluorescence photophore. Results from GluMetrics (Irvine, CA, USA)[17] indicate that this technology has the potential to be more accurate than the current glucose oxidase-based sensors in the hypoglycemic range. One possibility in the future would be to combine two different glucose sensing technologies on a single platform, allowing for redundancy in the glucose measurements and sensing technology that has complimentary regions of greater sensor accuracy (glucose oxidase-based sensors in the hyperglycemic range and fluorescent sensors in the hypoglycemic range).

Current needle-like continuous glucose sensors pass through the skin, so there is always the potential for an infection at the insertion site. Current sensors have a transmitter attached to them once they are inserted. The transmitter provides a source of energy to power the sensor, as well as allowing transmission of the glucose signal to a receiver using a radiofrequency (RF) signal. These sensors often take from 2 to 10 hours to stabilize to the local interstitial environment before they generate a reasonably accurate glucose signal. Because of the differences in interstitial and blood glucose levels when glucose values are changing rapidly, it is generally considered better to calibrate the sensor when blood glucose levels are stable (ideally when changes are <0.5 mg/dL/min).[18] Unfortunately, when patients enter their first calibration value, they are blind to the data from their continuous glucose sensor and their glucose rate of change. After their initial calibration, they are able to see their glucose trends and assess their rate of change before entering subsequent calibration values. The calibration system could be improved significantly if sensors internally evaluated the stability of the glucose signal and only requested calibration values when the glucose signal was stable.

There remain multiple factors that affect the patient's use of the sensors. Because sensors require a continuous source of power, the transmitter cannot be detached from the sensor for any length of time, or the sensor must be recalibrated. One of the biggest user issues with these devices has been the adhesive required to secure the sensor and transmitter to the skin. The adhesives can be irritating to some wearers, and others will develop a true tape allergy. A big issue for prolonged sensor wear (>3 days) is maintaining the adhesive. For those who use continuous SQ insulin infusions (CSII), there are two insertion sites (one for the insulin infusion cannula and one for the sensor) and two areas for potential tape-related issues. Wearing the tape repeatedly in the same area can temporarily disrupt the usual skin barriers to infection. Future devices may be able to combine a continuous glucose sensor with an insulin infusion set into one platform adhering to the skin.

One way to avoid the topical skin issues associated with adhesives is to implant the sensor. Implanted sensors are attractive to patients, since they are not visible; they do not have to insert a needle-like sensor under their skin repeatedly, and they do not interfere with daily activities such as showering, swimming, or exercising. There is one published report of long-term implanted subcutaneous continuous sensors.[19] The sensors were surgically implanted into the abdomen under local anesthesia. Two months after implantation, 13 of the 15 implanted sensors were functioning and had a mean absolute relative difference of 25% when compared with YSI (Yellow Springs Instrument Glucose Analyzer [Yellow Springs, OH, USA]) glucose levels. For implanted devices to be acceptable they will probably need to function for at least 1 year once they are implanted, and ideally their insertion and removal could be performed in a physician's office and not require a surgical referral. Another approach would be an intravascular continuous glucose sensor. This technology initially was developed by Dr David Gough,[20] and similar technology has been used in clinical trials conducted by Medtronic MiniMed (Northridge, CA, USA) in France[21] and the United States. This sensor has about a 20-minute delay in reported glucose levels, which has created difficulties when trying to integrate the sensor information into an artificial pancreas.

CLINICAL POINTERS IN THE USE OF CGM SENSORS TODAY

Recent studies have demonstrated that when subjects are wearing CGM devices 5 to 7 days a week they can improve their A1c levels without increasing their risk of hypoglycemia, and this benefit can be maintained over 12 months with continued sensor wear.[22,23] This benefit was seen across all age groups as long as they wore the sensor at least 5 to 6 days a week. The main predictors for success in using a CGM at the onset of the JDRF trial was the age of the subject (adults were more successful than adolescents) and the number of home glucose tests subjects were doing before entering the study (those reporting at least 6 tests a day were more successful).[24] Wearing a CGM does not automatically improve diabetes control; it takes effort to observe glucose patterns and make adjustments to the diabetes routine. The number of glucose tests subjects were doing before entering the study is probably a surrogate maker for their interest in managing their diabetes. Until the loop is closed, CGM performs as a behavior modification tool and provides alarms for hyper- and hypoglycemia.

Currently CGM use is approved only for adjunctive use in the United States. CGM is to be used only in conjunction with traditional blood glucose testing, and all treatment decisions should be based on blood glucose test results. Intermittent finger stick blood glucose monitoring often is described as a snapshot of diabetes control, and CGM is likened to a movie that provides dynamic information about glucose control. Perhaps the most exciting components of CGM use are the trend data it provides. This additional information about the rate and direction of glucose change is very important. Take the model of blood glucose testing. A finger stick blood glucose (BG) test of 90 mg/dL is considered a safe glucose level; now add the trend data that show the glucose is going down at a rate of 2 mg/dL/min, which means in 20 minutes the glucose may be at or below 50 mg/dL. This additional knowledge may prompt a different response, and in fact the trend data provided by CGM data may be used to prevent the glucose from dropping below or rising above the individual's glucose targets. All of the currently FD-DA-approved CGM systems used in the United States have user programmable low and high glucose threshold alarms. These alarms can be programmed to alert the user when the glucose drops below or rises above the individually set thresholds.

Although trend data are helpful for the user in day-to-day life, for health care providers (HCPs) distinct advantages of CGM use are the complete glucose profiles it provides. Current CGM systems have software that is available to download and view information on glucose control, including reports showing the modal day and statistics. This information, especially the data on nocturnal glycemic patterns, can be used in combination with the blood glucose levels to guide treatment decisions with a higher degree of confidence. The CGM tool then can be used as an adjunctive means of assessing how effective any therapy changes may be.

Advantages of CGM use include

CGM provides a more complete glucose picture
Adds trend data that helps predict where the glucose is headed
Provides constant feedback on how multiple variables impact glucose control
The immediacy of the feedback helps identify causality of glycemic variations
When combined with BG data, allows for more confidence in therapy management
Alarms, if acted on, can result in increased time within target and fewer glycemic excursions
Trend/prospective data may be used to prevent glucose from dropping below or rising above target.

Challenges to CGM use include

Similar to the model for insulin pump instruction, RT-CGM instruction may be best accomplished by well-trained diabetes educators who guide patients
Expense to patient and providers
Wearability
Teaching patients how to use the data
Unrealistic patient expectations. CGM is not an artificial pancreas but does provide a wealth of information to which the user can respond
Setting alarms and alerts to maximize utility and minimize patient burden
Time and support for intensive diabetes management and CGM often is poorly reimbursed.[25]

Strategies to overcome challenges include

Using group medical visits to educate patients about CGM technology and potentially for follow-up
Trial use of a CGM system before purchase may help patients and providers make a more informed decision about using the technology and how likely they are to wear it
For assistance with reimbursement, the JDRF Web site (http://www.jdrf.org/index.cfm?page_id=106514)
offers guidance for seeking CGM coverage and provides information about select insurance carriers and CGM coverage policies
Access CWD Insurance Forum to learn about what has worked well for others seeking reimbursement
(http://forums.childrenwithdiabetes.com/forumdisplay.php?f=57/)
Utilize online patient teaching resources like the Continuous Glucose Monitoring School Online created by members of the JDRF sensor study group
(http://cgmteaching.jaeb.org)
The tool includes:
Basic information on CGM technology
Device-specific teaching modules
Guidelines and exercises for using CGM data
Suggestions on how to integrate data algorithms into care.

Key CGM Education for Patients

Initially starting patients on CGM can be challenging, as they often are made aware of glucose trends of which they were previously unaware. Remind patients that perfection is not usually attainable, but the goal of CGM use is continued improvement.[26]

CGM is adjunctive technology, and patients still will need to perform blood glucose tests to calibrate the system and to use as the basis for therapy decisions. They will need to understand
The pharmacodynamics and role of basal/meal insulin coverage
The difference between interstitial glucose and BG, and this difference will be more pronounced when the BG is changing rapidlyIt is not realistic to expect the BG and CGM values to be identical all the time
Data interpretation (done with HCP team with retrospective analysis of results)
How to use trend data (real-time data) in combination with the BG data
Adjust insulin doses based on the glucose trend.[27]

In the authors' experience, ideal CGM candidates are patients who:

Are prepared to see the data
Are willing/able to make changes based on the data
Are willing to wear the CGM system.

PUMPS

CSII or insulin infusion pumps have been commercially available for almost 30 years.[28] Since the initial pumps were developed, there have been progressive improvements in their software features and improvements in their size and the insulin infusion sets. Most pumps are attached to the subject using an infusion set catheter. A newer pump (a patch or pod pump) eliminates the need for infusion set tubing and manual insertion of the infusion set catheter. Two such pumps are the OmniPod (Insulet, Bedford, MA, USA) and Solo Micro Pump (Medingo, Tampa, FL, USA). Current pump software features include the ability to calculate different carbohydrate to insulin ratios and different insulin sensitivities for correction doses at different times of the day. They also feature a calculation of residual insulin activity following an insulin bolus. Most pumps now can automatically receive data from a glucose meter (by RF, or they have a glucose meter built into the pump), so glucose values do not need to be manually entered. Conscientious pump users often can achieve very good glycemic control if they monitor their blood glucose frequently, adjust their insulin doses based on an accurate assessment of the quantity and type of meals they are eating, and compensate for the effect of physical activity on glucose levels. This may require a prolonged bolus (square wave) for foods that are absorbed gradually, and often requires a premeal bolus of insulin before eating, especially in the morning, and temporary changes in basal infusion rates to account for physical activity. If the user also makes additional adjustments for activity level, even better control can be achieved. Dose delivery, however, needs to be activated by the user. As with all chronic, life-long conditions, the problem is the human factor, with people remembering to give an insulin bolus before all meals, and knowing the amount of carbohydrate, protein, and fat in the meal, and how rapidly the food will be absorbed. In a review on downloaded pump data at the Barbara Davis Center, 65% of adolescents were missing at least one meal bolus a week, and their HbA1c was 0.8% higher than those not missing a meal bolus.[29]

A pump with the ability to store and deliver more than one hormone would better mimic islet physiology and its mechanism of glucose control. Even the option of two hormones, for instance the addition of the counter-regulatory hormone such as glucagon, would be an added countermeasure to prevent hypoglycemia. In fact, Dr. Edward Damiano and Firas El-Khatib have conducted studies using pigs and a dual-infusion system and model predictive control, where small doses of glucagon are given to prevent impending hypoglycemia. They found that glucagon was stable in an insulin infusion pump attached to the pig for at least 7 days.[30] The onset of action of subcutaneous glucagon was very rapid, allowing for quick prevention of possible hypoglycemia. This therapy, of course, depends on the patient having adequate glycogen stores. Epinephrine also has been tried in the treatment of hypoglycemia, but has been relatively ineffective.[31] Amylin, or islet amyloid polypeptide, also can be added to delay gastric emptying, resulting in a slower rate of glucose change following a meal, since meals with their rapid rate of change present the greatest challenge to an SQ insulin/SQ sensor closed loop.

Advantages of pump use include

Provides flexibility of dose delivery
More closely mimics pancreas physiology
Accuracy of dose calculation
Recorded data of insulin delivery
Lower incidence of severe hypoglycemic events[32]
Improved quality of life, particularly in the pediatric population[33]
Improved A1c[32]
Decreased glycemic variability
Possible cost effectiveness since lowers incidence of complications.[34]

Challenges to pump use include

Similar to the model for CGM, insulin pump instruction may be best accomplished
by well-trained diabetes educators who guide patients
Expense to the patient and providers
Wearability
Unrealistic patient expectations—the pump is not an AP and must be activated by
the user for delivery of insulin at mealtimes
Time and support for intensive diabetes management and pump use often are
poorly reimbursed
Possibility of infusion set failures
Possibility of weight gain.

Strategies to Overcome Challenges Include

Using group medical visits to educate patients about CGM technology and potentially for follow-up
Trial use of various types of insulin pumps before switching from multiple daily
injections (MDI) may help make a more informed decision about using the technology and how likely patients are to use it
Most insurance plans will cover the cost of a pump if there is proper documentation
Utilize online and each manufacturer's pump training program.

Key Pump Education for Patients

Initially starting patients on an insulin pump may be challenging, as they are given
a large possibility of insulin dose options. Before switching a patient from MDI,
be sure
The patient is able to wear a device continuously on the body
There is mastery of carbohydrate counting
Acknowledgment that pump therapy will intensify diabetes management
Remind patients that perfection is not usually attainable immediately, and doses
may continually need to be adjusted continually.
They also need to understand the pharmacodynamics and role of basal and meal
insulin coverage.

In the authors' experience, many patients who are on MDI and use real-time CGM
become frustrated with the insulin delivery options using MDI and switch to pump
therapy to allow easier meal coverage, more frequent correction doses, and the ability
to use dual wave boluses to cover a meal.

INFUSION SETS

Currently, infusion sets are generally used for 3 days, whereas continuous glucose sensors are generally functional for 5[6,35] to 7 days. Patients would prefer to have one device attached to their body that could serve as both the sensor and insulin infusion pump. For both to be merged onto a common platform, it would require a longer duration of insulin infusion set function, or the ability to insert several infusion sites on or into a common sensor platform. Another proposal is to use microneedle arrays[36] to deliver intradermal insulin.

INSULIN

One of the problems with the current rapid-acting insulins is that they are relatively slow for the purposes of a closed loop. The reach half their maximum activity in 20 minutes and do not reach full activity for 45 minutes.[37] When this is coupled with a 12- to 30-minute delay in the algorithm detecting the onset of a meal (based on the rate of change of glucose levels),[38] meal delivery of insulin becomes very difficult. This can be partially compensated for by having the patient give a premeal bolus of insulin, but then it is no longer a closed-loop system. Another approach would be to use an insulin with a more rapid onset of action. This can be accomplished by keeping the insulin in a monomeric (instead of hexameric) state. A new insulin developed by Biodel (Danbury, CT, USA) (ViaJect insulin) keeps the insulin in a monomeric state by chelating zinc, which allows a more rapid onset of insulin action, reaching peak activity about 10 to 15 minutes earlier than current analog short-acting insulins.[39] Other possible solutions would be to change the insulin delivery so that it is provided to a more vascular area, or the insulin could be delivered into the peritoneal cavity, where some of the insulin would be absorbed directly through the portal circulation. MiniMed has developed an implanted insulin pump using U-400 insulin and intraperitoneal insulin delivery. The greatest experience with this infusion system has been in France,[40] but there are currently no plans to market this system in the United States.

ALGORITHMS

Control algorithms are, by definition, designed and tuned based on a model of how a system works, ranging from the simple (knowledge of whether a manipulated input increases or decreases the output) to the complex (sets of nonlinear partial differential equations). This range trades off ease of design and implementation and possibly robustness to uncertainty with performance and ability to fine-tune and learn. These trade-offs become increasingly challenging when delays separate action and effect. Currently available insulin pumps use simple algorithms to incorporate current glucose levels into suggestions for bolus doses (the bolus calculator or bolus wizard features). With the availability of glucose trend from continuous glucose sensors, more sophisticated algorithms can be developed.

The simplest form of a partial closed-loop system would be for the delivery of insulin to be suspended when the patient is hypoglycemic and not responding to alarms. MiniMed has developed such a system, the Veo Pump, which is currently only available in Europe. When the glucose is below the hypoglycemic threshold (determined by the patient) and the patient does not respond to the alarm, insulin delivery is stopped for 2 hours.

The next step would be to stop insulin delivery based on predictive alarms (ie, the subject would not need to be hypoglycemic before basal insulin delivery is attenuated or stopped). This would be particularly important overnight, when subjects fail to respond to over 70% of alarms.[41] In a clinical research center setting where basal insulin infusion rates were increased to induce hypoglycemia, predictive algorithms that triggered a suspension of basal insulin prevented hypoglycemia 75% of the nights when hypoglycemia was predicted to occur.[42,43] These algorithms could trigger a pump shut-off without wakening the patient, thereby also decreasing the incidence of sleep disruption due to alarms. In the authors' reviews of nighttime CGM monitoring during which a seizure occurred during the night, hypoglycemia was recorded on the sensor for a minimum of 2.25 hours before a seizure,[44] so with this safety window, a pump shut-off over the night should prevent most episodes of nocturnal seizures and dead-in-bed (4 hours of nocturnal hypoglycemia[45]), unless a large dose of insulin had been given before bed. Another retrospective approach would be to have a computer program review 3 to 6 days of CGM and pump data looking for patterns. This can be done by dividing the day into 3-hour windows, with windows beginning when a meal bolus has been given. Time blocks beyond the meal blocks can be used for adjustment of basal insulin infusion rates. For a patient is using an insulin infusion pump, this can be accomplished by downloading both the sensor and pump information into a common file. If there is a consistent trend seen over multiple days, this could generate a recommendation to the patient to change either a basal rate or a carbohydrate-to-insulin ratio for a particular meal. These suggested doses would be more accurate than what physicians initially calculate and would allow for testing of algorithms before fully closing the loop. A third partial approach to closing the loop would be to have an algorithm incorporated into the insulin infusion pump that includes glucose rate of change information as well as insulin action profiles into the bolus calculator. This would allow adjustment of meal bolus doses and basal infusion rates based on glucose trend analysis as well as glycemic targets, but the final decision on insulin delivery is done by the user.

Another partial approach to a closed-loop system would be to have a control-to-range algorithm that would only be active when blood glucose levels are projected to be above a user-defined upper target (perhaps 160 to180 mg/dL) or below a lower target (perhaps 70 to 80 mg/dL). The JDRF AP consortium is planning studies in the next year on a control-to-range algorithm in a clinical research center setting, and the JDRF also has signed an agreement with Animas to bring such an algorithm to the market in 4 years.

To create a fully functional AP, there must be an algorithm that determines insulin delivery. Several algorithms have been proposed including a proportional-integral-derivative (PID) algorithm,[46] model predictive control,[47–49] and adaptive neural networks.[50] The first of these models to be tested in people has been the PID algorithm.[3] At each point in time, the controller assesses how far the current glucose is from the desired glucose (proportional), the rate of change in glucose (derivative), and how long the glucose has remained above or below target (integral). In these CRC studies on 10 subjects with type 1 diabetes who were on the AP for 30 hours, the PID controller achieved excellent control overnight, but there was mild hyperglycemia following meals, particularly breakfast, and a tendency for hypoglycemia 4 to 6 hours following meal insulin delivery.[3] These issues can be partly addressed by using a feed-forward algorithm where a partial meal bolus is given 5 to 15 minutes before the meal (ie, a hybrid closed loop). This approach initially was tested at Yale and resulted in a significant improvement in postprandial hyperglycemia.[51] The basal rate also can be decreased several hours after a meal to compensate for the insulin onboard from the meal bolus. With extended hyperglycemia, the integral component can become significant, and only can be decreased by a corresponding area under the curve below the target. To prevent this from happening, constraints can be placed on the insulin infusion rates using techniques such as reset windup.[52]

In model predictive control (MPC), the controller has a model of expected glucose values and responses to insulin that may vary by time of day (dawn phenomenon), meal events, and changes in insulin sensitivity. At each point in time the model compares the predicted glucose with the actual glucose, and the model then is updated with a new prediction horizon. At each step, the model takes into account the previous history of glucose measurements and insulin delivery, and the model may be updated to learn from discrepancies between actual and predicted values; then the optimization is repeated. How to best update the model to correct for model mismatch is one of the major challenges to MPC. MPC has been used in a simulated patient,[47] and there have been some short-term studies in people.[53,54] It should be noted that MPC is a basic strategy or concept, but any number of model types can be used, with many different methods of performing the optimization. Classic MPC uses a fixed linear model, but there have been many formulations using nonlinear models,[55] including artificial neural networks.[56] A nice feature of an optimization-based approach is that different weighting on the control objective can be used depending on whether the glucose is entering hyperglycemia or hypoglycemia conditions. Also, multiobjective optimization techniques can be used to rank order the important objective; for example, the highest ranked objective might be to avoid hypoglycemia.

POTENTIAL FUTURE APPLICATIONS OF A CLOSED-LOOP SYSTEM

One of the most promising uses for CGM and a closed-loop system may be in the intensive care unit (ICU). Tight glycemic control in the ICU has produced dramatic improvements in morbidity and mortality.[57] A glucose sensor that provides glucose information to the subject every few minutes (real-time CGM) has functioned well in an ICU setting even with variable changes in the core body temperature, use of inotropes, and body wall edema.[58] When intravenous glucose infusions are provided at a steady rate, the blood glucose fluctuations associated with oral absorption of meals is avoided. In an ICU setting, insulin is delivered intravenously, which significantly improves the pharmacodynamics of insulin delivery in a closed-loop system, since it has a more rapid onset of action and a shorter duration of action. The ICU may therefore be one of the initial settings where closed-loop delivery of insulin using a continuous glucose sensor will be implemented.

Another use would be to prevent continued glucotoxicity. Islet glucotoxicity occurs at the onset of type 1 diabetes and even occurs with type 2 diabetes. When β-cells are stimulated by hyperglycemia, they express increased levels of β-cell antigens[59–65] and are more susceptible to damage by cytokines.[66–69] One potential use of a closed-loop system would be at the onset of diabetes to limit glucotoxicity. The effectiveness of this therapy was demonstrated by studies done by Shah and colleagues[70] using a Biostater for 2 weeks at the onset of diabetes to preserve c-peptide secretion. Prevention of glucotoxicity at the time of transplantation also could prolong the life of the transplanted islets.

Strict metabolic control of blood glucose levels should be beneficial in many situations in the future treatment of diabetes. Initial applications will need to be in a research setting, with further expansion into ICUs and other inpatient settings. Eventually these studies may provide the basis for the FDA to approve the use of closed loop for daily outpatient use.

SUMMARY

Even with constant vigilance, current diabetes therapy does not prevent the fluctuations in blood glucose values. The most motivated patients find it difficult to achieve good control, with a hemoglobin A1c less 7% over multiple years, even with the currently available insulin infusion pumps and CGM systems. A closed-loop insulin delivery system could significantly decrease the patient burden of managing diabetes and should decrease the risks of both hyper- and hypoglycemia.

However, there are multiple factors that eventually will determine the feasibility of an ambulatory, outpatient closed-loop system. The system will have to be safe, and have a very low incidence of significant hypoglycemia. Currently children with an HbA1c of 6.8% spend about 15 minutes each day with glucose values less than 50 mg/dL and about 5 minutes each day with glucose values less than 40 mg/dL according to Free-Style Navigator CGM readings.[71] These children had no severe hypoglycemic events recorded. A closed-loop system should do better than this, and there should be no values less than 50 mg/dL for its use to be considered safe.

An initial closed-loop system ready for clinical use may have only limited goals (eg, automatically decreasing or stopping insulin delivery to prevent hypoglycemia rather than aiming for complete normalization of glucose values). Later models will control nocturnal glucose levels and postprandial hyperglycemia. Much of the progress will be based on demonstrating safety of the proposed algorithms, but much additional work needs to also occur in making the devices unobtrusive, comfortable, and easy to wear and use, perhaps integrating them into smart phones.

REFERENCES

1. Writing Team for the Diabetes Control and Complications Trial/Epidemiology of Diabetes Interventions and Complications Research Group. Sustained effect of intensive treatment of type 1 diabetes mellitus on development and progression of diabetic nephropathy: the Epidemiology of Diabetes Interventions and Complications (EDIC) study. JAMA 2003;290:2159–67.
2. Petitti DB, Klingensmith GJ, Bell RA, et al. Glycemic control in youth with diabetes: the SEARCH for diabetes in Youth Study. J Pediatr 2009;155:668–72.
3. Steil GM, Rebrin K, Darwin C, et al. Feasibility of automating insulin delivery for the treatment of type 1 diabetes. Diabetes 2006;55:3344–50.
4. Diabetes Research in Children Network (DIRECNET) Study Group. The accuracy of the CGMS in children with type 1 diabetes: results of the diabetes research in children network (DirecNet) accuracy study. Diabetes Technol Ther 2003;5: 781–9.
5. Tansey MJ, Beck RW, Buckingham BA, et al. Accuracy of the Modified Continuous Glucose Monitoring (CGMS) sensor in an outpatient setting: results from a Diabetes Research in Children Network (DirecNet) Study. Diabetes Technol Ther 2005;7:109–14.
6. Wilson DM, Beck RW, Tamborlane WV, et al. The accuracy of the FreeStyle navigator continuous glucose monitoring system in children with type 1 diabetes. Diabetes Care 2007;30:59–64.
7. DirecNet, Buckingham B, Beck RW, et al. Continuous glucose monitoring in children with type 1 diabetes. J Pediatr 2007;151:388–93.
8. Monnier L, Mas E, Ginet C, et al. Activation of oxidative stress by acute glucose fluctuations compared with sustained chronic hyperglycemia in patients with type 2 diabetes. JAMA 2006;295:1681–7.
9. Brownlee M, Hirsch IB. Glycemic variability: a hemoglobin A1c-independent risk factor for diabetic complications. JAMA 2006;295:1707–8.
10. Kilpatrick ES, Rigby AS, Atkin SL. The effect of glucose variability on the risk of microvascular complications in type 1 diabetes. Diabetes Care 2006;29:1486–90.

11. Khalil OS. Noninvasive glucose measurement technologies: an update from 1999 to the dawn of the new millennium. Diabetes Technol Ther 2004;6:660–97.
12. Keenan DB, Mastrototaro JJ, Voskanyan G, et al. Delays in minimally invasive continuous glucose monitoring devices: a review of current technology. Society 2009;3:1207–14.
13. Nielsen JK, Djurhuus CB, Gravholt CH, et al. Continuous glucose monitoring in interstitial subcutaneous adipose tissue and skeletal muscle reflects excursions in cerebral cortex. Diabetes 2005;54:1635–9.
14. Mauras N, Beck RW, Ruedy KJ, et al. Lack of accuracy of continuous glucose sensors in healthy, nondiabetic children: results of the Diabetes Research in Children Network (DirecNet) accuracy study. J Pediatr 2004;144:770–5.
15. Fox L, Beck R, Xing D, et al. Variation of interstitial glucose measurements assessed by continuous glucose monitors in healthy, nonobese, nondiabetic individuals. Diabetes Care 2010;33:1297–9.
16. Keenan DB, Cartaya R, Mastrototaro JJ. Accuracy of a new real-time continuous glucose monitoring algorithm. Society 2010;4:111–8.
17. Zisser H, Jovanovic L, Khan U, et al. Accuracy of a novel intravascular fluorescent continuous glucose sensor in an 8-hour Outpatient Clinic Feasibility Study. Diabetologia 2009;52:363.
18. Buckingham BA, Kollman C, Beck R, et al. Evaluation of factors affecting CGMS calibration. Diabetes Technol Ther 2006;8:318–25.
19. Garg SK, Schwartz S, Edelman SV. Improved glucose excursions using an implantable real-time continuous glucose sensor in adults with type 1 diabetes. Diabetes Care 2004;27:734–8.
20. Armour JC, Lucisano JY, McKean BD, et al. Application of chronic intravascular blood glucose sensor in dogs. Diabetes 1990;39:1519–26.
21. Renard E, Costalat G, Bringer J. From external to implantable insulin pump, can we close the loop? Diabetes Metab 2002;28. 2S19–2S25.
22. O'Connell MA, Donath S, O'Neal DN, et al. Glycaemic impact of patient-led use of sensor-guided pump therapy in type 1 diabetes: a randomised controlled trial. Diabetologia 2009;52:1250–7.
23. Tamborlane W, Beck R, Laffel L. Continuous glucose monitoring and type 1 diabetes. N Engl J Med 2009;360:191.
24. Beck RW, Buckingham B, Miller K, et al. Factors predictive of use and of benefit from continuous glucose monitoring in type 1 diabetes. Diabetes Care 2009;32:1947–53.
25. Gilliam LK, Hirsch IB. Practical aspects of real-time continuous glucose monitoring. Diabetes Technol Ther 2009;11(Suppl 1):S75–82.
26. Hirsch IB, Armstrong D, Bergenstal RM, et al. Clinical application of emerging sensor technologies in diabetes management: consensus guidelines for continuous glucose monitoring (CGM). Diabetes Technol Ther 2008;10:232–44 [quiz: 245–6].
27. Buckingham B, Xing D, Weinzimer S, et al. Use of the DirecNet Applied Treatment Algorithm (DATA) for diabetes management with a real-time continuous glucose monitor (the FreeStyle Navigator). Pediatr Diabetes 2008;9:142–7.
28. Felig P, Tamborlane W, Sherwin RS, et al. Insulin-infusion pump for diabetes. N Engl J Med 1979;301:1004–5.
29. Burdick J, Chase HP, Slover RH, et al. Missed insulin meal boluses and elevated hemoglobin A1c levels in children receiving insulin pump therapy. Pediatrics 2004;113:e221–4.
30. El-Khatib FH, Jiang J, Gerrity RG, et al. Pharmacodynamics and stability of subcutaneously infused glucagon in a type 1 diabetic Swine model in vivo. Diabetes Technol Ther 2007;9:135–44.

31. Monsod TP, Tamborlane WV, Coraluzzi L, et al. Epipen as an alternative to glucagon in the treatment of hypoglycemia in children with diabetes. Diabetes Care 2001;24:701–4.

32. Misso ML, Egberts KJ, Page M, et al. Continuous subcutaneous insulin infusion (CSII) versus multiple insulin injections for type 1 diabetes mellitus. Cochrane Database Syst Rev 2010;1:CD005103.

33. Nuboer R, Borsboom GJ, Zoethout JA, et al. Effects of insulin pump vs. injection treatment on quality of life and impact of disease in children with type 1 diabetes mellitus in a randomized, prospective comparison. Pediatr Diabetes 2008;9:291–6.

34. Cummins E, Royle P, Snaith A, et al. Clinical effectiveness and cost-effectiveness of continuous subcutaneous insulin infusion for diabetes: systematic review and economic evaluation. Health Technol Assess 2010;14:1–208.

35. Weinstein RL, Schwartz SL, Brazg RL, et al. Accuracy of the 5-day FreeStyle navigator continuous glucose monitoring system: comparison with frequent laboratory reference measurements. Diabetes Care 2007;30:1125–30.

36. Nordquist L, Roxhed N, Griss P, et al. Novel microneedle patches for active insulin delivery are efficient in maintaining glycaemic control: an initial comparison with subcutaneous administration. Pharm Res 2007;24:1381–8.

37. Mudaliar SR, Lindberg FA, Joyce M, et al. Insulin aspart (B28 asp-insulin): a fast-acting analog of human insulin: absorption kinetics and action profile compared with regular human insulin in healthy nondiabetic subjects. Diabetes Care 1999; 22:1501–6.

38. Dassau E, Bequette BW, Buckingham BA, et al. Detection of a meal using continuous glucose monitoring: implications for an artificial beta-cell. Diabetes Care 2008;31:295–300.

39. Steiner SS, Hompesch M, Pohl R, et al. Pharmacokinetics and phrmacodynamics of insulin VIAject and regular human insulin when injected subcutneously directly before a meal in patients with type1 diabetes. Diabetes 2007;56:A9.

40. Renard E. Implantable closed-loop glucose-sensing and insulin delivery: the future for insulin pump therapy. Curr Opin Pharmacol 2002;2:708–16.

41. Buckingham B, Block J, Burdick J, et al. Response to nocturnal alarms using a real-time glucose sensor. Diabetes Technol Ther 2005;7:440–7.

42. Buckingham B, Chase H, Dassau E, et al. Prevention of nocturnal hypoglycemia using predictive alarm algorithms and insulin pump suspension. Diabetes Care 2010;33:1249–54.

43. Buckingham B, Cobry E, Clinton P, et al. Preventing hypoglycemia using predictive alarm algorithms and insulin pump suspension. Diabetes Technol Ther 2009; 11:93–7.

44. Buckingham B, Wilson DM, Lecher T, et al. Duration of nocturnal hypoglycemia prior to seizures. Diabetes Care 2008;31:2110–2.

45. Tanenberg RJ, Newton CA, Drake AJ. Confirmation of hypoglycemia in the dead-in-bed syndrome as captured by a retrospective continuous glucose monitoring system. Endocr Pract 2010;16:244–8.

46. Steil GM, Rebrin K, Janowski R, et al. Modeling beta-cell insulin secretion—implications for closed-loop glucose homeostasis. Diabetes Technol Ther 2003;5: 953–64.

47. Parker RS, Doyle FJ 3rd, Peppas NA. A model-based algorithm for blood glucose control in type I diabetic patients. IEEE Trans Biomed Eng 1999;46:148–57.

48. Dua P, Doyle FJ 3rd, Pistikopoulos EN. Model based blood glucose control for type 1 diabetes via parametric programming. IEEE Trans Biomed Eng 2006; 53(8):1478–91.

49. Parker RI, Doyle 3rd FJ. Advanced Model Predictive Control (MPC) for type 1 diabetic patient blood glucose control. In: Proceedings of the American Control Conference. 2000. p. 3483–7.
50. Trajanoski Z, Regittnig W, Wach P. Simulation studies on neural predictive control of glucose using the subcutaneous route. Comput Methods Programs Biomed 1998;56:133–9.
51. Weinzimer SA, Steil GM, Swan KL, et al. Fully automated closed-loop insulin delivery versus semiautomated hybrid control in pediatric patients with type 1 diabetes using an artificial pancreas. Diabetes Care 2008;31:934–9.
52. Bequette BW. Process control: modeling, design and simulation. Upper Saddle River (NJ): Prentice Hall; 2003.
53. Schaller HC, Schaupp L, Bodenlenz M, et al. On-line adaptive algorithm with glucose prediction capacity for subcutaneous closed loop control of glucose: evaluation under fasting conditions in patients with type 1 diabetes. Diabet Med 2006;23:90–3.
54. Plank J, Blaha J, Cordingley J, et al. Multicentric, randomized, controlled trial to evaluate blood glucose control by the model predictive control algorithm versus routine glucose management protocols in intensive care unit patients. Diabetes Care 2006;29:271–6.
55. Bequette BW. Nonlinear control of chemical processes: a review. Ind Eng Chem Res 1991;30:1391–413.
56. Kuure-Kinsey MR, Cutright R, Bequette BW. Computationally efficient neural predictive control based on a feedforward architecture. In: 2006 American Control Conference. Minneapolis (MN), 2006.
57. van den Berghe G, Wouters P, Weekers F, et al. Intensive insulin therapy in the critically ill patients. N Engl J Med 2001;345:1359–67.
58. Piper HG, Alexander JL, Shukla A, et al. Real-time continuous glucose monitoring in pediatric patients during and after cardiac surgery. Pediatrics 2006;118:1176–84.
59. McCulloch DK, Barmeier H, Neifing JL, et al. Metabolic state of the pancreas affects end-point titre in the islet cell antibody assay. Diabetologia 1991;34:622–5.
60. Hao W, Li L, Mehta V, et al. Functional state of the beta cell affects expression of both forms of glutamic acid decarboxylase. Pancreas 1994;9:558–62.
61. Hagopian WA, Karlsen AE, Petersen JS, et al. Regulation of glutamic acid decarboxylase diabetes autoantigen expression in highly purified isolated islets from *Macaca nemestrina*. Endocrinology 1993;132:2674–81.
62. Aaen K, Rygaard J, Josefsen K, et al. Dependence of antigen expression on functional state of beta-cells. Diabetes 1990;39:697–701.
63. Kampe O, Andersson A, Bjork E, et al. High-glucose stimulation of 64,000-Mr islet cell autoantigen expression. Diabetes 1989;38:1326–8.
64. Bjork E, Kampe O, Andersson A, et al. Expression of the 64 kDa/glutamic acid decarboxylase rat islet cell autoantigen is influenced by the rate of insulin secretion. Diabetologia 1992;35:490–3.
65. Bjork E, Kampe O, Karlsson FA, et al. Glucose regulation of the autoantigen GAD65 in human pancreatic islets. J Clin Endocrinol Metab 1992;75:1574–6.
66. Mehta V, Hao W, Brooks-Worrell BM, et al. The functional state of the beta cell modulates IL-1 and TNF-induced cytotoxicity. Lymphokine Cytokine Res 1993;12:255–9.
67. Mellado-Gil JM, Aguilar-Diosdado M. Assay for high glucose-mediated islet cell sensitization to apoptosis induced by streptozotocin and cytokines. Biol Proced Online 2005;7:162–71.

68. Mellado-Gil JM, Aguilar-Diosdado M. High glucose potentiates cytokine- and streptozotocin-induced apoptosis of rat islet cells: effect on apoptosis-related genes. J Endocrinol 2004;183:155–62.

69. Maedler K, Storling J, Sturis J, et al. Glucose- and interleukin-1beta-induced beta-cell apoptosis requires Ca2+ influx and extracellular signal-regulated kinase (ERK) 1/2 activation and is prevented by a sulfonylurea receptor 1/inwardly rectifying K+ channel 6.2 (SUR/Kir6.2) selective potassium channel opener in human islets. Diabetes 2004;53:1706–13.

70. Shah SC, Malone JI, Simpson NE. A randomized trial of intensive insulin therapy in newly diagnosed insulin-dependent diabetes mellitus. N Engl J Med 1989;320:550–4.

71. Weinzimer S, Xing D, Tansey M, et al. FreeStyle navigator continuous glucose monitoring system use in children with type 1 diabetes using glargine-based multiple daily dose regimens: results of a pilot trial Diabetes Research in Children Network (DirecNet) Study Group. Diabetes Care 2008;31:525–7.

Complications of Type 1 Diabetes

L. Yvonne Melendez-Ramirez, MD, Robert J. Richards, MD,
William T. Cefalu, MD*

KEYWORDS

- Type 1 Diabetes • Complications
- Retinopathy • Heart disease

The prevalence of diabetes is increasing worldwide, and the concern regarding the number of new cases of diabetes relates to the development of chronic complications. It has been recognized for years that the complications are a cause of considerable morbidity and mortality worldwide and as such, negatively affect the quality of life in individuals with diabetes with an increase in disability and death.[1] Specifically, the complications of diabetes have been classified as either microvascular (ie, retinopathy, nephropathy and neuropathy) or macrovascular (ie, cardiovascular disease [CVD], cerebrovascular accidents, and peripheral vascular disease) (**Table 1**). In the United States, diabetes is the leading cause of blindness and kidney failure in adults aged 20 to 74 years and is implicated in approximately 60% of nontraumatic amputations. Adults with diabetes have an increased frequency and mortality from cardiovascular disease. The total estimated financial burden of diabetes was $174 billion in 2007 and the cost to care for individuals with diabetes will only continue to increase dramatically given the projected increase of 165% in new cases by the year 2050.[1,2]

In Type 1 Diabetes (T1D), the role of glycemic control in contributing to chronic complications is not questioned and has been well established in epidemiologic observations and prospective clinical studies. Complications are thought to be mainly related to the degree of and length of exposure to hyperglycemia as assessed by objective markers of glycemic control (ie, hemoglobin A1c [HbA1c] levels). As such, standards of care are in place that are aimed to reduce the incidence and progression of these complications by initiating early, aggressive treatment aimed at maintaining a level of HbA1c as close to normal as possible as shown by the Diabetes Control and Complications Trial (DCCT).[3,4] Yet, despite tighter control of hyperglycemia, it

Support: None.

Joint Program on Diabetes, Endocrinology and Metabolism, Louisiana State University Health Sciences Center School of Medicine, New Orleans, and the Pennington Biomedical Research Center, Baton Rouge, LA, USA

* Corresponding author. Section of Endocrinology, Department of Medicine, Louisiana State University School of Medicine, 1542 Tulane Avenue, New Orleans, LA 70112.

E-mail address: william.cefalu@pbrc.edu

Endocrinol Metab Clin N Am 39 (2010) 625–640
doi:10.1016/j.ecl.2010.05.009
0889-8529/10/$ – see front matter © 2010 Elsevier Inc. All rights reserved.

Table 1 Complications of diabetes			
Ophthalmologic	**Neuropathic**	**Nephropathic**	**Cardiovascular**
Retinopathy	**Sensory neuropathy**	**Microalbuminuria**	**Coronary heart**
Moderate	Acute sensory	**Macroalbuminuria**	**disease**
nonproliferative	neuropathy	**Chronic kidney**	**Cerebrovascular**
retinopathy	Chronic sensorimotor	**disease**	**disease**
Mild	diabetic peripheral		**Peripheral vascular**
nonproliferative	neuropathy		**disease**
retinopathy	**Focal and multifocal**		
Severe	**neuropathies**		
nonproliferative	**Autonomic neuropathy**		
retinopathy	Cardiovascular		
Proliferative	autonomic		
retinopathy	neuropathy		
Glaucoma	Gastrointestinal		
Cataracts	neuropathy		
	Genitourinary		
	neuropathy		

is apparent that other factors contribute to the development beyond glycemic control in many individuals.[4] For example, the role of proinflammatory and procoagulation cascades as well as genetic variability and how they interact with the metabolic abnormalities is being further elucidated in the development of the vascular complications of diabetes. A deeper understanding of these mechanisms will eventually translate into clinical interventions that will further impact the prevention of diabetes complications. A listing of complications related to T1D and clinical practice recommendations to address the complications have been published in detail.[3] For purposes of this article, the authors focus on a brief review of the major complications.

BIOCHEMICAL AND MOLECULAR PATHWAYS OF DAMAGE

Given the data from prospective clinical research trials, elevated glucose levels are thought to be the most important etiologic factor in the pathogenesis of microvascular damage in T1D.[4–7] It can be argued that all cells of the body are exposed to elevated glucose levels in T1D; however, not all cells develop the changes associated with vascular injury. The cells of the capillary endothelium of the retina, the mesangial cell in the glomerulus, and the Schwann cells of the peripheral nerves are vulnerable to the elevated extracellular concentration of glucose because they cannot efficiently regulate the transport of glucose into the cell, leading to intracellular hyperglycemia, which induces intracellular mechanisms that result in damage.[8] The mechanisms by which glucose induces the biochemical and metabolic changes that cause abnormalities in the tissues, such as increasing endothelial permeability resulting in protein and plasma extravasation, are not completely understood. Several mechanisms to explain the development of the microangiopathy seen in diabetes have been proposed. In an interesting review of the topic, Brownlee[8] has reported on the mechanisms by which 4 biochemical and molecular pathways contribute to hyperglycemia-induced tissue damage. These pathways were described as involving increased polyol flux, formation of advanced glycation end products, activation of protein kinase C (PKC), and increased flux through the hexosamine pathway.[8] Even though the previously mentioned pathways were established in the pathogenesis of diabetic complications and multiple animal experimental studies showed that inhibition of the individual pathways resulted in prevention of microvascular damage to the cells of the nerves, retina, and kidney, clinical trials where single pathways were blocked proved to be disappointing.[8–12] Also, how these pathways interacted or were activated in relation to the common injury of hyperglycemia was not understood. However, a hypothesis unifying all these pathways as a common downstream effect of overproduction of superoxide-anion by the mitochondrial electron transport chain was proposed (**Fig. 1**).[8]

METABOLIC MEMORY

One of the strongest predictors of microvascular complications during the DCCT was the A1c value at study entry, which reflected the glycemic control before randomization. It was suggested that prior glycemic control exerted a long-term effect on the development of diabetic complications.[5] Following the active clinical intervention of the DCCT, the cohort was followed longitudinally as the DCCT/EDIC (Epidemiology of Diabetes Interventions and Complications).[13] During the DCCT/EDIC cohort follow-up study, a statistically significant decrease in the rate of microvascular and cardiovascular complications was noted in the previously intensively treated cohort years after the completion of the DCCT. This decrease occurred despite the fact

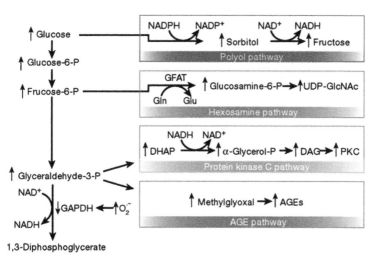

Fig. 1. Potential mechanism by which hyperglycemia-induced mitochondrial superoxide overproduction activates 4 pathways of hyperglycemic damage. Excess superoxide partially inhibits the glycolytic enzyme, GAPDH, thereby diverting upstream metabolites from glycolysis into pathways of glucose overutilization. This overutilization results in increased flux of dihydroxyacetone phosphate (DHAP) to DAG, an activator of PKC, and of triose phosphates to methylglyoxal, the main intracellular advanced glycation end product (AGE) precursor. Increased flux of fructose-6-phosphate to UDP-N-acetylglucosamine increases modification of proteins by O-linked N-acetylglucosamine (GlcNAc) and increased glucose flux through the polyol pathway consumes NADPH and depletes GSH. (*From* Brownlee M. Biochemistry and molecular cell biology of diabetic complications. Nature 2001;414:813–20; with permission.)

that there was no significant difference between measured A1c levels between treatment groups during the observation period.[4,5,7,14] The convergence of the A1c during the observational period essentially meant that any difference in the rate of development of complications between the two groups would be the result of the early differences in glucose control achieved during the DCCT. The concept that an improvement in glycemic control that is observed many years earlier results in a significant reduction in the development of complications when assessed many years later is supported by DCCT and DCCT/EDIC data in T1D and has been termed *metabolic memory*.[15]

MICROVASCULAR COMPLICATIONS
Retinopathy

One of the more disabling complications affecting quality of life for individuals with diabetes is the progressive loss of vision resulting from diabetic retinopathy. Diabetic retinopathy is a highly specific vascular complication of both Type 1 and Type 2 diabetes and the prevalence is highly associated to the duration of diabetes.[16] Unfortunately, this condition appears to represent the most frequent cause of new cases of blindness among adults aged 20 to 74 years.[16]

Stages and development

The development of retinopathy has been described as occurring in at least 4 stages.[17] It is described that at the initial stage microaneurysms (ie, small areas of balloon-like swelling in the retina's tiny blood vessels) occur. This stage is referred to as mild nonproliferative retinopathy. As the disease progresses, some blood vessels that nourish the retina are blocked leading to moderate nonproliferative retinopathy. As the process continues, many more blood vessels are blocked, depriving several areas of the retina with their blood supply. These areas of the retina send signals to the body to grow new blood vessels for nourishment leading to a stage referred to as severe nonproliferative retinopathy. The final and most advanced stage is referred to as proliferative retinopathy.[17] At this advanced stage, the growth of new blood vessels occur secondary to the signals sent by the retina for nourishment. Unfortunately, the new vessels that are formed grow along the retina. However, given that they are abnormal in that they have thin fragile walls, they are predisposed to leak blood.[16,17] At this stage, if there is no successful intervention, bleeding from vessels can leak into the center of the eye resulting in severe vision loss and blindness can be a resulting outcome. It has been described that fluid can also leak into the center of the macula, making the macula swell and blurring vision (ie, macular edema). Macular edema is reported to occur at any stage of diabetic retinopathy. In addition to the previously mentioned conditions, other eye conditions, such as cataracts and glaucoma, occur earlier and more frequently in people with diabetes.[16]

As previously outlined, the duration of disease is associated with the prevalence of retinopathy. However, several other clinical factors increase the risk. As discussed in the subsequent section, chronic hyperglycemia is a major factor and intensive therapy to improve glycemia is a major objective.[18] In addition to hyperglycemia, the prevalence of retinopathy appears to be related to both nephropathy[19] and hypertension.[20] To evaluate the relationship to clinical and metabolic factors, Klein and colleagues[21] examined the 25-year cumulative progression and regression of diabetic retinopathy (DR). Observations suggested that progression of DR was more likely with less severe DR, male sex, higher glycosylated hemoglobin, an increase in glycosylated hemoglobin level, and an increase in diastolic blood pressure level from the baseline to the 4-year follow-up.[21] An increased risk of incidence of proliferative diabetic retinopathy was associated with higher glycosylated hemoglobin, higher systolic blood

pressure, proteinuria, greater body mass index at baseline, and an increase in the glycosylated hemoglobin between the baseline and 4-year follow-up examinations.
Lower glycosylated hemoglobin and male sex, as well as decreases in glycosylated
hemoglobin and diastolic blood pressure during the first 4 years of follow-up, were
associated with improvement in DR.[21]

Screening
One of the more important aspects of care for individuals with T1D is the timely detection and treatment of underlying eye conditions. As such, it is imperative that providers
are vigilant regarding standards of care as related to suggested screening guidelines.
Standards of care in this regard have been recommended by the American Diabetes
Association[3,16] (ADA) in its yearly *Clinical Practice Guidelines*. The current recommendations as suggested by the ADA are that adults and children aged 10 years or older
with T1D have an initial dilated and comprehensive eye examination by an ophthalmologist or optometrist within 5 years after the onset of diabetes.[16] Examinations should
be performed by an ophthalmologist or optometrist who is knowledgeable and experienced in diagnosing the presence of diabetic retinopathy and is aware of its management. It is also recommended that subsequent examinations be repeated annually.
The suggested examinations may be less frequent (ie, every 2–3 years following one
or more normal eye evaluations by a qualified provider).[16]

Management
The successful treatment of retinopathy should be based on treating the underlying
metabolic conditions that contribute to the development of the retinopathy and effectively treating the specific abnormalities identified in the eye. As such, intensive diabetes management with the goal of achieving near normoglycemia is considered
one of the most important aspects of treatment. Improvement in glycemia has clearly
been shown to prevent or delay the onset and progression of diabetic retinopathy in
individuals with both Type 1 and Type 2 diabetes.[4–7,22,23] Given these findings, the
provider caring for patients with T1D will suggest insulin regimens that may include
multiple injections on a background of basal therapy or may suggest insulin pump
therapy if indicated. Clinical regimens that address both premeal and postmeal
glucose are needed to achieve the desired glycemic goals. Patients and providers
should have a clear understanding of the suggested A1c goal and communication
should be in place with the diabetes support team to achieve the goal. In addition
to glycemia, addressing blood pressure is recommended to decrease the progression
of retinopathy.[24]

A second aspect of prevention and treatment of retinopathy is to effectively address
any specific abnormality already present in the eye. Specifically, the provider should
promptly refer patients with any level of macular edema, severe nonproliferative diabetic retinopathy (NPDR), or any proliferative diabetic retinopathy (PDR) to an ophthalmologist who is knowledgeable and experienced in the management and treatment of
diabetic retinopathy.[16] Diabetic retinopathy may occur first in the peripheral retina,
which can only be adequately examined by an eye professional. The patient requires
dilation and the examiner must use the hand lens. Laser photocoagulation may be
indicated in the treatment for the individual with T1D.

It is now well established that laser photocoagulation surgery has considerable efficacy
in the effective prevention of diabetic retinopathy. In this regard, both the Diabetic Retinopathy Study (DRS) and the Early Treatment Diabetic Retinopathy Study (ETDRS),[25,26]
two large scale clinical trials, provide considerable data supporting the tremendous clinical benefits of photocoagulation surgery. In the DRS,[25] Panretinal photocoagulation

surgery reduced the risk of severe vision loss from PDR from 15.9% in untreated eyes to 6.4% in treated eyes. It appeared that the greatest benefit was observed among subjects whose baseline evaluation revealed high-risk characteristics, such as disc neovascularization or vitreous hemorrhage.[25] Panretinal laser surgery is primarily recommended for eyes with PDR approaching or having high-risk characteristics.

Another major trial (ETDRS[26]) established the benefit of focal laser photocoagulation surgery in eyes with macular edema. This study demonstrated a reduction of doubling of the visual angle (eg, 20/50–20/100) from 20% in untreated eyes to 8% in treated eyes. The ETDRS also verified the benefits of panretinal photocoagulation for high-risk PDR, but not for mild or moderate NPDR. In older-onset patients with severe NPDR or less-than-high-risk PDR, the risk of severe vision loss or vitrectomy was reduced 50% by early laser photocoagulation surgery at these stages.

Thus, the results of both trials demonstrate that laser photocoagulation surgery was beneficial in reducing the risk of further vision loss. However, the data suggest that laser photocoagulation was generally not beneficial in reversing already diminished acuity. These observations are critically important and given the fact that patients who have findings consistent with retinopathy or macular edema may be asymptomatic, the importance of screening, early detection, and effective treatment can have a significant effect to improve quality of life for the individual with T1D by preventing further vision loss.

As outlined earlier, there have been tremendous advances made in the intervention and management of retinopathy in individuals with T1D. However, it still appears that the cumulative rates of diabetic retinopathy and incidence of diabetic retinopathy is high. Specifically, Klein and colleagues[21] reported high 25-year cumulative rates of progression of DR and incidence of PDR (ie, 25-year cumulative rate of progression of DR was 83%, progression to PDR was 42%, and improvement of DR was 18%).[27] However, they also reported lower risk of prevalent PDR in more recently diagnosed persons, which possibly reflects improvement in care over the period of the study.[21] Additional evidence that management strategies may be working to reduce progression to diabetic retinopathy has come from a meta-analysis reported by Wong and colleagues.[27] A total of 28 studies comprising 27,120 subjects with diabetes (mean age 49.8 years) were included. After 4 years, pooled incidence rates for PDR and severe vision loss (SVL) were 11.0% and 7.2%, respectively. Rates were lower among participants in 1986 to 2008 than in 1975 to 1985. After 10 years, similar patterns were observed. Participants in the 1986 to 2008 studies had lower proportions of PDR and non-PDR at all time points than participants in 1975 to 1985 studies. The investigators concluded that since 1985, patients with diabetes have lower rates of progression to PDR and SVL. These findings may reflect an increased awareness of retinopathy risk factors; earlier identification and initiation of care for patients with retinopathy; and improved medical management of glucose, blood pressure, and serum lipids. Differences in baseline characteristics, particularly in the prevalence and severity of retinopathy, could also have contributed to these temporal differences.[27]

Nephropathy

Another major complication of diabetes that develops secondary to metabolic abnormalities is diabetic nephropathy. Nephropathy has been reported to occur in 20% to 40% of patients with diabetes and is the single leading cause of end-stage renal disease.[16,28] Generally, diabetic nephropathy is defined on clinical grounds as an increased urinary albumin excretion in the absence of other renal diseases.[16] As currently suggested, the earliest stage of diabetic nephropathy in T1D is microalbuminuria defined as albumin excretion of 30 to 299 mg/24 h, and is a marker for development of nephropathy in Type 2 diabetes.[16] Microalbuminuria is important on clinical grounds because it is also a well-established marker of increased CVD risk.[29,30] A more advanced stage of nephropathy (ie, macroalbuminuria) represents persistent albuminuria in the range of greater than or equal to 300 mg/24 h.[16] End-stage renal disease is increased if patients with microalbuminuria progress to albumin excretion rates consistent with macroalbuminuria.[16]

Diabetes nephropathy is known to be associated with increased risk of death, mainly from cardiovascular causes.[28] As is now well established, hyperglycemia, hypertension, and genetic predisposition are the main risk factors for the development of diabetic nephropathy.[28] In addition, other risk factors, such as elevated serum lipids, smoking, and dietary protein intake, provide a contribution.[16,28] The importance of the recognition of nephropathy at each stage of albuminuria is related to clinical characteristics. Specifically, Gross and colleagues[28] provided suggested clinical characteristics to be expected at each stage of observed urine albumin excretion (**Table 2**). Given the clinical significance of the findings, it is imperative that providers understand the screening guidelines for detection of nephropathy.

Screening
To screen for diabetic kidney disease, urine albumin excretion is considered the essential test and cornerstone of diagnosis. Currently, for patients with T1D, it is recommended that the provider obtain a urine albumin excretion in individuals with T1D

Table 2
Diabetic nephropathy stages

Cutoff Values of Urine Albumin for Diagnosis and Main Clinical Characteristics

Stages	Albuminuria Cutoff Values	Clinical Characteristics
Microalbuminuria	20–199 µg/min	Abnormal nocturnal decrease of blood pressure and increased blood pressure levels
	30–299 mg/24 h	Increased triglycerides, total and LDL cholesterol, and saturated fatty acids
	30–299 mg/g[a]	Increased frequency of metabolic syndrome components
		Endothelial dysfunction
		Association with diabetic retinopathy, amputation, and cardiovascular disease
		Increased cardiovascular mortality
		Stable GFR
Macroalbuminuria[b]	≥200 µg/min	Hypertension
	≥300 mg/24 h	Increased triglycerides and total and LDL cholesterol
	>300 mg/g[a]	Asymptomatic myocardial ischemia
		Progressive GFR decline

Abbreviations: GFR, glomerular filtration rate; LDL, low-density lipoprotein.
[a] Spot urine sample.
[b] Measurement of total proteinuria (≥500 mg/24 h or ≥430 mg/L in a spot urine sample) can also be used to define this stage.
Data from Gross JL, de Azevedo MJ, Silveiro SP, et al. Diabetic nephropathy: diagnosis, prevention, and treatment. Diabetes Care 2005;28(1):164–76.

starting 5 years after diagnosis or earlier in the presence of puberty or poor metabolic control.[16] Screening for microalbuminuria can be performed by measurement of the albumin-to-creatinine ratio in a random spot collection. A serum creatinine should also be obtained at least annually in all adults with diabetes regardless of the degree of urine albumin excretion and is used to estimate glomerular filtration rate (GFR) and to stage the level of chronic kidney disease.

In the past, GFR has been measured by specific techniques, such as inulin clearance, ^{51}Cr-ethylenediaminetetraacetic acid, ^{125}I-iothalamate, and iohexol.[31] In addition, the clearance of endogenous creatinine has been commonly used although there are recognized limitations.[32] In clinical practice, GFR can be estimated by prediction equations that take into account serum creatinine concentration and some or all of the following variables: age, sex, race, and body size.[28] Estimated GFR (eGFR) is commonly co-reported by laboratories or can be estimated using formulae, such as the Modification of Diet in Renal Disease (MDRD) study equation.[33] Specifically, the recommended equation by the National Kidney Foundation is that of the MDRD, which calculates GFR as follows: GFR (ml $\cdot$ min^{-1} $\cdot$ 1.73 m^{-2}) = 186 $\times$ (serum creatinine [mg/dl]$^{-1.154}$ $\times$ age [years]$^{-0.203}$ $\times$ [0.742 if female] $\times$ [1.210 if African American]).[33] Another way to calculate GFR is by the Cockroft-Gault equation (ie, creatinine clearance [ml/min] = [(140 $-$ age (years)] $\times$ weight [kg]/[72 $\times$ serum creatinine (mg/dl) $\times$ (0.85 if female)]).[34] Recent reports have indicated that the MDRD is more accurate for the diagnosis and stratification of chronic kidney disease (CKD) in patients with diabetes than the Cockcroft-Gault formula.[34] The level of GFR, in addition to information on abnormal urine albumin excretion, can then be used to stage the degree of CKD (**Table 3**).

Management

The screening procedures previously outlined are important when one considers whether the treatment regimen will be primarily one of prevention of kidney disease or one that will consist of aggressive treatment to prevent further progression of kidney disease. The general principles involved for the prevention of diabetic nephropathy are effective treatment of its known risk factors contributing to diabetic nephropathy (ie, hypertension, hyperglycemia, smoking, and dyslipidemia).[16,28] If patients are found

Table 3
Stages of chronic kidney disease

Stage	Description	GFR (ml/min per 1.73 m^2 Body Surface Area)
1	Kidney damage[a] with normal or increased GFR	$\geq$90
2	Kidney damage[a] with mildly decreased GFR	60–89
3	Moderately decreased GFR	30–59
4	Severely decreased GFR	15–29
5	Kidney failure	<15 or dialysis

[a] Kidney damage defined as abnormalities on pathologic, urine, blood, or imaging tests.
Data from American Diabetes Association. Standards of medical care in diabetes - 2010. Diabetes Care 2010;33:S11–63; and Levey AS, Coresh J, Balk E, et al. National Kidney Foundation. National Kidney Foundation practice guidelines for chronic kidney disease: evaluation, classification, and stratification. Ann Intern Med 2003;139:137–47.

to have evidence of nephropathy, the goal of treatment would then be one to prevent the progression from micro- to macroalbuminuria, to attenuate the decline of renal function in patients with macroalbuminuria, and to reduce the occurrence of cardiovascular events. In general, the strategy for treatment is similar to the strategies of prevention, but involve multiple and more intensive strategies.[28] The goals of management include achieving the best metabolic control (A1c <7%), treating hypertension (<130/80 mmHg or <125/75 mmHg if proteinuria is >1.0 g/24 h and increased serum creatinine), using drugs with blockade effect on the renin-angiotensin-aldosterone system, and treating dyslipidemia (low-density lipoprotein [LDL] cholesterol <100 mg/dL).[16] These strategies appear to be effective for preventing the development of microalbuminuria, in delaying the progression to more advanced stages of nephropathy, and in reducing cardiovascular mortality in patients with Type 1 and Type 2 diabetes.

Intensive blood glucose control The value of intensive blood glucose control cannot be understated in the management of patients when trying to prevent progression to microalbuminuria or progression of microalbuminuria. Landmark studies, such as the Diabetes Control and Complications trial, have demonstrated that A1c levels less than 7% are associated with decreased risk for clinical and structural manifestations of diabetic nephropathy in patients with Type 1 diabetes.[4–7] Intensive treatment of diabetes reduced the incidence of microalbuminuria by 39%. The benefit of the intensive intervention in patients randomized to strict glycemic control appeared to have a long-lasting effect. Specifically, there was a reduction of approximately 40% in the risk for development of microalbuminuria and hypertension 7 to 8 years after the end of the DCCT.[35] Thus, based on the evidence, insulin regimens should be designed to achieve the best glucose control while minimizing hypoglycemia in patients. As suggested for individuals with retinopathy, use of intensive insulin regimens (ie, basal/bolus therapy) with multiple insulin injections or insulin pumps needs to be strongly considered.

Intensive blood pressure control Effective treatment of blood pressure abnormalities is also a major strategy for both prevention and treatment of nephropathy. Treatment of hypertension, as well described, has been shown to reduce the risk of cardiovascular and microvascular events in patients with diabetes. With specific regard to individuals with T1D, about 40% of patients with Type 1 diabetes with normoalbuminuria have been reported to have blood pressure levels greater than 140/90 mmHg.[28] But hypertension is common in patients with diabetes, even when renal involvement is not present.[28]

The American Diabetes Association has also outlined in detail the recommendations for treatment of high-normal blood pressure (systolic or diastolic blood pressure consistently above the 90th percentile for age, sex, and height). It is currently recommended that patients with diabetes be treated to a systolic blood pressure less than 130 mm Hg and to a diastolic blood pressure less than 80 mmHg.[16] According to the published guidelines, patients with a systolic blood pressure of 130 to 139 mmHg or a diastolic blood pressure of 80 to 89 mmHg may be given lifestyle therapy alone for a maximum of 3 months. If after 3 months the targets are not achieved, patients should be advanced to treatment with pharmacologic agents. Lifestyle therapy for hypertension consists of weight loss if patients are overweight, and incorporating a Dietary Approaches to Stop Hypertension (DASH)-style dietary pattern, including reducing sodium and increasing potassium intake, moderation of alcohol intake, and increased physical activity.[16] It has also been recommended by the ADA that patients with more severe hypertension (systolic blood pressure ≥ 140 mmHg or diastolic blood pressure

$\geq$ 90 mmHg) at diagnosis or follow-up should receive pharmacologic therapy in addition to lifestyle therapy.

Current recommendations suggest that therapy for patients with diabetes and hypertension be paired with a regimen that includes either an angiotensin-converting (ACE) inhibitor or an angiotensin II receptor blocker (ARB). If one class is not tolerated, the other should be substituted.[16] If needed to achieve blood pressure targets, consideration of diuretics may be in order and prescribed based on efficacy given the measured GFR. As is well known for treatment of hypertension, multiple drug therapy (2 or more agents at maximal doses) may be required to achieve blood pressure targets.[16] In addition to effective glucose and blood pressure control, it has also been suggested to reduce protein intake to 0.8 to 1.0 g/kg body wt^{-1}/day^{-1} in individuals with diabetes and the earlier stages of CKD and to 0.8 g/kg body wt^{-1}/day^{-1} in the later stages of CKD.[16] Also, when ACE inhibitors, ARBs, or diuretics are used it is important to monitor serum creatinine and potassium levels for the development of acute kidney disease and hyperkalemia. Finally, the provider caring for patients with T1D should consider referral to a specialist experienced in diabetic nephropathy when there is uncertainty about the etiology of kidney disease, if there are difficult management issues, or if advanced kidney disease is present.[16]

Neuropathy

The diabetic neuropathies represent a heterogeneous group of disorders and the specific neuropathic abnormality can present with diverse clinical manifestations. Neuropathies may be present clinically as either focal or diffuse processes. The most common neuropathic disorders are chronic sensorimotor diabetic peripheral neuropathy (DPN) and autonomic neuropathy.[16] As any provider who cares for individuals with T1D will attest, DPN is viewed an extremely common disorder. Clearly, because of the degree and type of presentation, estimates of the prevalence will vary, but it is reported that at least 20% of adult patients with diabetes may present with at least one manifestation of DPN.[36] The etiologies of DPN are multiple, but the condition has been associated with several modifiable and nonmodifiable risk factors, including the degree of hyperglycemia, lipids, blood pressure, and diabetes duration.[36] The prevalence data for diabetic autonomic neuropathy (DAN) has been reported to range from 1.6% to 90% and clearly is dependent on the test used to assess the condition. In addition, the differences in populations examined and type and stage of disease play major roles in defining the prevalence.[36] As reported, risk factors for the development of DAN include diabetes duration, age, and long-term poor glycemic control. DAN is also associated with factors predisposing to macrovascular events (ie, hypertension and dyslipidemia).

Screening

The recognition and effective treatment of neuropathy is important at preventing further loss in sensory function and improving the quality of life for patients with T1D. The reasons for doing so are multiple but include the fact that up to half of individuals with DPN may be asymptomatic, and as such, may be at high risk for injury to the foot.[36] It is recognized that amputations are increased following a foot injury, so early recognition and management is crucial. Current recommendations suggest that providers screen all patients for distal symmetric polyneuropathy at diagnosis and at least annually thereafter using simple clinical tests. Specifically, it is recommended that the provider assess patients with use of tests, such as pinprick sensation, vibration perception (using a 128-Hz tuning fork), 10-g monofilament pressure sensation at the distal plantar aspect of both great toes and metatarsal joints, and assessment of ankle reflexes.[16,36] It has been reported that by using combinations of more than one test, sensitivity in detecting DPN can be as high as 87%.[36] Further, it is important to note that a loss of 10-g monofilament perception and reduced vibration perception may actually predict foot ulcers.[36] Electrophysiological testing is rarely needed, except in situations where the clinical features are atypical.[16]

For the individual with T1D, screening for signs and symptoms of autonomic neuropathy should be instituted at 5 years after the diagnosis.[37] Further, autonomic neuropathy can potentially involve most, if not all, systems in the body. Thus, the specific symptoms and signs of autonomic dysfunction should be evaluated with a careful history, and appropriately assessed and documented during the physical examination. As suggested, special testing may not be needed and may not affect management or outcomes.[37] Cardiovascular autonomic neuropathy is the most clinically important form of diabetic autonomic neuropathy because it is clearly a risk factor for cardiovascular disease.[38] A suggested diagnosis may be made clinically by demonstrating resting tachycardia (>100 bpm) or orthostasis changes in blood pressure. Gastrointestinal neuropathies should be evaluated with detailed history that may uncover symptoms suggestive of esophageal enteropathy and gastroparesis. For example, patients should be specifically questioned regarding symptoms, such as bloating after meals, explosive diarrhea and alternating constipation, and vomiting of previously ingested food. If gastroparesis is suspected, gastric emptying studies using double-isotope scintigraphy may be considered but in many cases, the test results may correlate poorly with clinical symptoms.[37] Diabetic autonomic neuropathy may present clinically with symptoms suggestive of genitourinary tract disturbances. For example, erectile dysfunction or retrograde ejaculation in men may be caused by diabetic autonomic neuropathy. Recurrent urinary tract infections, pyelonephritis, incontinence, or a palpable bladder may indicate the need for an evaluation of bladder dysfunction.

Management

Diabetic peripheral neuropathy Given the tremendous morbidity that can be caused secondary to significant clinical neuropathy, one of the primary strategies in the management of the individual with T1D is the prevention of neuropathy. We now have definitive evidence from landmark studies, such as the DCCT, that the risk for DPN and autonomic neuropathy can be significantly decreased with improved glycemic control over a sustained time.[4-6] Unfortunately, unlike for glycemic control, there is a paucity of data regarding control of other risk factors and prevention of neuropathy in T1D. But in general, improved lipid and blood pressure control, smoking cessation, and avoidance of excessive alcohol consumption are already recommended as preventive strategies for other diabetic complications.[16,36,37]

If patients are found to have DPN, the first step is not different from the overall management strategy for retinopathy and nephropathy because the primary goal is to obtain optimal glycemic control.[36,39,40] Although there is not definitive evidence from clinical trials and data is obtained from observational studies, it is thought that control of extreme blood glucose fluctuations, in addition to improved glycemic control, may reduce neuropathic symptoms.[16,37] There are also practice recommendations suggesting that patients with DPN may benefit clinically from pharmacologic intervention. Examples of drugs that have been used have been tricyclic drugs, such as amitriptyline, nortriptyline, and imipramine. Although tricyclic drugs may be useful, the side effects may limit their use and compliance. Anticonvulsants, such as gabapentin, carbamazepine and pregabalin, have been shown to be effective. Gabapentin is shown to be effective for neuropathic pain and is reported to be one of the most commonly prescribed anticonvulsants for this purpose. Pregabalin has also been confirmed to be useful in painful diabetic neuropathy in a randomized controlled trial.[41] In addition, the 5-Hydroxytryptamine and norepinephrine uptake inhibitor duloxetine is now indicated for use in DPN,[16] and substance P inhibitor capsaicin cream has also been used. It is important to note that with the exception of duloxetine and pregabalin, none of the other pharmacologic classes are specifically licensed for the management of painful DPN.

Autonomic neuropathy The treatments for autonomic neuropathy are generally geared to the specific organ and tissue affected. For example, clinical symptoms, such as postural hypotension and dizziness, may be treated with mechanical measures or a trial of pharmacologic agents. Gastroparesis may be treated with frequent small meals and prokinetic agents. Erectile dysfunction may be treated with psychological counseling, sildenafil, vardenafil, tadalafil, prostaglandin E1 injection, device, or prosthesis.[16] Given the multiple abnormalities and the complexity of the condition, the reader is strongly encouraged to consult the latest recommendations by the American Diabetes Association.[16]

MACROVASCULAR COMPLICATIONS

In contrast to microvascular disease, macrovascular complications have been less studied and less is known about the specific determinants of disease particular to T1D. However, as observed for individuals with Type 2 diabetes mellitus, macrovascular complications in T1D impart significant morbidity and mortality. In contrast to the general population, the macrovascular complications in T1D occur much earlier in life, have a more diffuse, accelerated course and have a higher mortality, especially in those aged less than 40 years.

There are several studies that have been published over the recent years that provide an estimate of the incidence of cardiovascular disease in T1D. In the Pittsburgh Epidemiology of Diabetes Complications study (EDC), men and women with T1D were shown to have a similarly increased risk of premature coronary artery disease (CAD), although risk factors (predictors) appeared to vary by both sex and type of CAD manifestation.[42] It was also confirmed how clinically important renal abnormalities were as a predictor, especially in men.[43] In addition, hypertension, smoking, and dyslipidemia were observed to be CAD predictors in T1D.[43] One of the more interesting findings as suggested from the Pittsburgh EDC study and the DCCT was the observation that insulin resistance, the hallmark of Type 2 diabetes, may also relate to CAD risk in T1D.[44,45] Specifically, the data suggested all factors predicting total CAD or angina have been linked to insulin resistance.[42]

Other studies have demonstrated the risk for CVD is also increased for a primarily African American cohort with T1D.[46] Six-year incidence of any CVD was significantly associated with older age and longer duration of diabetes when assessed at baseline.[46] In addition, it was established that baseline older age, higher body mass index, higher diastolic blood pressure, proteinuria, retinopathy severity, and being depressed were significant and independent risk factors for incidence of any CVD in this cohort. Thus, it is apparent that regardless of race, CVD risk appears to be high in individuals with T1D.[46]

Evaluation and Management

As recently reviewed,[47] the approach to glycemic control and its primary effect on CVD outcomes was stated to be controversial. However, the observations suggest clear benefit over a long-term period of observation resulting from intensive management of glycemia as evidenced from the DCCT/EDIC.[48] In fact, a 57% reduction in cardiovascular events was noted. As reviewed by Orchard and Costacou,[47] it was suggested that glycemia plays a significant role in the early atherogenic development of lesions, a conclusion consistent with recent evidence from the Veterans Affairs Diabetes Trial (VADT) in Type 2 diabetes, showing that any cardiovascular mortality benefit from intensification of glycemic therapy is limited to those diagnosed with diabetes 15 or fewer years earlier.

An important management strategy for individuals with T1D is the control of traditional risk factors as would be expected in the management for individuals with Type 2 diabetes. As previously outlined, traditional risk factors appear to assist the clinician in deciding what patients with T1D are at risk. Evidence of this comes from observations from the EURODIAB study.[49] Specifically, clinical risk factors, such as waist-hip ratio, blood pressure, and dyslipidemia, contributed to the overall cardiovascular mortality as did the presence of the complications (eg, albuminuria, retinopathy, neuropathy).[49] As reviewed, a major limitation for management of CVD in T1D is that there is no risk engine developed in the general population or in individuals with Type 2 diabetes that is appropriate for T1D because of the younger age of diabetes onset and interactions with complications, especially renal disease.[47,50] However, work is under way on developing a T1D cardiovascular disease risk engine.[47]

It has been suggested that other factors, such as genetic variation, may help identify susceptible individuals in being predisposed to CVD. In recent years, there has been great excitement with the haptoglobin (Hp) genotype.[47] This genotype may help characterize susceptible individuals with Type 2 diabetes.[47,51] The potential role of this genotype was evaluated in individuals with T1D as part of the Pittsburgh EDC study of childhood onset T1D.[52] It was observed that after statistical adjustment for traditional CVD risk factors, a 2-fold greater risk was observed for individuals noted to carry the Hp 2-2 genotype as compared with those carrying the Hp 1-1. Clearly, such data provides exciting new possibilities that allow a clinician to assess risk for individuals with T1D.

When one now considers what subject with T1D is at risk, we still have considerable gaps in knowledge. However, over the past few years there have been significant new findings. We do know that individuals with T1D with abnormalities in traditional risk factors must be considered at high risk, and in particular, the presence of retinopathy and neuropathy increases the risk for CVD. It is also suggested that certain genotypes now put patients at increased risk. For the clinician to design a regimen to reduce risk, intensive glycemic control is clearly indicated as is control of dyslipidemia and blood pressure.

REFERENCES

1. Zhao Y, Ye W, Boye KS, et al. Healthcare charges and utilization associated with diabetic neuropathy: impact of Type 1 diabetes and presence of other diabetes-related complications and comorbidities. Diabet Med 2009;26(1):61–9.
2. Boyle JP, Honeycutt AA, Venkat Narayan KM, et al. Projection of diabetes burden through 2050: impact of changing demography and disease prevalence in the U.S. Diabetes Care 2001;24:1936–40.
3. American Diabetes Association. Executive summary: standards of medical care in diabetes - 2010. Diabetes Care 2010;33:S4–10.
4. Diabetes Control and Complications Trial/Epidemiology of Diabetes Interventions and Complications (DCCT/EDIC) Research Group. Modern-day clinical course of type 1 diabetes mellitus after 30 years' duration: the diabetes control and complications trial/epidemiology of diabetes interventions and complications and Pittsburgh epidemiology of diabetes complications experience (1983–2005). Arch Intern Med 2009;169(14):1307–16.

5. The Writing Team for the Diabetes Control and Complications Trial/Epidemiology of Diabetes Interventions and Complications Research Group. Effect of intensive therapy on the microvascular complications of type 1 diabetes mellitus. JAMA 2002;287(19):2563–9.

6. The Diabetes Control and Complications Trial Research Group. The effect of intensive treatment of diabetes on the development and progression of long-term complications in insulin-dependent diabetes mellitus. N Engl J Med 1993; 329:977–86.

7. Diabetes Control and Complications Trial/Epidemiology of Diabetes Interventions and Complications Research Group. Prolonged effect of intensive therapy on the risk of retinopathy complications in patients with type 1 diabetes mellitus: 10 years after the diabetes control and complications trial. Arch Ophthalmol 2008; 126(12):1707–15.

8. Brownlee M. Biochemistry and molecular cell biology of diabetic complications. Nature 2001;414:813–20.

9. Degenhardt TP, Thorpe SR, Baynes JW. Chemical modification of proteins by methylglyoxal. Cell Mol Biol 1998;44:1139–45.

10. Nakamura S, Makita Z, Ishikawa S, et al. Progression of nephropathy in spontaneous diabetic rats is prevented by OPB-9195, a novel inhibitor of advanced glycation. Diabetes 1997;46:895–9.

11. Maisonpierre PC, Suri C, Jones PF, et al. Angiopoietin-2, a natural antagonist for Tie2 that disrupts in vivo angiogenesis. Science 1997;277:55–60.

12. Tanaka S, Avigad G, Brodsky B, et al. Glycation induces expansion of the molecular packing of collagen. J Mol Biol 1988;203:495–505.

13. Epidemiology of Diabetes Interventions and Complications (EDIC) Research Group. Design, implementation, and preliminary results of a long-term follow-up of the Diabetes Control and Complications Trial cohort. Diabetes Care 1999; 22:99–111.

14. Kilpatrick ES, Rigby AS, Atkin SL. The diabetes control and complications trial: the gift that keeps giving. Nat Rev Endocrinol 2009;5:537–45.

15. Lind M, Odén A, Fahlén M, et al. The shape of the metabolic memory of HbA1c: re-analysing the DCCT with respect to time-dependent effects. Diabetologia 2010;53(6):1093–8.

16. American Diabetes Association. Standards of medical care in diabetes - 2010. Diabetes Care 2010;33:S11–63.

17. Frank RN. Diabetic retinopathy. N Engl J Med 2004;350:48–58.

18. Klein R. Hyperglycemia and microvascular and macrovascular disease in diabetes. Diabetes Care 1995;18:258–68.

19. Estacio RO, McFarling E, Biggerstaff S, et al. Overt albuminuria predicts diabetic retinopathy in Hispanics with NIDDM. Am J Kidney Dis 1998;31:947–53.

20. Leske MC, Wu SY, Hennis A, et al. Barbados Eye Study Group. Hyperglycemia, blood pressure, and the 9-year incidence of diabetic retinopathy: the Barbados Eye Studies. Ophthalmology 2005;112:799–805.

21. Klein R, Knudtson MD, Lee KE, et al. The Wisconsin Epidemiologic Study of Diabetic Retinopathy: XXII the twenty-five-year progression of retinopathy in persons with type 1 diabetes. Ophthalmology 2008;115(11):1859–68.

22. UK Prospective Diabetes Study (UKPDS) Group. Effect of intensive blood-glucose control with metformin on complications in overweight patients with type 2 diabetes (UKPDS 34). Lancet 1998;352:854–65.

23. UK Prospective Diabetes Study (UKPDS) Group. Intensive blood-glucose control with sulphonylureas or insulin compared with conventional treatment

and risk of complications in patients with type 2 diabetes (UKPDS 33). Lancet 1998;352:837–53.

24. UK Prospective Diabetes Study Group. Tight blood pressure control and risk of macrovascular and microvascular complications in type 2 diabetes: UKPDS 38. BMJ 1998;317:703–13.

25. The Diabetic Retinopathy Study (DRS) Research Group. Preliminary report on the effects of photocoagulation therapy: DRS Report #1. Am J Ophthalmol 1976;81: 383–96.

26. Early Treatment Diabetic Retinopathy Study Research Group. Photocoagulation for diabetic macular edema. Early Treatment Diabetic Retinopathy Study report number 1. Arch Ophthalmol 1985;103:1796–806.

27. Wong TY, Mwamburi M, Klein R, et al. Rates of progression in diabetic retinopathy during different time periods: a systematic review and meta-analysis. Diabetes Care 2009;32(12):2307–13.

28. Gross JL, de Azevedo MJ, Silveiro SP, et al. Diabetic nephropathy: diagnosis, prevention, and treatment. Diabetes Care 2005;28(1):164–76.

29. Garg JP, Bakris GL. Microalbuminuria: marker of vascular dysfunction, risk factor for cardiovascular disease. Vasc Med 2002;7:35–43.

30. Klausen K, Borch-Johnsen K, Feldt-Rasmussen B, et al. Very low levels of micro-albuminuria are associated with increased risk of coronary heart disease and death independently of renal function, hypertension, and diabetes. Circulation 2004;110:32–5.

31. Gaspari F, Perico N, Remuzzi G. Measurement of glomerular filtration rate. Kidney Int Suppl 1997;63:S151–4.

32. Friedman R, De Azevedo MJ, Gross JL. Is endogenous creatinine clearance still a reliable index of glomerular filtration rate in diabetic patients? Braz J Med Biol Res 1988;21:941–4.

33. Levey AS, Bosch JP, Lewis JB, et al. A more accurate method to estimate glomerular filtration rate from serum creatinine: a new prediction equation. Modification of Diet in Renal Disease Study Group. Ann Intern Med 1999; 130:461–70.

34. Rigalleau V, Lasseur C, Perlemoine C, et al. Estimation of glomerular filtration rate in diabetic subjects: Cockcroft formula or modification of Diet in Renal Disease study equation? Diabetes Care 2005;28:838–43.

35. Writing Team for the Diabetes Control and Complications Trial/Epidemiology of Diabetes Interventions and Complications Research Group. Sustained effect of intensive treatment of type 1 diabetes mellitus on development and progression of diabetic nephropathy: the Epidemiology of Diabetes Interventions and Compli-cations (EDIC) study. JAMA 2003;290:2159–67.

36. Boulton AJ, Vinik AI, Arezzo JC, et al. American Diabetes Association. Diabetic neuropathies: a statement by the American Diabetes Association. Diabetes Care 2005;28:956–62.

37. Vinik AI, Maser RE, Mitchell BD, et al. Diabetic autonomic neuropathy. Diabetes Care 2003;26:1553–79.

38. Appel LJ, Moore TJ, Obarzanek E, et al. A clinical trial of the effects of dietary patterns on blood pressure. DASH Collaborative Research Group. N Engl J Med 1997;336:1117–24.

39. Boulton AJM, Malik RA, Arezzo JC, et al. Diabetic somatic neuropathies (tech-nical review). Diabetes Care 2004;27:1458–86.

40. Boulton AJM, Gries FA, Jervell JA. Guidelines for the diagnosis and outpatient management diabetic peripheral neuropathy. Diabet Med 1998;15:508–14.

41. Rosenstock J, Tuchman M, LaMoreaux L, et al. Pregabalin for the treatment of painful diabetic neuropathy: a double-blind, placebo-controlled trial. Pain 2004; 110:628–38.

42. Orchard TJ, Olson JC, Erbey JR, et al. Insulin resistance-related factors, but not glycemia, predict coronary artery disease in type 1 diabetes: 10-year follow-up data from the Pittsburgh Epidemiology of Diabetes Complications Study. Diabetes Care 2003;26(5):1374–9.

43. Forrest KYZ, Becker DJ, Kuller LH, et al. Are predictors of coronary heart disease and lower extremity arterial disease in type 1 diabetes the same? A prospective study. Atherosclerosis 2000;148:159–69.

44. Erbey JR, Kuller LH, Becker DJ, et al. The association between a family history of type 2 diabetes (NIDDM) and coronary artery disease in a type 1 diabetes (IDDM) population. Diabetes Care 1998;21:610–4.

45. Purnell JQ, Hokanson JE, Marcovina SM, et al. Effect of excessive weight gain with intensive therapy of type 1 diabetes on lipid levels and blood pressure. JAMA 1998;280:140–6.

46. Roy MS, Peng B, Roy A. Risk factors for coronary disease and stroke in previously hospitalized African-Americans with Type 1 diabetes: a 6-year follow-up. Diabet Med 2007;24(12):1361–8.

47. Orchard TJ, Costacou T. When are type 1 diabetic patients at risk for cardiovascular disease? Curr Diab Rep 2010;10(1):48–54.

48. Nathan DM, Cleary PA, Backlund JY, et al, Diabetes Control and Complications Trial/Epidemiology of Diabetes Interventions and Complications (DCCT/EDIC) Study Research Group. Intensive diabetes treatment and cardiovascular disease in patients with type 1 diabetes. N Engl J Med 2005;353:2643–53.

49. Soedamah-Muthu SS, Chaturvedi N, Witte DR, et al, EURODIAB Prospective Complications Study Group. Relationship between risk factors and mortality in type 1 diabetic patients in Europe: the EURODIAB Prospective Complications Study (PCS). Diabetes Care 2008;31:1360–6.

50. Zgibor JC, Piatt GA, Ruppert K, et al. Deficiencies of cardiovascular risk prediction models for type 1 diabetes. Diabetes Care 2006;29:1860–5.

51. Levy AP, Hochberg I, Jablonski K, et al, Strong Heart Study. Haptoglobin genotype is an independent risk factor for cardiovascular disease in individuals with diabetes: the Strong Heart Study. J Am Coll Cardiol 2002;40:1984–90.

52. Costacou T, Ferrell RE, Orchard TJ. Haptoglobin genotype and renal disease progression in type 1 diabetes. Diabetes 2008;57:1702–6.

Hypoglycemia in Type 1 Diabetes Mellitus

Philip E. Cryer, MD[a,b,*]

KEYWORDS

- Hypoglycemia • Diabetes
- Defective glucose counter-regulation
- Hypoglycemia unawareness
- Hypoglycemia-associated autonomic failure in diabetes

THE LIMITING FACTOR IN GLYCEMIC CONTROL

The clinical problem of hypoglycemia in diabetes has been summarized[1] and discussed in detail.[2] Because it reduces microvascular complications[3]—retinopathy, nephropathy, and neuropathy—and may reduce macrovascular complications,[4] glycemic control is generally in the best interest of people with type 1 diabetes mellitus (T1DM). Iatrogenic hypoglycemia, however, is the limiting factor in the glycemic management of T1DM.[1,2] It (1) causes recurrent morbidity in most people with T1DM and is sometimes fatal, (2) impairs defenses against subsequent hypoglycemia and therefore causes a vicious cycle of recurrent hypoglycemia, and (3) precludes maintenance of euglycemia over a lifetime of diabetes and thus full realization of the benefits of glycemic control. Euglycemia is not an appropriate glycemic goal in the vast majority of people with T1DM.[1,2] Perhaps a reasonable goal is the matching of exogenous insulin actions and circulating glucose availability that results in the lowest

The author's original research cited was supported, in part, by National Institutes of Health grants R37 DK27085, MO1 RR00036 (now UL1 RR24992), P60 DK20579, and T32 DK07120 and a fellowship award from the American Diabetes Association.

Disclosures: This article was written shortly after the publication of the author's book, *Hypoglycemia in Diabetes: Pathophysiology, Prevalence, and Prevention,* American Diabetes Association, Alexandria, Virginia, 2009.[2] Therefore, much of the factual and interpretive content here is the same, as is no small part of the phraseology.

The author has served as a consultant to several pharmaceutical or device firms, including Amgen Inc, Johnson & Johnson, MannKind Corp, Marcadia Biotech, Medtronic MiniMed Inc, Merck and Co, Novo Nordisk A/S, Takeda Pharmaceuticals North America, and TolerRx Inc, in recent years. He does not receive research funding from, hold stock in, or speak for any of these firms.

[a] Department of Medicine, Washington University School of Medicine, Campus Box 8127, 660 South Euclid Avenue, St Louis, MO 63110, USA

[b] Barnes-Jewish Hospital, St Louis, MO, USA

* Department of Medicine, Washington University School of Medicine, Campus Box 8127, 660 South Euclid Avenue, St Louis, MO 63110.

E-mail address: pcryer@wustl.edu

mean glycemia (eg, hemoglobin A_{1C} [HbA_{1C}]) that causes no severe hypoglycemia, permits continued awareness of hypoglycemia, and produces a tolerable number of episodes of symptomatic hypoglycemia.

INCIDENCE AND IMPACTS OF HYPOGLYCEMIA IN T1DM

Iatrogenic hypoglycemia is a fact of life for people with T1DM.[1,2] They suffer untold numbers of episodes of asymptomatic hypoglycemia. In one study of subcutaneous glucose sensing in T1DM, glucose levels were less than or equal to 70 mg/dL (3.9 mmol/L) 1.5 hours per day (ie, 6.3% of the time).[5] In a study involving nocturnal plasma glucose measurements every 15 minutes in T1DM, glucose levels were less than 70 mg/dL in 57% (12 of 21) of the patients.[6] Many of these episodes are asymptomatic but they are not benign because they impair physiologic and behavioral defenses against subsequent hypoglycemia.[1,2] People with T1DM suffer an average of two episodes of symptomatic hypoglycemia per week—thousands of such episodes over a lifetime of diabetes. They suffer an average of approximately one episode of severe, at least temporarily disabling, hypoglycemia, often with seizure or coma, per year.[1,2]

Falling plasma glucose concentrations normally signal a series of responses, including a decrease in insulin secretion as glucose levels decline within the physiologic range, increases in glucagon and epinephrine secretion as glucose levels fall below the physiologic range, and a more intense sympathoadrenal response with symptoms at plasma glucose levels of 50 to 55 mg/dL (2.8–3.0 mmol/L).[1,2] Neurogenic (autonomic) symptoms (catecholamine-mediated or adrenergic: tremor, palpitations, and anxiety/arousal; and acetylocholine-mediated or cholinergic: sweating, hunger, and paresthesias) are the result of the perception of physiologic changes caused by sympathoadrenal, largely sympathetic neural,[7] activation.[8] Neuroglycopenic symptoms (cognitive impairments, behavioral changes, and psychomotor abnormalities and at lower glucose levels seizure and coma) are the result of brain glucose deprivation per se. The glycemic thresholds for these responses are dynamic.[1,2] They shift to higher plasma glucose concentrations in people with poorly controlled T1DM[9,10] and to lower plasma glucose concentrations in those with well-controlled T1DM.[10]

Functional brain failure caused by hypoglycemia is typically corrected after the plasma glucose concentrations is raised.[1,2,11] Rarely, hypoglycemia causes sudden, presumably cardiac arrhythmic, death or, if it is prolonged and profound, brain death.[11–13] Early reports suggested that 2% to 4% of deaths of people with diabetes are the result of hypoglycemia.[1,2] More recent reports indicate that 6% to 10% of deaths of people with T1DM are caused by hypoglycemia.[14–16] Regardless of the exact rates, the existence of iatrogenic mortality is alarming.

DEFINITION OF HYPOGLYCEMIA IN T1DM

The American Diabetes Association (ADA) Workgroup on Hypoglycemia defined hypoglycemia in people with diabetes as "all episodes of abnormally low plasma glucose concentration that expose the individual to potential harm."[17] That includes episodes of asymptomatic hypoglycemia because those impair defenses against subsequent hypoglycemia.[1,2] It is not possible to state a specific plasma glucose concentration that defines hypoglycemia because the glycemic thresholds for symptoms, among other manifestations, are dynamic.[9,10] Nonetheless, the ADA Workgroup recommended that people with T1DM become concerned about the possibility of hypoglycemia at a self-monitored (or glucose sensing device–estimated) plasma glucose concentration of less than or equal to 70 mg/dL (3.9 mmol/L).[17] The rationale for that cutoff value is that, within the error of these measurements, 70 mg/dL approximates the lower limit of the postabsorptive plasma glucose concentration range and the glycemic threshold for activation of glucose counter-regulatory systems and is the highest low level reported to reduce counter-regulatory responses to subsequent hypoglycemia in nondiabetic individuals.[17] That recommendation does not mean, however, that patients should always self-treat at a glucose level of less than or equal to 70 mg/dL (3.9 mmol/L).[18] The options include repeating the measurement in the near term (or observing the trend with a device), avoiding a critical task such as driving, ingesting carbohydrates, and using the information to adjust the subsequent therapeutic regimen.

The ADA Workgroup also suggested a classification of hypoglycemia in diabetes.[17] That includes (1) severe hypoglycemia (an event requiring assistance of another person to raise glucose levels and promote neurologic recovery), (2) documented symptomatic hypoglycemia (symptoms plus low glucose), and (3) asymptomatic hypoglycemia (low glucose without symptoms) as well as (4) probable symptomatic hypoglycemia (symptoms without a glucose estimate) and (5) relative hypoglycemia (symptoms with glucose levels that are not low but are approaching that level).

PHYSIOLOGY OF GLUCOSE COUNTER-REGULATION

The physiologic defenses against falling plasma glucose (**Fig. 1**) concentrations in nondiabetic individuals include (1) decrements in pancreatic β-cell insulin secretion, (2) increments in pancreatic α-cell glucagon secretion, and, absent the latter, (3) increments in adrenomedullary epinephrine secretion.[1,2,19] Lower insulin levels favor increased glucose production, which is also stimulated by glucagon and epinephrine. Epinephrine also limits glucose use and mobilizes gluconeogenic precursors; it normally inhibits insulin secretion although it cannot do so in many patients with T1DM.[19] The behavioral defense is carbohydrate ingestion prompted by symptoms that are largely sympathoadrenal, predominantly sympathetic neural,[1,2,7–19] in origin. All of these defenses are typically compromised in people with T1DM.[1,2,20,21]

PATHOPHYSIOLOGY OF GLUCOSE COUNTER-REGULATION IN T1DM

All insulin preparations are pharmacokinetically imperfect. Thus, episodes of therapeutic hyperinsulinemia occur from time to time in T1DM (see **Fig. 1; Fig. 2**). These cause declining plasma glucose concentrations that may, if not effectively countered, result in hypoglycemia. Absolute therapeutic insulin excess of sufficient magnitude can cause an isolated episode of hypoglycemia despite intact glucose counter-regulatory defenses (see **Fig. 2**).[1,2] But, hypoglycemia is more commonly the result of the interplay of relative or mild-to-moderate absolute therapeutic insulin excess and compromised physiologic and behavioral defenses against falling plasma glucose concentrations in T1DM (see **Figs. 1** and **2**).[1,2,20,21]

Defective Glucose Counter-regulation and Hypoglycemia Unawareness

In established T1DM, the first and second physiologic defenses against hypoglycemia—a decrease in insulin and an increase in glucagon—are lost, and the third physiologic defense—an increase in epinephrine—is often attenuated.[1,2,20,21] Loss of the endogenous insulin response is the result of β-cell failure, the basic cause of T1DM. Loss of the glucagon response[22] is also likely the result of β-cell failure[1,2] because a decrease in β-cell secretion of insulin, perhaps among other secretory products, in concert with hypoglycemia, normally signals increased α-cell glucagon secretion.[23,24] Although it can be caused by recent antecedent hypoglycemia,[25] by

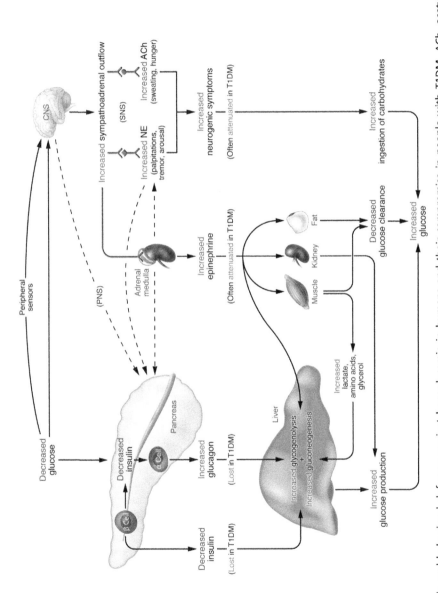

Fig. 1. Physiologic and behavioral defenses against hypoglycemia in humans and their compromise in people with T1DM. ACh, acetylcholine; NE, norepinephrine; PNS, parasympathetic nervous system; SNS, sympathetic nervous system. (*From* Cryer PE. Mechanisms of sympathoadrenal failure and hypoglycemia in diabetes. J Clin Invest 2006;116(6):1471; with permission of the American Society for Clinical Investigation.)

Hypoglycemia-Associated Autonomic Failure

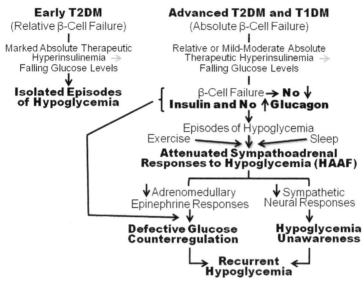

Fig. 2. Schematic diagram of defective glucose counter-regulation and hypoglycemia unawareness and the unifying concept of hypoglycemia-associated autonomic failure in T1DM. (*From* Cryer PE. Exercise-related hypoglycemia-associated autonomic failure. Diabetes 2009;58(9):1952; with permission of the American Diabetes Association.)

prior exercise, or by sleep,[1,2] the mechanism of the attenuated sympathoadrenal response to falling glucose levels is not known.[1,2] In the setting of therapeutic hyperinsulinemia and falling plasma glucose concentrations and absent insulin and glucagon secretory responses, the attenuated epinephrine response causes the clinical syndrome of defective glucose counter-regulation,[1,2,21,25] which is associated with a 25-fold[26] or greater[27] increased risk of severe iatrogenic hypoglycemia. The attenuated sympathoadrenal response, largely attenuation of its sympathetic neural component,[7] causes the clinical syndrome of hypoglycemia unawareness (or impaired awareness of hypoglycemia) and, thus, loss of the behavioral defense, carbohydrate ingestion.[1,2,21] Hypoglycemia unawareness is associated with a 6-fold increased risk of iatrogenic hypoglycemia.[28]

Hypoglycemia-Associated Autonomic Failure

The concept of hypoglycemia-associated autonomic failure (HAAF) in diabetes[1,2,11,21] (see **Fig. 2**) posits that recent antecedent hypoglycemia, or prior exercise or sleep, causes defective glucose counter-regulation (by attenuating increments in epinephrine in the setting of absent decrements in insulin and absent increments in glucagon during subsequent hypoglycemia) and hypoglycemia unawareness (by attenuating sympathoadrenal and resulting neurogenic symptom responses during subsequent hypoglycemia) and, thus, a vicious cycle of recurrent hypoglycemia. Perhaps the most convincing evidence of the clinical relevance of HAAF is the finding—originally in three independent laboratories[29–32]—that as little as 2 to 3 weeks of scrupulous avoidance of hypoglycemia reverses hypoglycemia unawareness and improves the deficient epinephrine component of defective glucose counter-regulation in most affected patients.

The mechanism of the attenuated sympathoadrenal response to falling plasma glucose concentrations, the key feature of HAAF, are unknown. Theories include effects of a systemic mediator, such as cortisol, on the brain; an increase in blood-to-brain transport of a metabolic fuel, such as glucose, among others; altered hypothalamic mechanisms; and activation of an inhibitory cerebral network mediated through the thalamus.[1,2,33]

RISK FACTORS FOR HYPOGLYCEMIA IN T1DM
Conventional Risk Factors

The conventional risk factors for hypoglycemia in diabetes are based on the premise that relative or absolute therapeutic hyperinsulinemia is the sole determinant of risk.[1,2,34] Relative—to low rates of glucose influx into the circulation or high rates of glucose efflux out of the circulation—or absolute therapeutic hyperinsulinemia occurs when (1) insulin doses are excessive, ill-timed, or of the wrong type; (2) exogenous glucose delivery is decreased (as after missed meals or during the overnight fast or when glucose absorption is delayed, as in gastroparesis or decreased as in celiac disease); (3) glucose use is increased (as during and shortly after exercise); (4) endogenous glucose production is decreased (as after alcohol ingestion); (5) sensitivity to insulin is increased (as during the middle of the night or after weight loss, improved fitness, or improved glycemic control); or (6) insulin clearance is decreased (as with renal failure). These risk factors must be considered carefully when hypoglycemia is a problem. Aside from the first, however, they explain only a minority of episodes of hypoglycemia.[35]

Risk Factors for HAAF

Risk factors for HAAF[1–4] include (1) the degree of absolute endogenous insulin deficiency; this determines the extent to which insulin levels do not decrease and glucagon levels do not increase as glucose levels fall in response to therapeutic hyperinsulinemia; (2) a history of severe hypoglycemia, hypoglycemia unawareness, or both as well as recent antecedent hypoglycemia, prior exercise, or sleep. A history of severe hypoglycemia documents, and that of hypoglycemia unawareness implies, recent antecedent hypoglycemia, which, like prior exercise or sleep, causes attenuated sympathoadrenal and symptomatic responses to subsequent hypoglycemia, the key feature of HAAF; (3) aggressive glycemic therapy per se (lower HbA_{1C} levels, lower glycemic goals); hypoglycemia can occur in patients with any HbA_{1C} level; nonetheless, lower mean glycemia is a risk factor for hypoglycemia. Studies with a control group treated to a higher HbA_{1C} consistently report a higher rate of hypoglycemia in patients treated to a lower HbA_{1C}.[1–3] That does not mean that glycemic control cannot be improved and the risk of iatrogenic hypoglycemia minimized in individual people with T1DM.[1,2,34]

MINIMIZING THE RISK OF HYPOGLYCEMIA IN T1DM

Minimizing the risk of hypoglycemia in T1DM involves the practice of hypoglycemia risk factor reduction.[1,2,34,36,37] That includes four steps: (1) acknowledge the problem, (2) apply the principles of aggressive glycemic therapy, (3) consider the conventional risk factors for hypoglycemia, and (4) consider the risk factors indicative of HAAF in diabetes.

Acknowledge the Problem

Patient concerns about the reality, or the possibility, of hypoglycemia can be a barrier to glycemic control.[38] Some patients are reluctant to raise the issue despite those concerns. Therefore, the issue of hypoglycemia should be addressed in every contact with a person with T1DM. In addition to questioning patients and examining the self-monitoring of blood glucose (SMBG) log (and any glucose sensing record), it is often helpful to question close associates of patients.

Apply the Principles of Aggressive Glycemic Therapy

The principles of aggressive glycemic therapy, which have been reviewed else-where,[1,2,34,36,37] include (1) patient education and empowerment; (2) frequent SMBG (and in some instances glucose sensing); (3) flexible and appropriate insulin, among other, regimens; (4) individualized glycemic goals; and (5) ongoing professional guidance and support.

Patient education and empowerment

Contemporary regimens for the treatment of T1DM are complex[34,36,37] and the glycemic management of T1DM becomes more challenging over time.[39] Successful glycemic management is largely dependent on the skills and decisions of a well-informed person with diabetes. Patient education and empowerment are fundamentally important.

In addition to the key relationship between exogenous insulin action and glucose availability in the circulation and the basic survival skills of diabetes, people with T1DM need to learn about the anticipation, recognition, and treatment of hypoglycemia.[40,41] They need to know the common symptoms, and their most meaningful symptoms, of hypoglycemia, how to treat (and not overtreat) hypoglycemia, and the risk factors for hypoglycemia. Close associates need to learn how to recognize severe hypoglycemia and how to administer glucagon. Patients need to know that increasing episodes of hypoglycemia signal an increasing likelihood of future, even more severe, hypoglycemia[41] and how to apply SMBG (and glucose sensing) data to the adjustment of their subsequent regimen.

Frequent SMBG (and in some instance continuous glucose sensing)

Patients with T1DM should perform SMBG regularly and whenever they suspect hypoglycemia.[1,2] It is particularly important for them to check their glucose level before performing a critical task, such as driving. SMBG permits documentation of hypoglycemia (or hyperglycemia), allows patients to correlate their symptoms and glucose levels, and provides information that may lead to regimen adjustments that prevent hypoglycemia.[41] Continuous glucose sensing should reduce the risk of hypoglycemia without compromising glycemic control because it informs patients whether or not the glucose level is stable, rising, or falling. There seems to be steady progress with the devices, although compelling evidence of net benefit remains to be reported.[5,42] Ultimately, a continuous glucose monitoring device will be a component of a closed-loop insulin replacement system.

Flexible and appropriate insulin, among other, regimens

Although a variety of combinations are used, contemporary insulin therapy of T1DM is basically a basal-bolus approach using multiple daily injection (MDI) of insulin or continuous subcutaneous insulin infusion. The use of a long-acting basal insulin analog (glargine or detemir) rather than NPH insulin in an MDI regimen reduces at least the incidence of nocturnal hypoglycemia, perhaps that of total and symptomatic hypoglycemia, in T1DM.[43,44] The use of a rapid acting prandial insulin analog (lispro, aspart, or glulisine) rather than regular insulin reduces the incidence of nocturnal hypoglycemia in T1DM.[43,44] Albeit conceptually attractive, the superiority of continuous subcutaneous insulin infusion with an insulin analog over MDI with insulin analogs with respect to the incidence of hypoglycemia at comparable levels of glycemic control remains to be established convincingly.[45,46] That is also the case in pregnant women with diabetes.[47]

Iatrogenic hypoglycemia often occurs at night, specifically during sleep.[3,6,35,48,49] In one study, one quarter of youth with T1DM suffered nocturnal hypoglycemia.[49] In another study, more than half of adults with T1DM had nocturnal plasma glucose levels less than 70 mg/dL (3.9 mmol/L).[6] Nighttime is typically the longest interval between SMBG and between eating and is the time of maximal sensitivity to insulin. Furthermore, sleep causes a further reduced sympathoadrenal response to hypoglycemia.[50,51] Thus, sleeping patients with T1DM have further reduced epinephrine responses to hypoglycemia,[5,51] the key feature of defective glucose counterregulation, and reduced arousal from sleep,[51,52] a form of hypoglycemia unawareness. They have sleep-related HAAF[1,2,51] and are at high risk for hypoglycemia.[6,49] Approaches to the prevention of nocturnal hypoglycemia include the use of insulin analogs[43,44] (discussed previously). Other approaches include attempts to provide sustained delivery of exogenous carbohydrate throughout the night.[1,2,6] Those include bedtime snacks and bedtime administration of uncooked cornstarch, both of which have been found to only shift episodes of hypoglycemia to later in the night.[6] Alternative approaches to the prevention of nocturnal hypoglycemia include attempts to provide sustained delivery of endogenous glucose throughout the night. Those include bedtime oral administration of the epinephrine-simulating β_2-adrenergic agonist, terbutaline,[6,53] and overnight glucagon infusion. Both are effective, albeit at the risk of hyperglycemia, but neither has been subjected to suitably powered randomized controlled trials to determine if they provide net benefit (ie, less hypoglycemia without deterioration of glycemic control). As described previously, afternoon exercise is also a potential cause of nocturnal hypoglycemia.[1,2,49,54–57]

Exercise increases glucose use (by exercising muscle) but decrements in insulin and increments in glucagon normally prevent hypoglycemia.[54] Largely because insulin levels do not decrease, hypoglycemia occurs commonly during or shortly after exercise in people with T1DM.[54,55] Although that risk is generally recognized, the risk of late postexercise hypoglycemia[49,54–57] is less widely appreciated. Late postexercise hypoglycemia in T1DM typically occurs 6 to 15 hours after strenuous exercise and is, therefore, often nocturnal.[56] In one study, approximately half of youth with T1DM suffered nocturnal hypoglycemia after afternoon exercise whereas only approximately one quarter of that group suffered nocturnal hypoglycemia in the absence of afternoon exercise.[49] Exercise reduces sympathoadrenal responses to hypoglycemia several hours later in T1DM.[54,57] Thus, people with T1DM often develop exercise-related HAAF and suffer late postexercise hypoglycemia.[1,2,54]

The vast majority of episodes of hypoglycemia in people with T1DM are iatrogenic, but those individuals can suffer from hypoglycemia caused by mechanisms other than insulin treatment.[58]

Individualized glycemic goals

Given the benefits of glycemic control in T1DM,[3,4] mean glycemia as close to the nondiabetic range as can be accomplished safely is in patients' best interest.[1,2] That is generally an HbA$_{1C}$ of less than 7.0%.[59,60] Although that goal often can be accomplished relatively early in T1DM,[39] it is sometimes not possible to achieve that level without excessive hypoglycemia. It should be recalled that there is long-term benefit from reducing HbA$_{1C}$ from higher to lower, although still above desirable, levels.[61] Ultimately, in individuals with limited life expectancy or functional capacity in whom glycemic control is unlikely to be beneficial,[60,62] a higher glycemic goal becomes reasonable. Perhaps a reasonable generic goal is the lowest mean glycemia that causes no severe hypoglycemia, permits continued awareness of hypoglycemia, and produces a tolerable number of episodes of symptomatic hypoglycemia.

Ongoing professional guidance and support

Because the glycemic management of T1DM is empiric, caregivers should work with each individual patient over time to find the best methods of glycemic control for that individual at a given stage in the evolution of his or her diabetes.[1,2] Patient support is best provided by a team that includes professionals trained in, and dedicated to, translation of the standards of care[59] into the care of individual patients.

Consider the Conventional Risk Factors for Hypoglycemia

As discussed previously, conventional risk factors for hypoglycemia include the dose, timing, and type of the insulin preparations used and conditions in which exogenous glucose delivery or endogenous glucose production is decreased, glucose use or insulin sensitivity is increased, or insulin clearance is decreased.[1,2] They result in relative or absolute therapeutic hyperinsulinemia. Each must be considered carefully when hypoglycemia is a real or a potential problem.

Consider the Risk Factors Indicative of HAAF

As detailed previously, risk factors indicative of HAAF include the degree of absolute endogenous insulin deficiency, a history of severe hypoglycemia, hypoglycemia unawareness, or both, as well as a relationship between hypoglycemia and recent antecedent hypoglycemia, prior exercise or sleep, and lower glycemic goals.[1,2] The degree of endogenous insulin deficiency is, of course, beyond the caregiver's control. Unless the cause is readily correctable, a history of severe hypoglycemia should prompt a fundamental change in the regimen that causes reduced insulin action, increased glucose availability, or both at the time of the earlier episode. Otherwise, the likelihood of another episode of severe hypoglycemia is high.[41,48] With a history of hypoglycemia unawareness, a 2- to 3-week trial of scrupulous avoidance of hypoglycemia is advisable because that may restore awareness.[29–32] When that was incorporated into a structured educational program, approximately half of the patients reported restored awareness of hypoglycemia 1 year later.[63] Finally, a history of nocturnal hypoglycemia, late postexercise hypoglycemia, or both should prompt regimen adjustments that reduce insulin action, increase glucose availability, or both at the appropriate time.

TREATMENT OF HYPOGLYCEMIA IN T1DM
Oral Self-Treatment

Most episodes of asymptomatic or symptomatic hypoglycemia are effectively self-treated with glucose tablets or carbohydrate containing juice, soft drinks, candy, other snacks, or a meal by the person with T1DM[1,2] (20 g, repeated in 15 to 20 minutes if necessary, is a reasonable dose of carbohydrate).[64] Because the glycemic response is transient,[64] a subsequent more substantial snack or meal is generally advisable.

Parenteral Treatment

When hypoglycemic patients are unable or, because of neuroglycopenia, unwilling to take carbohydrate orally, parenteral therapy is necessary. That is often glucagon injected subcutaneously or intramuscularly by an associate of a patient who has been trained to recognize severe hypoglycemia and treat it with glucagon. The usual glucagon dose of 1.0 mg in adults causes substantial, albeit transient, hypergly-cemia[64] and can cause nausea or even vomiting. Smaller doses (eg, 150 μg), repeated if necessary, have been found effective without side effects in adolescents with T1DM.[65] Glucagon is ineffective in glycogen-depleted individuals (eg, after a binge of alcohol ingestion). Intravenous glucose (25 g initially) is the standard parenteral therapy in a medical setting. Because the response is transient, a subsequent intrave-nous glucose infusion is usually needed and a meal should be provided as soon as a patient is able to ingest it.

SUMMARY OF RECOMMENDATIONS

Because mean glycemia as close to the nondiabetic range as can be accomplished safely is in the best interest of patients with T1DM, it follows that caregivers should attempt to match insulin actions and circulating glucose availability at all times under all conditions so as to avoid severe hypoglycemia, hypoglycemia unawareness, and intolerable symptomatic hypoglycemia while maintaining a meaningful degree of gly-cemic control. Thus, the following are recommended (the strength of the evidence for these recommendations is *A* for randomized controlled trials and meta-analysis and *B* for other evidence):

1. Acknowledge the problem of hypoglycemia in T1DM (B)
2. Apply the principles of aggressive glycemic therapy
   - Patient education and empowerment (B)
   - Frequent SMBG (and in some instance continuous glucose sensing) (B)
   - Flexible and appropriate insulin (and other) regimens, including insulin analogs (A) and consideration of the special issues of nocturnal and early and late post-exercise hypoglycemia (B)
   - Individualized glycemic goals (B)
   - Ongoing professional guidance and support (B)
3. Consider the conventional risk factors for hypoglycemia in T1DM.
   - Insulin dose, timing, and type (A)
   - Glucose influx is decreased or efflux is increased (B)
   - Sensitivity to insulin is increased or glucose clearance is decreased (B)
4. Consider the risk factors for HAAF in T1DM.
   - The degree of endogenous insulin deficiency (B)
   - A history of severe hypoglycemia, hypoglycemia unawareness, or both as well as any relationship with recent antecedent hypoglycemia, prior exercise, or sleep (B)
   - Lower HbA1C levels (A).

Although the approach to the problem of hypoglycemia will likely become more successful as more is learned about the mechanisms of hypoglycemia in T1DM, elim-ination of hypoglycemia from the lives of people with T1DM will probably be accom-plished by the development of new treatment methods that provide plasma glucose–regulated insulin replacement or secretion.

ACKNOWLEDGMENTS

The author is grateful for the contributions of postdoctoral fellows and the skilled nursing, technical, dietary, and data management/statistical assistance of the staff of the Washington University General Clinical Research Center. Janet Dedeke prepared this manuscript.

REFERENCES

1. Cryer PE. The barrier of hypoglycemia in diabetes. Diabetes 2008;57(12): 3169–76.
2. Cryer PE. Hypoglycemia in diabetes. Pathophysiology, prevalence and prevention. Alexandria (VA): American Diabetes Association; 2009.
3. The Diabetes Control and Complications Trial Research Group. The effect of intensive treatment of diabetes on the development and progression of long-term complications in insulin-dependent diabetes mellitus. N Engl J Med 1993; 329(14):977–86.
4. Diabetes Control and Complications Trial/Epidemiology of Diabetes Interventions and Complications (DCCT/EDIC) Study Research Group. Intensive diabetes treatment and cardiovascular disease in patients with type 1 diabetes. N Engl J Med 2005;353(25):2643–53.
5. Juvenile Diabetes Research Foundation Continuous Glucose Monitoring Study Group. The effect of continuous glucose monitoring in well-controlled type 1 diabetes. Diabetes Care 2009;32(8):1378–83.
6. Raju B, Arbelaez AM, Breckenridge SM, et al. Nocturnal hypoglycemia in type 1 diabetes: an assessment of preventive bedtime treatments. J Clin Endocrinol Metab 2006;91(6):2087–92.
7. DeRosa MA, Cryer PE. Hypoglycemia and the sympathoadrenal system: neurogenic symptoms are largely the result of sympathetic neural, rather than adrenomedullary, activation. Am J Physiol Endocrinol Metab 2004;287(1):E32–41.
8. Towler DA, Havlin CE, Craft S, et al. Mechanism of awareness of hypoglycemia. Perception of neurogenic (predominantly cholinergic) rather than neuroglycopenic symptoms. Diabetes 1993;42(12):1791–8.
9. Boyle PJ, Schwartz NS, Shah SD, et al. Plasma glucose concentrations at the onset of hypoglycemic symptoms in patients with poorly controlled diabetes and in nondiabetics. N Engl J Med 1988;318(23):1487–92.
10. Amiel SA, Sherwin RS, Simonson DC, et al. Effect of intensive insulin therapy on glycemic thresholds for counterregulatory hormone release. Diabetes 1988;37(7): 901–7.
11. Cryer PE. Hypoglycemia, functional brain failure, and brain death. J Clin Invest 2007;117(4):868–70.
12. Heller SR. Sudden death and hypoglycaemia. Diabetic Hypoglycemia 2008;1(2): 2–7. Available at: www.hypodiab.com. Accessed October 10, 2008.
13. Adler GK, Bonyhay I, Failing H, et al. Antecedent hypoglycemia impairs autonomic cardiovascular function: implications for rigorous glycemic control. Diabetes 2009;58(2):360–6.
14. Diabetes Control and Complications Trial/Epidemiology of Diabetes Interventions and Complications Study Research Group. Long-term effect of diabetes and its treatment on cognitive function. N Engl J Med 2007;356(18):1842–52.
15. Feltbower RG, Bodansky HJ, Patterson CC, et al. Acute complications and drug misuse are important causes of death for children and young adults with type 1 diabetes: results from the Yorkshire Register of diabetes in children and young adults. Diabetes Care 2008;31(5):922–6.
16. Skrivarhaug T, Bangstad HJ, Stene LC, et al. Long-term mortality in a nationwide cohort of childhood-onset type 1 diabetic patients in Norway. Diabetologia 2006; 49(2):298–305.
17. American Diabetes Association Workgroup on Hypoglycemia. Defining and reporting hypoglycemia in diabetes. Diabetes Care 2005;28(5):1245–9.

18. Cryer PE. Preventing hypoglycaemia: what is the appropriate glucose alert value? Diabetologia 2009;52(1):35–7.
19. Cryer PE. The prevention and correction of hypoglycemia. In Handbook of physiology. Section 7, The endocrine system. In: Jefferson LS, Cherrington AD, editors, The endocrine pancreas and regulation of metabolism, vol. II. New York: Oxford University Press; 2001. p. 1057–92.
20. Cryer PE. Mechanisms of sympathoadrenal failure and hypoglycemia in diabetes. J Clin Invest 2006;116(6):1470–3.
21. Dagogo-Jack SE, Craft S, Cryer PE. Hypoglycemia-associated autonomic failure in insulin-dependent diabetes mellitus. J Clin Invest 1993;91(3):819–28.
22. Gerich JE, Langlois M, Noacco C, et al. Lack of glucagon response to hypoglycemia in diabetes: evidence for an intrinsic pancreatic alpha cell defect. Science 1973;182(108):171–3.
23. Raju B, Cryer PE. Loss of the decrement in intraislet insulin plausibly explains loss of the glucagon response to hypoglycemia in insulin-deficient diabetes. Diabetes 2005;54(3):757–64.
24. Cooperberg BA, Cryer PE. Beta-cell-mediated signaling predominates over direct alpha-cell signaling in the regulation of glucagon secretion in humans. Diabetes Care 2009;32(12):2275–80.
25. Heller SR, Cryer PE. Reduced neuroendocrine and symptomatic responses to subsequent hypoglycemia after 1 episode of hypoglycemia in nondiabetic humans. Diabetes 1991;40(2):223–6.
26. White NH, Skor DA, Cryer PE, et al. Identification of type I diabetic patients at increased risk for hypoglycemia during intensive therapy. N Engl J Med 1983; 308(9):485–91.
27. Bolli GB, De Feo P, De Cosmo S, et al. A reliable and reproducible test for adequate glucose counterregulation in type I diabetes mellitus. Diabetes 1984; 33(8):732–7.
28. Geddes J, Schopman JE, Zammitt NN, et al. Prevalence of impaired awareness of hypoglycaemia in adults with Type 1 diabetes. Diabet Med 2008; 25(4):501–4.
29. Fanelli CG, Epifano L, Rambotti AM, et al. Meticulous prevention of hypoglycemia normalizes the glycemic thresholds and magnitude of most of neuroendocrine responses to, symptoms of, and cognitive function during hypoglycemia in intensively treated patients with short-term IDDM. Diabetes 1993;42(11): 1683–9.
30. Fanelli C, Pampanelli S, Epifano L, et al. Long-term recovery from unawareness, deficient counterregulation and lack of cognitive dysfunction during hypoglycaemia, following institution of rational, intensive insulin therapy in IDDM. Diabetologia 1994;37(12):1265–76.
31. Cranston I, Lomas J, Maran A, et al. Restoration of hypoglycaemia awareness in patients with long-duration insulin-dependent diabetes. Lancet 1994;344(8918): 283–7.
32. Dagogo-Jack S, Rattarasarn C, Cryer PE. Reversal of hypoglycemia unawareness, but not defective glucose counterregulation, in IDDM. Diabetes 1994; 43(12):1426–34.
33. Arbelaez AM, Powers WJ, Videen TO, et al. Attenuation of counterregulatory responses to recurrent hypoglycemia by active thalamic inhibition: a mechanism for hypoglycemia-associated autonomic failure. Diabetes 2008;5(2):470–5.
34. Cryer PE, Davis SN, Shamoon H. Hypoglycemia in diabetes. Diabetes Care 2003; 26(6):1902–12.

35. The Diabetes Control and Complications Trial Research Group. Epidemiology of severe hypoglycemia in the diabetes control and complications trial. Am J Med 1991;90(4):450–9.
36. Davis S, Alonso MD. Hypoglycemia as a barrier to glycemic control. J Diabetes Complications 2004;18(1):60–8.
37. Rossetti P, Porcellati F, Bolli GB, et al. Prevention of hypoglycemia while achieving good glycemic control in type 1 diabetes: the role of insulin analogs. Diabetes Care 2008;31(Suppl 2):S113–20.
38. Gonder-Frederick LA, Fisher CD, Ritterband LM, et al. Predictors of fear of hypoglycemia in adolescents with type 1 diabetes and their parents. Pediatr Diabetes 2006;7(4):215–22.
39. The UK, Hypoglycaemia Study Group. Risk of hypoglycaemia in types 1 and 2 diabetes: effects of treatment modalities and their duration. Diabetologia 2007; 50(6):1140–7.
40. Cox DJ, Kovatchev B, Koev D, et al. Hypoglycemia anticipation, awareness and treatment training (HAATT) reduces occurrence of severe hypoglycemia among adults with type 1 diabetes mellitus. Int J Behav Med 2004;11(4):212–8.
41. Cox DJ, Gonder-Frederick L, Ritterband L, et al. Prediction of severe hypoglycemia. Diabetes Care 2007;30(6):1370–3.
42. Juvenile Diabetes Research Foundation Continuous Glucose Monitoring Study Group. Continuous glucose monitoring and intensive treatment of type 1 diabetes. N Engl J Med 2008;359(14):1464–76.
43. Hirsch IB. Insulin analogues. N Engl J Med 2005;352(2):174–83.
44. Gough SCL. A review of human and analogue insulin trials. Diabetes Res Clin Pract 2007;77(1):1–15.
45. Fatourechi MM, Kudva YC, Murad MH, et al. Hypoglycemia with intensive insulin therapy: a systematic review and meta-analyses of randomized trials of continuous subcutaneous insulin infusion versus multiple daily injections. J Clin Endocrinol Metab 2009;94(3):729–40.
46. Bolli GB, Kerr D, Thomas R, et al. Comparison of a multiple daily insulin injection regimen (basal once-daily glargine plus mealtime lispro) and continuous subcutaneous insulin infusion (lispro) in type 1 diabetes: a randomized open parallel multicenter study. Diabetes Care 2009;32(7):1170–6.
47. Mukhopadhyay A, Farrell T, Fraser RB, et al. Continuous subcutaneous insulin infusion vs intensive conventional insulin therapy in pregnant diabetic women: a systematic review and metaanalysis of randomized, controlled trials. Am J Obstet Gynecol 2007;197(5):447–56.
48. The Diabetes Control and Complications Trial Research Group. Hypoglycemia in the Diabetes Control and Complications Trial. Diabetes 1997; 46(2):271–86.
49. Tsalikian E, Mauras N, Beck RW, et al. Impact of exercise on overnight glycemic control in children with type 1 diabetes mellitus. J Pediatr 2005;147(4): 528–34.
50. Jones TW, Porter P, Sherwin RS, et al. Decreased epinephrine responses to hypoglycemia during sleep. N Engl J Med 1998;338(23):1657–62.
51. Banarer S, Cryer PE. Sleep-related hypoglycemia-associated autonomic failure in type 1 diabetes: reduced awakening from sleep during hypoglycemia. Diabetes 2003;52(5):1195–203.
52. Schultes B, Jauch-Chara K, Gais S, et al. Defective awakening response to nocturnal hypoglycemia in patients with type 1 diabetes mellitus. PLoS Med 2007;4(2):e69.

53. Cooperberg BA, Breckenridge SM, Arbelaez AM, et al. Terbutaline and the prevention of nocturnal hypoglycemia in type 1 diabetes. Diabetes Care 2008; 31(12):2271–2.

54. Ertl AC, Davis SN. Evidence for a vicious cycle of exercise and hypoglycemia in type 1 diabetes mellitus. Diabetes Metab Res Rev 2004;20(2):124–30.

55. Tansey MJ, Tsalikian E, Beck RW, et al. The effects of aerobic exercise on glucose and counterregulatory hormone concentrations in children with type 1 diabetes. Diabetes Care 2006;29(1):20–5.

56. MacDonald MJ. Postexercise late-onset hypoglycemia in insulin-dependent diabetic patients. Diabetes Care 1987;10(5):584–8.

57. Sandoval DA, Guy DL, Richardson MA, et al. Effects of low and moderate antecedent exercise on counterregulatory responses to subsequent hypoglycemia in type 1 diabetes. Diabetes 2004;53(7):1798–806.

58. Cryer PE, Axelrod L, Grossman AB, et al. Evaluation and management of adult hypoglycemic disorders: an Endocrine Society Clinical Practice Guideline. J Clin Endocrinol Metab 2009;94(3):709–28.

59. American Diabetes Association. Standards of medical care in diabetes–2009. Diabetes Care 2009;32(Suppl 1):S13–61.

60. Skyler JS, Bergenstal R, Bonow RO, et al. Intensive glycemic control and the prevention of cardiovascular events: implications of the ACCORD, ADVANCE, and VA diabetes trials. Diabetes Care 2009;32(1):187–92.

61. Lachin JM, Genuth S, Nathan DM, et al. Effect of glycemic exposure on the risk of microvascular complications in the diabetes control and complications trial: revisited. Diabetes 2008;57(4):995–1001.

62. Huang ES, Zhang Q, Gandra N, et al. The effect of comorbid illness and functional status on the expected benefits of intensive glucose control in older patients with type 2 diabetes: a decision analysis. Ann Intern Med 2008;149(1): 11–9.

63. Hopkins D, Lawrence I, Mansell P, et al. Routine structured education reduces HbA1C and hypoglycemia and improves psychological health in patients with type 1 diabetes mellitus [abstract]. Diabetes 2008;57(Suppl 1):A37.

64. Wiethop BV, Cryer PE. Alanine and terbutaline in treatment of hypoglycemia in IDDM. Diabetes Care 1993;16(8):1131–6.

65. Haymond MW, Schreiner B. Mini-dose glucagon rescue for hypoglycemia in children with type 1 diabetes. Diabetes Care 2001;24(4):643–5.

Update on Transplanting Beta Cells for Reversing Type 1 Diabetes

R. Paul Robertson, MD

KEYWORDS

- Pancreas transplantation • Islet transplantation
- Type 1 diabetes • Beta cells

HISTORY OF PANCREAS AND ISLET TRANSPLANTATION

The first successful pancreas transplantation in two patients with type 1 diabetes mellitus was reported by Kelly and colleagues[1] from the University of Minnesota in 1967. One patient had postoperative complications, underwent removal of the graft, and soon thereafter died of pulmonary embolism. The other patient became normoglycemic within 6 days and remained so for 6 months. Not many more procedures were performed until 1978. By this time progress was being made because of improved surgical techniques for the procedure and the introduction of dramatically improved immunosuppressive regimens (cyclosporine and anti–T-cell agents) and selection of healthier recipients. From the 1980s through the early 2000s, clinical outcomes of pancreas transplantation steadily improved so that the procedure compared favorably with the results of other solid organ transplant procedures. Today graft survival rates after 3 years are generally in the range of 70% to 80% and patient survival rates are 90% or better (**Fig. 1**).[2] The history for islet transplantation is shorter. The first successful attempts also took place at the University of Minnesota and involved transplanting islets in patients who had undergone total pancreatectomy followed by crude isolation and then infusion of their islets into the liver via the portal venous route.[3] No immunosuppressive drugs were administered because this procedure involved autotransplantation rather than allotransplantation of islets. By 1995, the success rate for autoislet transplants (defined as insulin independence) was reported to be 74% for greater than 2 years post transplant if more than 300,000 islets (the normal pancreas is usually thought to contain 1,000,000 islets) were used for the infusion.[4] Attempts to render type 1 diabetic recipients insulin independent using the same approach were

This work was supported by Grant No. NIDDK RO1 39994 from the National Institutes of Health.
Division of Endocrinology and Metabolism, Pacific Northwest Diabetes Research Institute, University of Washington, 720 Broadway, Seattle, WA 98122, USA
E-mail address: rpr@pnri.org

Endocrinol Metab Clin N Am 39 (2010) 655–667
doi:10.1016/j.ecl.2010.05.010
0889-8529/10/$ – see front matter © 2010 Elsevier Inc. All rights reserved.

endo.theclinics.com

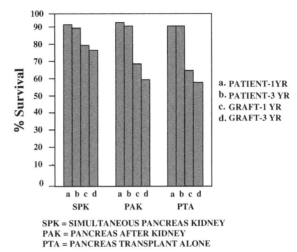

a. PATIENT-1YR
b. PATIENT-3 YR
c. GRAFT-1 YR
d. GRAFT-3 YR

SPK = SIMULTANEOUS PANCREAS KIDNEY
PAK = PANCREAS AFTER KIDNEY
PTA = PANCREAS TRANSPLANT ALONE

Fig. 1. Contemporary graft and recipient survival rates 1 and 3 years post pancreas transplant. (*Data from* Gruessner AC, Sutherland DE. Pancreas transplant outcomes for United States (US) and non-US cases as reported to the United Network for Organ Sharing (UNOS) and the International Pancreas Transplant Registry (IPTR) as of October 2002. Clin Transpl 2002:41–77.)

with alloislets largely unsuccessful until 2000 when Shapiro and colleagues[5] reported success in seven consecutive recipients at an average of 1 year post transplant in a series using an average of two islet infusions and a corticosteroid-free immunosuppressive regimen.

GRAFT SURVIVAL RATES

The most common approaches to pancreas transplantation are simultaneous pancreas and kidney (SPK), pancreas after kidney, and pancreas transplantation alone procedures in which the pancreas is placed into the pelvis. There the graft receives arterial blood supply from the iliac artery and its venous drainage is by a connection to the femoral vein of the recipient. This leads to a state of hyperinsulinemia because the normal first-pass hepatic catabolism of insulin is absent due to systemic drainage of the allograft by the femoral vein.[6] No adverse effects of this arrangement, however, have been reported. If anything, levels of lipids in transplant recipients are favorably affected, with lower levels of triglycerides and low-density lipoprotein cholesterol.[7–9] Exocrine products from a segment of the donor duodenum still attached to the allograft is used for drainage of exocrine pancreatic products into the urinary bladder or small bowel of the recipient. Graft survival rates have improved over time and vary with the type of transplantation procedure (see **Fig. 1**).[2] SPK graft survival rates are 70% to 80% at 3 years post transplantation, whereas pancreas after kidney and pancreas transplantation alone rates are generally 10% lower. The reasons for this may be that SPK is the procedure most commonly used and, therefore, the most familiar. A benefit of simultaneous kidney transplantation is that postoperative serum creatinine levels are used to monitor for early rejection, which results in antirejection treatment that also benefits the transplanted pancreas. Graft rejection rates for pancreatic islets are much more of a problem. The 100% success rate reported by the Edmonton group in 2000 deteriorated to 64% by 2 years[10] and 8% by 5 years

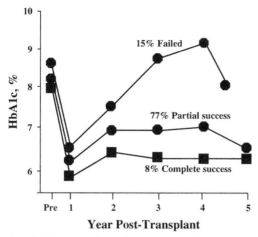

Fig. 2. Success rates for alloislet transplantation in type 1 diabetic recipients at the University of Alberta, Canada, up to 5 years post transplant. Complete success is defined as normal or nearly normal levels of HbA$_{1c}$ and not using insulin for treatment for diabetes. Partial success is defined as evidence for circulating C-peptide levels with use of insulin for treatment with good glycemic control. Failure is defined as lack of circulating C peptide and use of insulin for treatment with modest control of glycemia. (*Data from* Ryan EA, Paty BW, Senior PA, et al. Five-year follow-up after clinical islet transplantation. Diabetes 2005;54:2060–9.)

postoperatively (**Fig. 2**).[11] A large fraction of the recipients in this series, however, continued to have measurable levels of C peptide, indicating partial islet fraction despite the need for exogenous insulin treatment to control levels of hemoglobin A$_{1c}$ (HbA$_{1c}$). The corresponding data at 2 and 5 years for C-peptide positivity were 86% and 85%, respectively.[10,11] These C-peptide positive patients were also using appreciably less exogenous insulin for glucose management and were having many fewer hypoglycemic reactions. This interesting outcome is open to interpretation. One possibility is that some of the recipients who were having difficulties with hypoglycemia pretransplant were being overtreated with insulin and then became better managed (ie, used less insulin) after returning to insulin post transplant. Alternatively, another possibility is that the residually functioning islets were providing meaningful amounts of insulin and thereby contributing substantially to glycemic control. Subsequent information from publications by the Immune Tolerance Network and other groups of investigators using the Edmonton protocol for islet transplantation reported similar findings.[12–17]

PATIENT SURVIVAL RATES AND COMPLICATIONS OF TRANSPLANTATION

Patient survival rates for pancreas transplantation are generally greater than 90% 3 years post transplantation (see **Fig. 1**).[2] The steepest portion of the mortality curve is during the first several months after the procedure. It is unusual, however, for death to occur perioperatively or even within 3 months of transplantation. The unanswered question is what the death rate would be over 3 years in a group of diabetic patients with similar degrees of complications of the disease. This illustrates a fundamental problem with interpretation of studies of pancreas and, for that matter, islet transplantation. All series are basically uncontrolled, observational studies with no randomized or matched patient groups that correct for complications of diabetes independent of surgery. It is clear, however, that serious complications are encountered after pancreas transplantation. This is not a surprise nor is it unexpected that some of these problems are more likely in the setting of a patient with a serious chronic disease, such as diabetes, and with the added complication of systemic immunosuppression. A partial list of complications includes graft thrombosis; surgical wound infections; systemic infections; leakage of enteric secretions; graft pancreatitis, pseudocysts, and fistulas; intra-abdominal bleeding; and complications of immunosuppression, primarily increased prevalence of skin malignancies. Metabolic bone disease has been a major problem with older recipients who were treated with glucocorticoids chronically. The practice today is to avoid as much as possible using glucocorticoids for immunosuppression. The range of complications for islet transplantation is not nearly as extensive, which is one of the distinct advantages of this less-invasive procedure. Nonetheless, the initial series experienced bleeding and thrombosis episodes associated with hepatic puncture with the metal cannula used to advance the tubing intrahepatically for islet infusion.[5] Insufficient experience has been reported to calculate a meaningful mortality rate for islet transplantation, although no deaths have occurred among 325 recipients in the immediate peritransplantation period.[18]

PANCREAS AND ISLET CELL FUNCTION POST TRANSPLANT

Successful pancreas transplantation restores normal levels of fasting glucose and HbA_{1c} in a large majority of recipients (**Fig. 3**).[19] Should the graft fail, both values again rise into the diabetic range and insulin treatment is again given. Occasionally, pancreas graft failure is partial and recipients are treated as though they have type 2 diabetes mellitus. The reason for such good glycemic control in successful recipients is that glucose-induced insulin secretion is fully restored[6] and the acute insulin response to intravenous glucose correlates inversely with the fasting glucose level as seen in the normal and marginally diabetic populations.[19] Glucagon secretion, whose primary stimulus is hypoglycemia, is typically absent in type 1 diabetic subjects because this response is dependent on the presence of neighboring beta cells to provide an intraislet switch-off signal for glucagon release.[20,21] After pancreas transplantation, glucagon secretion during hypoglycemia from the allograft

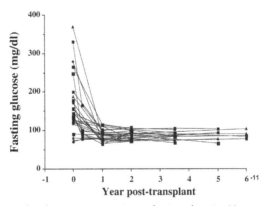

Fig. 3. Fasting glucose levels pre–pancreas transplant and up to 11 years post transplant in type 1 diabetic recipients. (*Data from* Robertson RP. Consequences on β-cell function and reserve after long-term pancreas transplantation. Diabetes 2004;53:633–44.)

fully restores this critical counterregulatory response (**Fig. 4**).[22] This response in turn stimulates glucose production by the liver, resulting in full counterregulation of low glucose levels as seen in nondiabetic individuals. In addition, the abnormally low epinephrine response to hypoglycemia typical of type 1 diabetes mellitus is improved and adds another important counterregulatory force directed toward restoration of normal glucose levels (**Fig. 5**).[22] From the recipients' point of view, the most gratifying results of successful pancreas transplantation is the return of symptom awareness for hypoglycemia (see **Fig. 5**). Patients who are recurrently hypoglycemic due to excessive insulin therapy lose their ability to recognize hypoglycemia via the usual symptoms of warmth, sweating, hunger, and decreased environmental awareness. This situation can be rectified by avoidance of hypoglycemia for 2 weeks. Replacement of exogenous insulin therapy by pancreas transplantation provides physiologic insulin secretion that virtually ceases when glucose levels reach the hypoglycemia range. This prevents hypoglycemia and restores symptom awareness of this condition. Pancreas transplantation can be especially valuable for the subgroup of diabetic patients who have autonomic nervous system dysfunction and gastroparesis because they are especially at risk for insulin-induced hypoglycemia. Successful islet transplantation also restores glucose-induced insulin secretion and achieves normal or nearly normal levels of fasting glucose and HbA_{1c},[5] thus removing the need for exogenous insulin treatment as well as recurrent hypoglycemia. Unlike pancreas transplantation, however, which clinically seems to work well or not work at all when the allograft undergoes rejection, islet transplantation seems to have a more complex range of outcomes in the range between complete success and complete failure. As indicated by the description of the results of the Edmonton and other trials (described previously), many recipients of islet transplants have partial successes (or partial failures) and remain C-peptide positive. These individuals usually again require

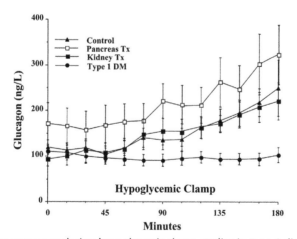

Fig. 4. Glucagon responses during hypoglycemic clamp studies in type 1 diabetic pancreas transplant recipients compared with nontransplanted type 1 diabetic subjects, nondiabetic control subjects, and nondiabetic kidney transplant subjects receiving the same immunosuppressive drugs as the pancreas transplant recipients. The glucagon responses in the normal control group and the pancreas transplantation group are virtually identical. Tx, transplant. (*Data from* Kendall DM, Rooney DP, Smets YF, et al. Pancreas transplantation restores epinephrine response and symptom recognition during hypoglycemia in patients with long-standing type I diabetes and autonomic neuropathy. Diabetes 1997;46:249–57.)

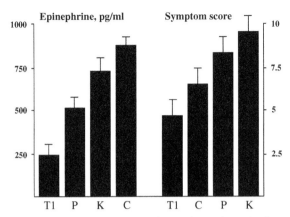

Fig. 5. Epinephrine and symptom responses during hypoglycemic clamp studies in the same groups referenced in **Fig. 4**. C, nondiabetic control group; K, kidney transplant group; P, pancreas transplant group; T1, type 1 diabetic group.

insulin treatment but many require much less than insulin they used previously and have many fewer episodes of hypoglycemia. In the context of hypoglycemia, an important difference between pancreas and islet transplants has been reported regarding alpha cell function. Whereas the alpha cells in the pancreas allograft secrete glucagon normally during hypoglycemia, the alpha cells in intrahepatic islet transplants do not (**Fig. 6**).[23,24] This is not due to damaged alpha cells, because intrahepatic islets have normal glucagon responses to intravenous arginine injection.[23] The reason for nonresponse to hypoglycemia has been reported to be due to increased intrahepatic glucose flux, especially during times of hypoglycemia and increased glucose production. This explanation suggests that the increased glucose levels in the environment of the transplanted islets blinds the intraislet alpha cells to

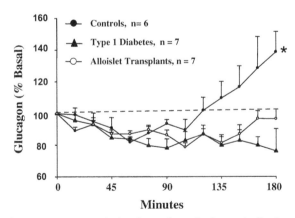

Fig. 6. Absent glucagon responses during hypoglycemic clamp studies in successful type 1 diabetic recipients of alloislet transplantation. (*From* Paty B, Ryan E, Shapiro AM, et al. Intrahepatic islet transplantation in type 1 diabetic patients does not restore hypoglycemic hormonal counterregulation or symptom recognition after insulin independence. Diabetes 2002;51(12):3428–34.)

the hypoglycemic signal it receives via the pancreatic arterioles during systemic hypoglycemia.[25]

IMPACT ON SECONDARY COMPLICATIONS OF DIABETES

Resolution of dysglycemia in patients with type 1 diabetes mellitus via successful pancreas and islet transplantation provides immediate relief from abnormal glucose excursions and the need for exogenous insulin treatment. More long-term benefits also accrue. The major secondary complications of diabetes can involve eyes, kidneys, nerves, blood vessels, and quality of life. Tight control of blood glucose levels by exogenous insulin results in decreased prevalence of these adverse outcomes.[26] Successful pancreas transplantation has been reported to have beneficial effects on eye disease. Although early studies failed to find retinal benefits,[27–29] more recently a study by Koznarova and colleagues[30] indicated that successful SPK versus successful kidney alone transplantation was associated with improved retinal outcomes. Inclusion of a pancreas in the transplant procedure was accompanied by significantly less retinal deterioration and less need for laser therapy in the group receiving a pancreas (**Fig. 7**).[30] Abnormal changes in kidneys that are specific to diabetes include decreased glomerular function and increased mesangium. Normal kidneys that are transplanted into diabetic recipients develop the same abnormalities as native kidneys, hence, the attractiveness of the SPK procedure, which has better kidney outcomes if the pancreas functions well. Fioretto and colleagues[31] reported results from native kidney biopsies showing marked decrease in basement membrane thinckening and glomerular mass 10 years after successful pancreas transplantation (**Fig. 8**). Motor and sensory neuropathies are the bane of many diabetic patients. Successful pancreas transplantation has consistently been associated with stabilization of neuropathies.[32–35] The work of Navarro and colleagues demonstrated arrest in

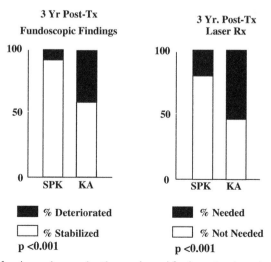

Fig. 7. Impact on fundoscopic examination and need for laser treatment of retinas in simultaneous kidney and pancreas versus kidney transplant recipients. The pancreas transplant group had less deterioration of fundoscopic examination and less need for laser treatment 3 years post transplant. KA, kidney alone; Rx, therapy; Tx, transplant. (*Data from* Koznarova R, Saudek F, Sosna T, et al. Beneficial effect of pancreas and kidney transplantation on advanced diabetic retinopathy. Cell Transplant 2000;9:903–8.)

Pre- transpl.   5 yrs. Post-transpl.   10 yrs. Post-transpl.

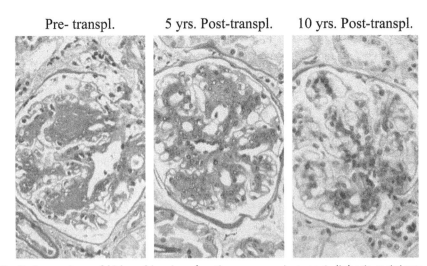

Fig. 8. Comparison of kidney biopsies of native pancreas in type 1 diabetic recipients of pancreas transplantation before, 5-years, and 10 years post transplant. The increased basement membrane thickness and increased mesangium characteristic of type 1 diabetes mellitus that was present pretransplant was still present at 5 years post transplant but greatly decreased at 10 years post transplant. (*Adapted from* Fioretto P, Steffes MW, Sutherland DE, et al. Reversal of lesions of diabetic nephropathy after pancreas transplantation. N Engl J Med 1998;339:69–75; with permission.)

progression of neuropathies by physical examination, motor and nerve conduction studies, and measurement of cardiorespiratory reflexes for 10 years post transplant.[32] Jukema and colleagues[36] have provided data indicating that successful pancreas transplantation stabilizes and in some cases reverses macrovascular disease in the carotid artery (**Fig. 9**). Many quality-of-life studies have been conducted in recipients

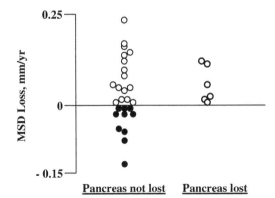

Fig. 9. Patency of coronary arteries in type 1 diabetic recipients of pancreas transplantation improved in 10 (*solid circles*) of 26 subjects retaining grafts for an average of 4 years. (*Data from* Jukema JW, Smets YF, van der Pijl JW, et al. Impact of simultaneous pancreas and kidney transplantation on progression of coronary atherosclerosis in patients with endstage renal failure due to type 1 diabetes. Diabetes Care 2002;25:906–11.)

of a transplanted pancreas.[37–39] Recipients consistently report that they prefer having had the surgery and the ongoing immunosuppression as the price for returning to normoglycemia and the avoidance of further secondary complications, especially hypoglycemia, as opposed to returning to insulin therapy. These results are independent of whether or not a kidney is included with the pancreas transplant. Not surprisingly, the patients who had worse quality of life before pancreas transplantation are more likely to improve their lives after transplantation. A particular case in point is the patient group with autonomic nervous system dysfunction. This subgroup has a particularly poor quality of life because of postural hypotension, diabetic diarrhea, gastroparesis, and recurrent, severe hypoglycemia. The later is related to gastroparesis, which results in highly variable transit of ingested food into the small bowel and consequent erratic absorption. This situation makes it almost impossible for patients to accurately estimate their insulin needs, which makes them at increased risk for hypoglycemia. Most sobering is the estimated death rate after this diagnosis has been made (ie, approximately 50% mortality 5 years post diagnosis). After successful pancreas transplantation, this figure changes to 10% mortality.[32] Many fewer data are available regarding chronic complications and quality of life before and after islet transplantation, and generally speaking, in the studies available, less time has elapsed between since islet transplantation was performed. A recent study published by Fiorina and colleagues,[40] however, reports long-term beneficial effect of islet transplantation on diabetic macro-/microangiopathy in type 1 diabetic kidney-transplanted patients. Toso and colleagues[41] have reported that quality of life, primarily relief of fear of hypoglycemia, improves after islet transplantation in proportion to the number of islet infusions received. Pancreas and islet transplantation are not considered as options for children because of the concern about immunosuppression intensifying their expected encounters with childhood infectious diseases. Autoislet transplantation in children undergoing pancreatectomy for pancreatitis, however, is not uncommon because they do not need immunosuppressive drugs.

PROBLEMS WITH IMMUNOSUPPRESSIVE DRUGS

Systemic immunosupression is required for organs and tissues from one human to thrive after transplantation to another human. The only exception to this rule is transplantation between identical twins.[42] Recipients undergo induction of immunosuppression a short time before the transplantation procedure and their immunosuppressed state is maintained thereafter by chronic administration of various drugs. All of the many drugs developed have significant side effects. A complete description of these is beyond the scope of this article. Independent of which drugs are used, however, the immunosuppressed state is generally associated with clinical problems. Chief among these are recurrent bacterial, viral, and fungal infections and the possibility of developing cancer, chiefly dermatologic. The beta cell itself is a special case. The therapeutic irony is that these drugs, which are given to protect transplanted pancreas and islets from undergoing rejection, also often have deleterious effects on beta cell function and insulin sensitivity. In particular, corticoids, cyclosporine, and tacrolimus have been associated with decreased insulin gene expression, insulin synthesis, and insulin secretion.[43] Sirolimus and mycophenolate mofetil have been associated with decreased insulin synthesis. This issue is exaggerated in the case of intrahepatic islet transplantation because the drugs are taken orally and after absorption develop high circulating concentrations in the liver.

PROBLEMS WITH TRANSPLANTATION SITES

From the beginning, the pelvic site for pancreas and kidney transplantation has been deemed satisfactory. The selection of the intrahepatic site for islet transplantation came from the original work of Kemp and colleagues.[44] They were the first to demonstrate that islet transplantation could regulate glucose levels in rodents made diabetic by streptozotocin. They also compared various transplantation sites and concluded that the liver was the most desirable. Since then, this has been the site favored for islet auto- and alloislet transplantation. The hepatic site has limitations, however. One of these is the need to puncture the liver transcutaneously to insert a catheter within the hepatic portal venous system, for islet infusion, which not infrequently is associated with intrahepatic bleeding and thrombosis. Another is the high concentration of toxins ingested from the environment, which is higher in the liver than in the systemic blood because of detoxification by the liver before entering the general circulation. The same is true for some immunosuppressive drugs that are taken orally and can be toxic for beta cell function. Another drawback from using the liver it that it prevents glucagon release from intrahepatic islets during hypoglycemia (discussed previously). These facts have led some to explore alternative sites (mostly in animals) for use, such as celiac artery, intravenous access to lung, intrapancreas, intramuscular, subcutaneous, thymus, testis, intracisterna magna, omental pouches, bowel surfaces, peritoneal cavity, spleen, bone marrow, and kidney capsule.[45]

PROBLEMS WITH SUPPLY AND DEMAND

The largest barrier to use of pancreas and islet transplantation is the seemingly insoluble problem that not enough Americans volunteer to be organ donors. It has been estimated that only approximately 6000 pancreases are available each year, and that perhaps 4000 might be suitable for pancreas and islet transplantation. That number dwindles further when complications are encountered during procurement and transportation of organs to transplantation sites. Approximately 1000 pancreas transplants and 750 islet infusions (an average of two for each recipient) are performed annually. Consequently, at best, both procedures could possibly be performed only twice as often. This has led to a great deal of pressure to identify beta cell surrogates that can be used rather than human islets. These include islets from animals, beta cell lines, and stem cells, none of which can currently be used. This problem led to the development of the successful use of pancreatic segments from living, related donors has been ongoing for several decades, mostly at the University of Minnesota. In this procedure, the donor undergoes hemipancreatectomy (distal pancreas) in a surgical suite adjoining another suite where the recipient is prepared for transplantation of the donated segment. Patient and graft survival rates are similar to those when whole pancreas transplantation is used. The additional benefits are that the donor, who is extensively tested for normal pancreatic islet function before the procedure, is nearby. Consequently, the recipient receives much fresher tissue that generally occurs compared to usage of an organ donated by an unknown donor who may be at a distance from the hospital site where the transplantation occurs. Testing of donors also provides relatively accurate assurance that they will not develop diabetes post donation. The best estimates are that one-half a healthy pancreas is fully capable of meeting the metabolic endocrine and exocrine needs of a donor. The only caveat is that donors must know to remain nonobese so they do not develop resistance to the action of insulin and consequent hyperglycemia.[46] If insulin resistance develops, donors can develop mild diabetes that requires treatment with oral agents or insulin, much like patients with type 2 diabetes mellitus.

SUMMARY

Successful beta cell replacement in humans with type 1 diabetes mellitus has been possible for over several decades by pancreas and more recently by pancreatic islet transplantation. Both are capable of restoring normoglycemia without exogenous insulin therapy and both have patient survival rates that are consistent with other organ transplantation procedures. Currently, transplanted pancreases have a longer survival rate that islets, but that may in large part be because islet transplantation became consistently successful at least 20 years later than was the case for pancreas transplantation. Both procedures restore normal glucose-induced insulin secretion, but only the transplanted pancreas restores hypoglycemia-induced glucagon secretion by virtue of the fact that islets are transplanted in the liver. Pancreas transplantation is accompanied by stabilization or improvement in the secondary complications of diabetes that involve eyes, kidneys, nerves, and large blood vessels. Initial reports suggest that these benefits may also accrue after islet transplantation, even if only partial success is achieved long term. Both procedures are followed by improvements in quality of life. The future goal is to discover suitable beta cell surrogates because of the problem of supply and demand for beta cell replacement of organs and islets.

REFERENCES

1. Kelly WD, Lillehei RC, Merkel FK, et al. Allotransplantation of the pancreas and duodenum along with the kidney in diabetic nephropathy. Surgery 1967;61: 827–37.
2. Gruessner AC, Sutherland DE. Pancreas transplant outcomes for United States (US) and non-US cases as reported to the United Network for Organ Sharing (UNOS) and the International Pancreas Transplant Registry (IPTR) as of October 2002. Clin Transpl 2002;41–77.
3. Najarian JS, Sutherland DE, Baumgartner D, et al. Total or near total pancreatectomy and islet autotransplantation for treatment of chronic pancreatitis. Ann Surg 1980;192:526–42.
4. Wahoff DC, Papalois BE, Najarian JS, et al. Autologous islet transplantation to prevent diabetes after pancreatic resection. Ann Surg 1995;222:562–75 [discussion: 575–69].
5. Shapiro AM, Lakey JR, Ryan EA, et al. Islet transplantation in seven patients with type 1 diabetes mellitus using a glucocorticoid-free immunosuppressive regimen. N Engl J Med 2000;343:230–8.
6. Diem P, Abid M, Redmon JB, et al. Systemic venous drainage of pancreas allografts as independent cause of hyperinsulinemia in type I diabetic recipients. Diabetes 1990;39:534–40.
7. La Rocca E, Secchi A, Parlavecchia M, et al. Lipid metabolism after successful kidney and pancreatic transplantation. Transplant Proc 1991;23:1672–3.
8. Larsen JL, Stratta RJ, Ozaki CF, et al. Lipid status after pancreas-kidney transplantation. Diabetes Care 1992;15:35–42.
9. Katz HH, Nguyen TT, Velosa JA, et al. Effects of systemic delivery of insulin on plasma lipids and lipoprotein concentrations in pancreas transplant recipients. Mayo Clin Proc 1994;69:231–6.
10. Ryan EA, Lakey JR, Paty BW, et al. Successful islet transplantation: continued insulin reserve provides long-term glycemic control. Diabetes 2002;51:2148–57.
11. Ryan EA, Paty BW, Senior PA, et al. Five-year follow-up after clinical islet transplantation. Diabetes 2005;54:2060–9.

12. Shapiro AM, Ricordi C, Hering BJ, et al. International trial of the Edmonton protocol for islet transplantation. N Engl J Med 2006;355:1318–30.

13. Froud T, Ricordi C, Baidal DA, et al. Islet transplantation in type 1 diabetes mellitus using cultured islets and steroid-free immunosuppression: Miami experience. Am J Transplant 2005;5:2037–46.

14. Toso C, Baertschiger R, Morel P, et al. Sequential kidney/islet transplantation: efficacy and safety assessment of a steroid-free immunosuppression protocol. Am J Transplant 2006;6:1049–58.

15. O'Connell PJ, Hawthorne WJ, Holmes-Walker DJ, et al. Clinical islet transplantation in type 1 diabetes mellitus: results of Australia's first trial. Med J Aust 2006; 184:221–5.

16. Cure P, Pileggi A, Froud T, et al. Improved metabolic control and quality of life in seven patients with type 1 diabetes following islet after kidney transplantation. Transplantation 2008;85:801–12.

17. Deng S, Markmann JF, Rickels M, et al. Islet alone versus islet after kidney transplantation: metabolic outcomes and islet graft survival. Transplantation 2009;88:820–5.

18. CITR Research Group. 2007 Update on allogeneic islet transplantation from the Collaborative Islet Transplant Registry (CITR). Cell Transplant 2009;18:753–67.

19. Robertson RP. Long-term pancreas transplantation: consequences on beta cell function and reserve. Diabetes 2004;53:633–45.

20. Banarer S, McGregor VP, Cryer PE. Intraislet hyperinsulinemia prevents the glucagon response to hypoglycemia despite an intact autonomic response. Diabetes 2002;51:958–65.

21. Zhou H, Tran PO, Yang S, et al. Regulation of alpha-cell function by the beta-cell during hypoglycemia in Wistar rats: the "switch-off" hypothesis. Diabetes 2004; 53:1482–7.

22. Kendall DM, Rooney DP, Smets YF, et al. Pancreas transplantation restores epinephrine response and symptom recognition during hypoglycemia in patients with long-standing type I diabetes and autonomic neuropathy. Diabetes 1997;46: 249–57.

23. Paty B, Ryan E, Shapiro AM, et al. Intrahepatic islet transplantation in type 1 diabetic patients does not restore hypoglycemic hormonal counterregulation or symptom recognition after insulin independence. Diabetes 2002;51(12):3428–34.

24. Rickels MR, Schutta MH, Mueller R, et al. Islet cell hormonal responses to hypoglycemia after human islet trasnplatation for type 1 diabetes. Diabetes 2006;54: 3206–11.

25. Zhou H, Zhang T, Bogdani M, et al. Intrahepatic glucose flux as a mechanism for defective intrahepatic islet alpha-cell response to hypoglycemia. Diabetes 2008; 57:1567–74.

26. DCCT Research Group. The effect of intensive treatment of diabetes on the development and progression of long-term complications in insulin-dependent diabetes mellitus. N Engl J Med 1993;329:977–85.

27. Ramsay RC, Goetz FC, Sutherland DE, et al. Progression of diabetic retinopathy after pancreas transplantation for insulin-dependent diabetes mellitus. N Engl J Med 1988;318:208–14.

28. Petersen MR, Vine AK. University of Michigan Pancreas Transplant Evaluation Committee: progression of diabetic retinopathy after pancreas transplantation. Ophthalmology 1990;97:496–502.

29. Scheider A, Meyer-Schwickerath E, Nusser J, et al. Diabetic retinopathy and pancreas transplantation: a 3-year follow-up. Diabetologia 1991;34(Suppl 1): S95–9.

30. Koznarova R, Saudek F, Sosna T, et al. Beneficial effect of pancreas and kidney transplantation on advanced diabetic retinopathy. Cell Transplant 2000;9:903–8.
31. Fioretto P, Steffes MW, Sutherland DE, et al. Reversal of lesions of diabetic nephropathy after pancreas transplantation. N Engl J Med 1998;339:69–75.
32. Navarro X, Kennedy WR, Loewenson RB, et al. Influence of pancreas transplantation on cardiorespiratory reflexes, nerve conduction, and mortality in diabetes mellitus. Diabetes 1990;39:802–6.
33. Aridge D, Reese J, Niehoff M, et al. Effect of successful renal and segmental pancreatic transplantation on peripheral and autonomic neuropathy. Transplant Proc 1991;23:1670–1.
34. Gaber AO, Cardoso S, Pearson S, et al. Improvement in autonomic function following combined pancreas-kidney transplantation. Transplant Proc 1991;23:1660–2.
35. Allen RD, Al-Harbi IS, Morris JG, et al. Diabetic neuropathy after pancreas transplantation: determinants of recovery. Transplantation 1997;63:830–8.
36. Jukema JW, Smets YF, van der Pijl JW, et al. Impact of simultaneous pancreas and kidney transplantation on progression of coronary atherosclerosis in patients with end-stage renal failure due to type 1 diabetes. Diabetes Care 2002;25:906–11.
37. Zehrer CL, Gross CR. Comparison of quality of life between pancreas/kidney and kidney transplant recipients: 1-year follow-up. Transplant Proc 1994;26:508–9.
38. Piehlmeier W, Bullinger M, Nusser J, et al. Quality of life in type 1 (insulin-dependent) diabetic patients prior to and after pancreas and kidney transplantation in relation to organ function. Diabetologia 1991;34(Suppl 1):S150–7.
39. Barrou B, Baldi A, Bitker MO, et al. Pregnancy after pancreas transplantation: report of four new cases and review of the literature. Transplant Proc 1995;27:3042–4.
40. Fiorina P, Folli F, Bertuzzi F, et al. Long-term beneficial effect of islet transplantation on diabetic macro-/microangiopathy in type 1 diabetic kidney-transplanted patients. Diabetes Care 2003;26:1129–36.
41. Toso C, Shapiro AM, Bowker S, et al. Quality of life after islet transplant: impact of the number of islet infusions and metabolic outcome. Transplantation 2007;84:664–6.
42. Sibley RK, Sutherland DE, Goetz F, et al. Recurrent diabetes mellitus in the pancreas iso- and allograft. A light and electron microscopic and immunohistochemical analysis of four cases. Lab Invest 1985;53:132–44.
43. Robertson RP. Islet transplantation as a treatment for diabetes – a work in progress. N Engl J Med 2004;350:694–705.
44. Kemp CB, Knight MJ, Scharp DW, et al. Effect of transplantation site on the results of pancreatic islet isografts in diabetic rats. Diabetologia 1973;9:486–91.
45. Merani S, Toso C, Emamaullee J, et al. Optimal implantation site for pancreatic islet transplantation. Br J Surg 2008;95:1449–61.
46. Robertson RP, Lanz KJ, Sutherland DE, et al. Relationship between diabetes and obesity 9 to 18 years after hemipancreatectomy and transplantation in donors and recipients. Transplantation 2002;73:736–41.

Index

Note: Page numbers of article titles are in **boldface** type.

A

A1c. See *Hemoglobin A1c (HbA1c).*
Absenteeism, with type 1 diabetes mellitus, 506–508
Adaptive neural network algorithm, for closed-loop systems, in type 1 diabetes mellitus management, 618–619
Adhesives, for continuous glucose monitors, 612
Age, type 1 diabetes mellitus development and, 484
Alarms, in closed-loop systems, for type 1 diabetes mellitus management, 617–618
Albumin excretion test, urine, for diabetic nephropathy, 632
Algorithms, control, for closed-loop systems, in type 1 diabetes mellitus management, 617–619
Alleles, in type 1 diabetes mellitus, nonobese diabetic mouse model vs. human, 548–552
    loci mapping of, 541, 544–547, 549–551
Alloislet transplantation. See *Islet transplantation.*
American Diabetes Association (ADA), blood pressure control recommendations of, 633–634
    hypoglycemia definition of, 642–643
    insulin therapy terminology of, 597
    retinopathy screening recommendations of, 629
American Diabetes Association (ADA) 2007 study, on type 1 diabetes mellitus, cost of illness data from, 501–502, 504, 506
    mortality data from, 507
Angiotensin II receptor blocker (ARB), for hypertension, with type 1 diabetes mellitus, 634
Angiotensin-converting (ACE) inhibitor, for hypertension, with type 1 diabetes mellitus, 634
Animal models, of disease, 541
    of type 1 diabetes mellitus. See also *Nonobese diabetic (NOD) mouse model.*
    intestinal microbiota and, 566–567
Antibodies, in autoimmunity, type 1 diabetes mellitus risk related to.
    See *Islet autoantibodies.*
    monoclonal, for type 1 diabetes mellitus, 531–532, 535
        nonobese diabetic mice preclinical trials on, 552–553
Anti-CD3, for type 1 diabetes mellitus, 531
    nonobese diabetic mice preclinical trials of, 552
Anti-CD20, for type 1 diabetes mellitus, 531
Anti-CD25, for type 1 diabetes mellitus, 531–532
Anticonvulsants, for diabetic peripheral neuropathy, 635–636
Antigen-presenting cells (APCs), in type 1 diabetes mellitus, nonobese diabetic mouse model vs. human, 548

Endocrinol Metab Clin N Am 39 (2010) 669–695
doi:10.1016/S0889-8529(10)00059-9
0889-8529/10/$ – see front matter © 2010 Elsevier Inc. All rights reserved.

endo.theclinics.com

Antigens, in type 1 diabetes mellitus, nonobese diabetic mouse model vs. human, 542–543
    risk prediction with, 516–518. See also *Islet autoantibodies.*
        cell-mediated immunity vs., 521
        early vs. late autoimmunization to, 519–520
        immune response profiles in, 520–521
        need for multiple, 517–518
        nonobese diabetic mouse model and, 543, 548
        progression patterns of, 521
Antigen-specific therapies, for type 1 diabetes mellitus, 517, 530–533
Anti-thymocyte globulin (ATG), for type 1 diabetes mellitus, 532–533
    granulocyte colony-stimulating factor with, 533
Artificial pancreas (AP), components of, 610
  control algorithms for, 617–619
Assays, for forensic prediction, of type 1 diabetes mellitus, high-quality, for quantifiable
    signals and diverse analytes, 516–517
      specificity and disease relevance of, 517–518
      target or cognate autoantigens in, 517, 553
Autoantibodies, type 1 diabetes mellitus risk related to. See *Islet autoantibodies.*
Autoimmune disease, type 1 diabetes mellitus as, beta cells and, **527–539**. See also
  Beta cell destruction.
    combined risk biomarkers of, 518–519
    for cost of illness analysis, 502–503
    genetic markers of, 514–516
    intestinal mucosal barrier–microbial interaction and, 566–568
    islet autoantibodies and, 516–518
    natural history of, 519–521
Autoislet transplantation, 664
Autonomic failure, in type 1 diabetes mellitus, glucose counter-regulation associated with,
    642–643, 645
        pancreas and islet transplantation impact on, 659–661
      hypoglycemia-associated, 645–646
Autonomic neuropathy, diabetic, biochemical and molecular pathways of, 626–627
    management of, 636
    occurrence of, 634
    screening for, 634–635

B

B cell response, in type 1 diabetes mellitus. See *Beta cell function/response.*
B2m molecule, in type 1 diabetes mellitus, 550
Bacille Calmette–Guérin (BCG), for type 1 diabetes mellitus, 530
Bacteria, intestinal, functions of, 564–565
    type 1 diabetes mellitus relationship to, **563–571**. See also *Microbiome.*
Basal insulin, 597–598
  contemporary regimens for, 582–583
  in aggressive glycemic therapy, 647
  inpatient management of, 599, 602, 605
Bayes' theorem, of clinical diagnosis, 517
Beta cell destruction, in type 1 diabetes mellitus, **527–539**
    intervention strategies for, anti-CD3 as, 531
      anti-CD20 as, 531

anti-CD25 as, 531–532
anti-thymocyte globulin as, 532–533
    granulocyte colony-stimulating factor with, 533
cell therapies as, 533–534
cytotoxic T-lymphocyte antigen-4 immunoglobulin as, 532
mycofenolate mofetil as, 531–532
nonobese diabetic mice preclinical trials on, 552–553
prevention vs., 527–530
using past lessons for future predictions, 534–536
islet autoimmunity response of, 520. See also *Islet autoantibodies.*
prevention strategies for, glutamic acid decarboxylase 65 as, 530
    insulin as, 529–530
    intervention vs., 527–529
    nonobese diabetic mice preclinical trials on, 552–553
    using past lessons for future predictions, 534–536
Beta cell function/response, in type 1 diabetes mellitus, defective glucose
    counter-regulation and, 643–645
        pancreas and islet transplantation impact on, 659–661
    nonobese diabetic mouse model vs. human, 542–543, 548
    risk prediction based on, 516
    SQ sensor–SQ insulin delivery system vs., 610. See also *Closed-loop system.*
Beta cell regeneration therapies, for type 1 diabetes mellitus, 535
Beta cell transplantation, for type 1 diabetes mellitus, **655–667**
    cellular function following, 658–661
    closed-loop system applications in, 619
    complications of, 657–658
    graft survival rates of, 656–657
    history of, 655–656
    immunosuppressive drug problems with, 663
    impact on secondary complications, 661–663
    patient survival rates of, 657
    summary overview of, 665
    supply and demand problems with, 664
    transplantation site problems with, 664
Biobreeding diabetes-prone (BBDP) rat model, of type 1 diabetes mellitus, intestinal
    microbiota alterations and, 566–567
        intestinal mucosal barrier–microbial interaction and, 566–568
Biochemical pathways, of type 1 diabetes mellitus-related damage, 626–627
Birth month, type 1 diabetes mellitus onset patterns related to, 486–487
Blood glucose level, pancreas and islet transplantation impact on, 658–661
    with type 1 diabetes mellitus, 641. See also *Hyperglycemia; Hypoglycemia.*
Blood glucose monitors/monitoring, for type 1 diabetes mellitus, 586–587
    contemporary meter designs for, 586–587
    continuous. See *Continuous glucose monitors/monitoring (CGM).*
    home techniques for, 490
    insulin pump therapy and, 585. See also *Closed-loop system.*
    lag time between readings and continuous glucose monitor readings, 611
    multidisciplinary team for, 574
    self-management with, during inpatient stay, 601
        hypoglycemia thresholds for, 642–643
        oral glucose supplements for, 649

Blood glucose (*continued*)
    self-monitoring component of, 586–587
        aggressive glycemic therapy and, 647
Blood pressure, in type 1 diabetes mellitus management, nephropathy prevention and, 633–634
    recommendations for, 576, 578
Body mass index (BMI), in type 1 diabetes mellitus, insulin therapy consideration of, 582, 584
Bolus, of insulin, 599
Brain failure, functional, with hypoglycemia, 642

    C

C peptide, in pancreas and islet transplantation, 619, 657, 659
Carbohydrates, for type 1 diabetes mellitus, 585–586
    as hypoglycemia treatment, 649
    closed-loop systems calculation of, 609, 619
    insulin ratio to, 598
Cardiovascular disease (CVD), as type 1 diabetes mellitus complication, 636–637
    autonomic neuropathy and, 635–636
    biochemical and molecular pathways of, 626–627
    evaluation of, 636–637
    incidence of, 636
    management of, 636–637
    pancreas and islet transplantation impact on, 662–663
    scope of, 489–490, 626, 636
    target ranges for care of, 574, 576, 578
Case management. See *Intensive case management.*
CD4+ T cells, in type 1 diabetes mellitus, nonobese diabetic mouse model vs. human, 543, 548
CD8+ T cells, in type 1 diabetes mellitus, nonobese diabetic mouse model vs. human, 543, 548
Celiac disease, with type 1 diabetes mellitus, 577
Cell therapies, for type 1 diabetes mellitus, 533–534
Cell-mediated immunity, in type 1 diabetes mellitus risk prediction, 521
    nonobese diabetic mice studies on, 553
Chance, in type 1 diabetes mellitus prediction, 515
Children, with type 1 diabetes mellitus, insulin analogues for, inpatient considerations with, 606
    meta-analyses of health outcomes of, 575, 579, 581
    target glucose values for, 600–601
    target HbA1c goals for, 609–610
Chronic kidney disease (CKD), with type 1 diabetes mellitus, stages of, 632, 634
Clinical diagnosis, of type 1 diabetes mellitus, Bayes' theorem applied to, 517
    month of, birth month patterns related to, 486–487
Closed-loop system, for type 1 diabetes mellitus management, **609–624**
    aggressive glycemic therapy and, 647
    continuous subcutaneous insulin infusion in, control algorithms for, 617–619
        delivery system for, infusion sets in, 617
            insulins in, 617
            overcoming challenges of, 616

patient education on, 616
pumps in, 615–616
future applications of, 619
limitations of current technology for, 610, 612
need for, 609–610
subcutaneous sensor in, 610–612
clinical pointers in use of, 613–614
patient education on, 614–615
summary overview of, 619–620
Cognate autoantigens, in type 1 diabetes mellitus risk prediction, 517
Combination insulin preparations, for type 1 diabetes mellitus, contemporary regimens for, 582–583
inpatient management of, 598
pharmacodynamic profiles of, 579, 596–597
Combination therapies, for reversal of type 1 diabetes mellitus, 531–532, 535
Complications, of pancreas and islet transplantation, 657–658
of type 1 diabetes mellitus, **625–640**
beta cell transplantation impact on, 661–663
biochemical pathways of damage, 626–627
blood sugar imbalances as. See *Hyperglycemia; Hypoglycemia.*
cardiovascular disease as, 636–637
costs of, 506
macrovascular, 636–637
medical costs of, 506
metabolic memory and, 627–628
microvascular, 628–636
molecular pathways of damage, 626–627
multidisciplinary team for, 574, 576–578
nephropathy as, 626, 630–634
neuropathy as, 626, 634–636
prevalence of, 489–490
retinopathy as, 626, 628–630
summary overview of, 625–626
Continuous glucose monitors/monitoring (CGM), for type 1 diabetes mellitus, 489–490, 610
accuracy of real-time, 611, 619
advantages of, 613
artificial pancreas and, 610
lag time between blood glucose readings and, 611
limitations of, 609–610
multidisciplinary team for, 574
overcoming challenges with, 614
self-monitoring component of, 586–587
for aggressive glycemic therapy, 647
subcutaneous sensor for, 610–612
clinical pointers in use of, 613–614
patient education on, 614–615
Continuous subcutaneous insulin infusion (CSII). See also *Insulin pump therapy.*
for type 1 diabetes mellitus, control algorithms for, 617–619
delivery system for, 610, 615–617. See also *Closed-loop system.*
infusion sets in, 617
insulins in, 617

Continuous subcutaneous (*continued*)
      overcoming challenges of, 616
      patient education on, 616
      pumps in, 615–616
   future applications of, 619
   inpatient management of, 599, 601–602, 604
   perioperative management of, 604
Control algorithms, for closed-loop systems, in type 1 diabetes mellitus management, 617–619
Control-to-range algorithm, for closed-loop systems, in type 1 diabetes mellitus management, 618
Conventional insulin therapy (CIT), 598
Coronary artery disease (CAD), as type 1 diabetes mellitus complication, 636
      pancreas and islet transplantation impact on, 662–663
Correction factor, 598
Correction insulin, 597–598
   perioperative use of, 604
   standard order sets for, 605
Cost of illness (COI) analysis, of type 1 diabetes mellitus, 500–509
      clinically derived definitions for, 503
      data availability for, 500–502
      description of, 500
      methods for estimating, 500–501
      patient identification for, 502–504
Cost-benefit analysis (CBA), of type 1 diabetes mellitus, 500
Cost-effectiveness analysis (CEA), of type 1 diabetes mellitus, 500
Cost-utility analysis (CUA), of type 1 diabetes mellitus, 500
Counter-regulation, of glucose, in type 1 diabetes mellitus. See *Glucose counter-regulation.*
C-peptide, in type 1 diabetes mellitus, 527, 530–531, 536, 553
      insulin regimens and, 583
Critically ill patients, with type 1 diabetes mellitus, closed-loop systems for, 619
      increase in insulin requirements with, 598, 602
      target glucose values for, 599–600
      transition from IV to SC insulin for, 604–605
CTLA-4 gene, in type 1 diabetes mellitus, 549, 551
Cytokines, in type 1 diabetes mellitus, intestinal mucosal barrier–microbial interaction and, 567–568
Cytotoxic T-lymphocyte antigen-4 immunoglobulin (CTLA-4), for type 1 diabetes mellitus, 532
      nonobese diabetic mice preclinical trials of, 552–553
Cytotoxic T-lymphocytes, in type 1 diabetes mellitus, interventions targeted at, 532
      nonobese diabetic mouse model vs. human, 543, 548

D

Daclizumab, for type 1 diabetes mellitus, 532
Data availability, for cost of illness analysis, on type 1 diabetes mellitus, 501–502
Decision tree approach, to type 1 diabetes mellitus risk prediction, 518–519
Dendritic cells (DCs), in type 1 diabetes mellitus, intestinal microbiota and, 568
      nonobese diabetic mouse model vs. human, 542, 548
      therapeutic applications of, 534

Dental examination, for type 1 diabetes mellitus, 577
Diabetes care team, for type 1 diabetes mellitus, 574, 585, 647, 649
Diabetes Control and Complications Trial (DCCT), type 1 diabetes mellitus findings of,
    488–490
        complications development and, 627–628
        HbA1c targets from, 626
        insulin therapy and, 582–584
        nutrition therapy and, 586
Diabetes mellitus (DM), latent autoimmune, cost of illness analysis of, 503
    "pre-type 1," prevention strategies for, 527–530
    type 1. See *Type 1 diabetes mellitus (T1D)*.
    type 2. See *Type 2 diabetes mellitus (T2D)*.
Diabetic ketoacidosis (DKA), with type 1 diabetes mellitus, in nonobese diabetic
    mouse model vs. human, 542
        inpatient management of, 595–596, 603–604
        insulin pump therapy and, 584–585
        sliding scale for insulin for, 598
Diagnostic month, of type 1 diabetes mellitus onset, birth month patterns related to,
    486–487
DIAMOND Project, on type 1 diabetes mellitus, 482–483
Diamyd. See *Glutamic acid decarboxylase 65 (GAD65)*.
Diet education, for type 1 diabetes mellitus, 585–586
        hypertension and, 633
Dietary Approaches to Stop Hypertension (DASH), 633–634
Disability costs, of type 1 diabetes mellitus, 507–508
Discharge planning, for type 1 diabetes mellitus, 606
Diuretics, for hypertension, with type 1 diabetes mellitus, 634
DNA analysis, of intestinal microbes, type 1 diabetes mellitus and, 563, 566–567
Duloxetine, for diabetic peripheral neuropathy, 636
Dyslipidemia, as type 1 diabetes mellitus complication, 490
        target ranges for care of, 576, 578

E

Economics, of type 1 diabetes mellitus, **499–512**
        cost of illness in, 500–509
            data availability for, 500–502
            description of, 500
            methods for estimating, 500–501
            patient identification for, 502–504
        general evaluation components for, 500
        indirect costs in, 506–508
        lifetime costs in, 508–509
        medical costs in, 504–506
        summary overview of, 499–500, 509–510
Education, for type 1 diabetes mellitus, on continuous glucose monitoring system,
    614–615
        on continuous subcutaneous insulin infusion, 616
        on diet, 585–586
            hypertension and, 633
        on glycemic control therapy, 647

Empowerment, of patient, for glycemic control, in type 1 diabetes mellitus, 647
Endothelial damage, with type 1 diabetes mellitus, 626–627
Environmental factors, of type 1 diabetes mellitus development, 487
    genetic risk markers and, 514–515
    islet autoimmunity and, 520–521
    microbes as, **563–571**. See also *Microbiome.*
Epidemiology, of type 1 diabetes mellitus, **481–497**
    age and, 484
    and retinopathy, 630
    clinical course trends, 488
    environmental factors, 487
        genetic risk markers and, 514–515
        islet autoimmunity and, 520–521
    gender and, 484
    genotype and, 486
    incidence of, 482–483
        temporal trends in, 483–484
    nutritional factors, 487
    prevalence of, 483
    prevalence of complications, 489–490
    race/ethnicity and, 484–486
    seasonality of onset and birth, 486–487
    summary overview of, 481–482, 490–491
    treatment and management trends, 488–489
Epistatic interactions, of alleles, in type 1 diabetes mellitus, nonobese diabetic
    mouse model vs. human, 551–552
Erectile dysfunction, with type 1 diabetes mellitus, 635–636
Euglycemia, 641
EUROBIAB ACE study, on type 1 diabetes mellitus, 482–484
Excercise-induced hypoglycemia, with type 1 diabetes mellitus, 648
Eye disease, with type 1 diabetes mellitus. See *Retinopathy.*

F

Family history, in type 1 diabetes mellitus risk prediction, 514–515, 519
Foot care, for type 1 diabetes mellitus, 577
Forensic prediction, of type 1 diabetes mellitus, 516–518
    assay specificity and disease relevance in, 517–518
    quantifiable signals and diverse analytes requiring high-quality assays in, 516–517
    target or cognate autoantigens in, 517, 553

G

Gabapentin, for diabetic peripheral neuropathy, 635–636
GAD65 autoantibodies, type 1 diabetes mellitus risk related to, 516
    early vs. late autoimmunization and, 520
    immune response patterns in, 520
Gastrointestinal (GI) tract, immune system of, microbiota and, 564–565.
    See also *Microbiome.*
        mucosa and. See *Mucosal immune system.*
        type 1 diabetes mellitus and, 565–566

neuropathies of, with type 1 diabetes mellitus, 635–636
  pancreas and islet transplantation impact on, 659, 663
Gender, type 1 diabetes mellitus development and, 484
Genes/genotype, of type 1 diabetes mellitus, as risk markers, 515–516
  for cardiovascular disease, 637
  development related to, 486–487
  nonobese diabetic mouse model of, 548–552
    insulin-dependent diabetes loci and, 541, 544–547, 549–551
Genetic markers, of type 1 diabetes mellitus risk, 514–516
  family history in, 514–515, 519
  major genes in, 515–516
Genitourinary tract disturbances, with type 1 diabetes mellitus, 635–636
Genome, human, evolution into superorganism, 564–565
Genome-wide association studies (GWASs), of type 1 diabetes mellitus, 548–552
  nonobese diabetic mouse model vs. human loci mapping with, 541, 544–547, 549–551
Glomerular filtration rate (GFR), in diabetic nephropathy, 632, 634, 661
Glucagon injection, for hypoglycemia, in type 1 diabetes mellitus, 649–650
Glucagon response, in type 1 diabetes mellitus, pancreas and islet transplantation impact on, 658–661
  with defective glucose counter-regulation, 643–645
Glucocorticoid-induced hyperglycemia, inpatient management of, 600, 603–605
Glucose control. See also *Glycemic control.*
  tight, clinical trials of, 595–596
    closed-loop systems for, 619
Glucose counter-regulation, in type 1 diabetes mellitus, pancreas and islet transplantation impact on, 659–661
  pathophysiology of, 643–646
    autonomic failure associated with, 643, 645
      hypoglycemia-associated, 645–646
      risk factors for, 642, 646
    defective, schematic diagram of, 643, 645
      with unawareness, 643, 645
        acknowledgment of, 646–647
  physiology of, 643–644
Glucose infusions, for hypoglycemia, in type 1 diabetes mellitus, 650
Glucose level. See *Blood glucose level.*
Glucose monitoring. See *Blood glucose monitors/monitoring.*
Glucose tablets, for hypoglycemia, in type 1 diabetes mellitus, 649
Glucotoxicity, prevention of continued, closed-loop systems for, 619
Glutamic acid decarboxylase 65 (GAD65), for type 1 diabetes mellitus prevention, 530
  in autoimmunity. See *GAD65 autoantibodies.*
Glycation end products, advanced, vascular damage related to, in type 1 diabetes mellitus, 627
Glycemic control, for type 1 diabetes mellitus, 488–489
  aggressive principles for, flexible and appropriate insulin regimens as, 647–648
    frequent blood glucose monitoring as, 647
    individualized goals as, 648–649
    ongoing professional guidance and support as, 574, 585, 647, 649
    patient education and empowerment as, 647
  cardiovascular disease and, 636–637, 641

Glycemic (*continued*)
    closed-loop system for, **609–624**. See also *Closed-loop system.*
    complications related to, 625–626
    failure factors of, 609–610
    limiting factor in, 641–642
    long-acting insulins and, 579–581
    nephropathy prevention with, 633
    neuropathy prevention with, 635–636
    nutrition and, 585
    pancreas and islet transplantation and, as success factor, 657
        restoration of good, 658–661, 663
    rapid-acting insulins and, 575, 580–581
    reduction of complications and, 489–490
    retinopathy prevention with, 629
    target ranges for, 574, 578
        for adults, 599–600
        for children, 600–601
        subcutaneous insulin adjustments and, 602
        with inpatient management, 599–601
Glycemic thresholds, for symptomatic hypoglycemia, 642
Graft survival rates, with pancreas transplantation, 656–657
Granulocyte colony-stimulating factor (GCSF), for type 1 diabetes mellitus, 533

H

H2-D^{dx} haplotype, in type 1 diabetes mellitus, 550
H2^{g7} haplotype, in type 1 diabetes mellitus, 549–550
H2-K^{wm7} haplotype, in type 1 diabetes mellitus, 550
Haptoglobin (Hp) genotype, cardiovascular disease and, 637
Hemoglobin A1c (HbA1c), in pancreas and islet transplantation, 657, 659
  in type 1 diabetes mellitus management, complications related to, 626–628
    continuous glucose monitoring and, 613
    hypoglycemia and, 646, 648
    inpatient considerations of, 601
    insulin pump therapy and, 583–585
    insulin regimens and, 582–583
    long-acting insulins and, 579–581
    mean, 488–489, 641–642
    nutrition and, 586
    rapid-acting insulins and, 575, 580–581
    target ranges for, 576, 578, 626
        by age group, 609–610
Hemolytic complement, in type 1 diabetes mellitus, nonobese diabetic
    mouse model vs. human, 542
Hepatic portal venous system, for islet transplantation, 664
Hexosamine pathway, of vascular damage, with type 1 diabetes mellitus, 627
History taking, family, in type 1 diabetes mellitus risk prediction, 514–515, 519
HLA DR-DQ genotype, type 1 diabetes mellitus risk related to, 514–515
    as combined biomarker, 518–519
    early autoimmunization and, 519
Home glucose monitoring, for type 1 diabetes mellitus, 490

Hospital inpatient costs, of type 1 diabetes mellitus, 504–506
Human genome, evolution into superorganism, 564–565
Human leukocyte antigens (HLAs), in type 1 diabetes mellitus, genetics of, 548.
    See also *HLA DR-DQ genotype.*
        linkage studies of, 549–550
        intestinal mucosal barrier–microbial interaction and, 567–568
        nonobese diabetic mouse model vs. human, 548
Human life, value of, in costs of type 1 diabetes mellitus, 501
Human Microbiome Project, 563
Humanized mice, for nonobese diabetic mouse model, of type 1 diabetes mellitus, 552
Hyperglycemia, as type 1 diabetes mellitus complication, 595
        continuous insulin infusions and, 599, 601
        glucocorticoids and, 603–605
        inpatient management of, **595–608**. See also *Inpatient management.*
        sliding scale for insulin for, 598
        vascular damage related to, 625–627
Hypertension, as type 1 diabetes mellitus complication, 490
        nephropathy management and, 633–634
Hypoglycemia, in type 1 diabetes mellitus, 490, **641–654**
        definition of, 642–643
        glucose counter-regulation and, pancreas and islet transplantation impact
            on, 658–661
            pathophysiology of, 643–646
                autonomic failure associated with, 645–646
                    risk factors for, 642, 646
                defective, schematic diagram of, 643, 645
                    with unawareness, 643, 645
                        acknowledgment of, 646–647
            physiology of, 643–644
        impacts of, 642
        incidence of, 642
        limiting factor in glycemic control and, 641–642
        management of, 649–650
            insulin pump therapy and, 584
            long-acting insulins and, 579–581
            oral self-treatment, 649
            parenteral treatment, 649–650
            rapid-acting insulins and, 575, 580–581
            reduction strategies in, 489–490
            sliding scale for insulin for, 598
            standard order sets for, 605
            summary of recommendations for, 650
            with inpatient insulin regimens, 595, 602
        minimizing risk of, 646–649
            acknowledge the problem, 646–647
            aggressive glycemic therapy for, 647–649
            consider conventional risk factors, 649
            consider HAAF risk factors, 649
        risk factors for, 646
            associated with autonomic failure, 642, 646
            conventional, 646

Hypoglycemia (*continued*)
    symptomatic episodes of, 642
        pancreas and islet transplantation impact on, 658–661
Hypoglycemia-associated autonomic failure (HAAF), in type 1 diabetes mellitus,
    pathophysiology of, 644–646
      risk factors for, 646
        minimizing, 649

I

IA-2 autoantibodies, type 1 diabetes mellitus risk related to, 516
    early autoimmunization and, 520
Iatrogenic hypoglycemia, with type 1 diabetes mellitus, 641–642, 646
    aggressive glycemic therapy for, 647–648
IDDM12 gene, in type 1 diabetes mellitus, 549
IDDM17 gene, in type 1 diabetes mellitus, 549
IgG autoantibodies, type 1 diabetes mellitus risk related to, 516
    early autoimmunization and, 519
Illness, in type 1 diabetes mellitus patients. See also *Critically ill patients.*
    increase in insulin requirements with, 598, 602, 604
    target glucose values for, 599–600
Immunity, in type 1 diabetes mellitus risk prediction, cell-mediated, 521
    insulin-proinsulin autoimmunity, 519–520
    to islet cells. See *Autoimmune disease; Islet autoantibodies.*
Immunology, of human gastrointestinal tract, microbiota and, 564–565
    type 1 diabetes mellitus and, 565–566
  of type 1 diabetes mellitus, nonobese diabetic mouse model vs. human, 542–543, 548
Immunomodulation therapies, for type 1 diabetes mellitus, 531–532, 534–536
    intestinal microbiota and, 568
    nonobese diabetic mice preclinical trials on, 552–553
Immunosuppressive drugs, for pancreas and islet transplantation, in type 1 diabetes
    mellitus, 663
  for type 1 diabetes mellitus, regimens of, 530, 535
Incidence, of type 1 diabetes mellitus, 482–483
    lifetime costs and, 508–509
    temporal trends in, 483–484
Indirect costs, of type 1 diabetes mellitus, 506–508
    yearly per capita summary of, 507–508
Inflammatory mediators, of intestinal mucosal barrier–microbial interaction,
    in type 1 diabetes mellitus, 567–568
Infusion sets, for continuous subcutaneous insulin infusions, 617
Injection-based regimens, of insulin therapy. See *Multiple daily injection (MDI).*
Inpatient management, of type 1 diabetes mellitus, **595–608**
    adjusting insulin regimen for, 601–602
    children's insulin requirements for, 606
    discharge planning with, 606
    glucocorticoids and, 603–605
    insulin management fundamentals for, 597–598
    insulin orders for, 605
    insulin pharmacokinetics and pharmacodynamics in, 596–597
    intravenous insulin administration for, 597, 603–604

transition to subcutaneous, 604–605
    perioperative insulin recommendations for, 604
    subcutaneous insulin administration for, 596, 598–602
        adjustment of, 601–602
        glycemic goals in, 599–601
        methods of, 598–599
        self-management of, 601
        transition from intravenous, 604–605
    summary overview of, 595–596, 606
    TPN and, 602–603
    tube feedings and, 601, 603
INS gene, in type 1 diabetes mellitus, 549
Insulin analogues, for type 1 diabetes mellitus, 574–575, 579–582
    contemporary regimens for, 582–583
    long-acting, 579, 582. See also *Long-acting insulins.*
    meta-analyses of health outcomes of, in adults, 575, 579–580
        in children, 575, 579, 581
    overview of, 574–575
    pharmacokinetics and pharmacodynamics of, 596–597, 643
        profiles of, 575, 579, 596
    rapid-acting, 575, 579. See also *Rapid-acting insulins.*
Insulin aspart, for type 1 diabetes mellitus, 596
Insulin autoantibodies (IAA), type 1 diabetes mellitus risk related to, 516
    early autoimmunization and, 519–520
    late autoimmunization and, 520
Insulin detemir, 596, 599, 603, 605, 647
Insulin gene, in type 1 diabetes mellitus, 549
Insulin glargine, 596, 599, 605, 647
Insulin glulisine, for type 1 diabetes mellitus, 596
Insulin lispro, for type 1 diabetes mellitus, 596–597
Insulin pump therapy, for type 1 diabetes mellitus, 489–490
    artificial pancreas and, 610
    contemporary management of, 583–585
    continuous subcutaneous. See *Continuous subcutaneous insulin infusion (CSII).*
        closed-loop system for. See *Closed-loop system.*
    inpatient management of, 599
    limitations of, 609–610
    multidisciplinary team for, 574
Insulin pumps, technological features of, 583–584
    continuous subcutaneous, 615–616
Insulin self-management, for type 1 diabetes mellitus, during inpatient stay, 601
    hypoglycemia thresholds for, 642–643
    oral glucose supplements for, 649
Insulin sensitivity factor (ISF), 598
Insulin therapy, for type 1 diabetes mellitus, 488, 490
    analogues for, 574–582
    as prevention strategy, 529–530
    contemporary regimens for, 582–583
    continuous, pumps for. See *Insulin pump therapy.*
        subcutaneous. See *Continuous subcutaneous insulin infusion (CSII).*
    flexible and appropriate, for aggressive glycemic therapy, 647–648

Insulin therapy (*continued*)
  hypoglycemia related to. See *Hypoglycemia.*
  inpatient management of, **595–608**. See also *Inpatient management.*
  intravenous. See *Intravenous insulin administration.*
  nonobese diabetic mice preclinical trials of, 552–553
  self-management during inpatient stay, 601
  sliding scale for, 598
  subcutaneous. See *Subcutaneous insulin administration.*
  terminology for, 597
Insulin-dependent diabetes mellitus 1 (IDDM1). See also *Type 1 diabetes mellitus (T1D).*
  genetics of, 548
    loci mapping, in nonobese diabetic mouse model, 541, 544–547, 549–551
Insulin-proinsulin autoimmunity, 519–520
Insulin-to-carbohydrate (I:C) ratio, 598
Insulitis, in type 1 diabetes mellitus, nonobese diabetic mouse model vs. human,
  542, 553
Intensive case management, for type 1 diabetes mellitus management, 574.
  See also *Critically ill patients.*
    closed-loop systems for, 619
    failure factors of, 609–610
    insulin regimens in, 582–583
    of nephropathy, 633–634
Internal organ sites, for islet transplantation, 664
Intestinal microbiota, functions of, 564–565
  type 1 diabetes mellitus relationship to, **563–571**. See also *Microbiome.*
Intestinal mucosa, immune system of. See *Mucosal immune system.*
Intravenous glucose, for hypoglycemia, in type 1 diabetes mellitus, 650
Intravenous insulin administration, for type 1 diabetes mellitus, inpatient management of,
  597, 603–604
    transition to subcutaneous, 604–605
Islet autoantibodies, in type 1 diabetes mellitus risk prediction, 516–518.
  See also *Autoimmune disease.*
    cell-mediated immunity vs., 521
    early vs. late autoimmunization to, 519–520
    immune response profiles in, 520–521
      nonobese diabetic mouse models and, 543, 548
    need for multiple, 517–518
    prevention and intervention strategies for, **527–539**. See also *Beta cell destruction.*
    progression patterns of, 521
Islet cells, in type 1 diabetes mellitus, destruction of, **527–539**.
  See also *Beta cell destruction.*
    function of. See *Beta cell function/response.*
    regeneration therapies for, 535
    transplantation of, **655–667**. See also *Islet transplantation.*
Islet infusions, post-transplantation, 664
Islet transplantation, for type 1 diabetes mellitus, cellular function following, 658–661
    complications of, 657–658
    history of, 655
    impact on secondary complications, 661–663
    problems with, 663–664
    survival rates with, 656–657

K

Ketotifen, for type 1 diabetes mellitus, 530
Kidney disease, as type 1 diabetes mellitus complication. See *Nephropathy.*
    transplantation for. See *Pancreas after kidney (PAK) transplantation.*
    chronic, stages of, 632, 634

L

Lag time, between blood glucose readings and continuous glucose monitor readings, 611
    for preprandial insulin, 602
Laser photocoagulation, for diabetic retinopathy, 629–630, 661
Latent autoimmune diabetes of the adult (LADA), cost of illness analysis of, vs.
    type 1 diabetes mellitus, 503
Lifetime costs, of type 1 diabetes mellitus, for new cohort of newly diagnosed patients, 509
    incidence- vs. prevalence-based, 508–509
Ligands, of toll-like receptors, intestinal microbiota and, in type 1 diabetes mellitus, 568
Lipid profile, in type 1 diabetes mellitus management, target ranges for, 576, 578
Liver, for islet transplantation, 664
Loci, insulin-dependent diabetes, in nonobese diabetic mouse model, 541, 544–547,
    549–551
Long-acting insulins, for type 1 diabetes mellitus, 579, 582
        contemporary regimens for, 582–583
        inpatient management of, 596, 599
        pharmacodynamic profile of, 575, 579, 596–597
Lymphocyte adhesion molecules, in type 1 diabetes mellitus, intestinal mucosal
    barrier–microbial interaction and, 567–568
Lymphopenia, in type 1 diabetes mellitus, nonobese diabetic mouse model vs. human,
    542–543

M

Macroalbuminuria, in diabetic nephropathy, 631, 633
Macrophages, in type 1 diabetes mellitus, nonobese diabetic mouse model vs. human,
    543, 548
Macrovascular complications, of type 1 diabetes mellitus, 490, 636–637.
    See also *Cardiovascular disease (CVD).*
        biochemical and molecular pathways of, 626–627
        glycemic control and, 636–637, 641
        pancreas and islet transplantation impact on, 662–663
Macular edema, diabetic retinopathy and, 629–630
Major histocompatibility complex (MHC) genotypes, in islet autoimmunity, 518, 520.
    See also *HLA DR-DQ genotype.*
    in type 1 diabetes mellitus, linkage studies of, 549–550
        nonobese diabetic mouse model vs. human, 542–543, 548
Medical claims, cost of illness data from, for type 1 diabetes mellitus, 503–504
Medical costs, of type 1 diabetes mellitus, 504–506
        yearly per capita summary of, 507–508
Medical errors, with insulin, 596
Medical Expenditures Panel Survey (MEPS), cost of illness data from, for type 1 diabetes
    mellitus, 501–503
            medical costs, 504–506

Medical nutrition therapy (MNT), for type 1 diabetes mellitus, 585–586
    closed-loop systems and, 609, 619
Medication costs, of type 1 diabetes mellitus, 504–506
Mesenchymal stem cell (MSC) therapy, for type 1 diabetes mellitus, 534
Messenger RNA (mRNA), in type 1 diabetes mellitus, 551
Metabolic memory, type 1 diabetes mellitus complications and, 627–628
Methodology, for cost of illness analysis, on type 1 diabetes mellitus, 500–501
Microalbuminuria, in diabetic nephropathy, 631, 633
Microbiome, intestinal, type 1 diabetes mellitus relationship to, **563–571**
    functions of, 564
    human superorganism and, 564–565
    microbiota alterations and, 566
    mucosal barrier–microbial interaction and, 566–568
    mucosal immunology and, 565–566
    nutrient interactions and immunity in, 568–569
    probiotics and, 568
    summary overview of, 563–564, 569
Microvascular diseases, as type 1 diabetes mellitus complication, 490, 628–636
    biochemical and molecular pathways of, 626–627
    glycemic control and, 629, 633, 635–636
    nephropathy as, 626, 630–634
    neuropathy as, 626, 634–636
    pancreas and islet transplantation impact on, 661–662
    retinopathy as, 626, 628–630
Mitochondrial reactive oxygen species, in type 1 diabetes mellitus, 550–551
Mitochondrial superoxide overproduction, type 1 diabetes mellitus complications related to, 627
Model predictive control (MPC) algorithm, for closed-loop systems, in type 1 diabetes mellitus management, 618–619
Molecular pathways, of type 1 diabetes mellitus-related damage, 626–627
Monoclonal antibodies, for type 1 diabetes mellitus, 531–532, 535
    nonobese diabetic mice preclinical trials on, 552–553
Mortality, as type 1 diabetes mellitus complication, 490
    ADA data on, 507
    cardiovascular disease and, 637
    cost of illness and, 501, 507–508
    nephropathy and, 631
    pancreas and islet transplantation impact on, 663
    with hypoglycemia, 642
Motor function, type 1 diabetes mellitus impact on, 634, 661. See also *Neuropathy.*
mt-ND2 gene, in type 1 diabetes mellitus, 549–550
mt-Nd2 gene, in type 1 diabetes mellitus, 550
Mucosal immune system, of human gastrointestinal tract, altered microbiota and, 566–567
    barrier–microbial interaction and, 566–568
    microbiota and, 564–565
    type 1 diabetes mellitus and, 565–566
Multidisciplinary team, for type 1 diabetes mellitus management, 574, 585, 647, 649
Multiple daily injection (MDI), of insulin therapy, for type 1 diabetes mellitus, 582–583
    aggressive glycemic therapy and, 647–648
    inpatient management of, 599
    insulin pump therapy vs., 584–585

Mycofenolate mofetil (MMF), for pancreas and islet transplantation, 663
    for type 1 diabetes mellitus, 531–532

N

National Health and Nutrition Examination Survey (NHANES), cost of illness data from,
    for type 1 diabetes mellitus, 502–503
National Health Care Surveys, cost of illness data from, for type 1 diabetes mellitus,
    501–502
National Health Interview Study (NHIS), cost of illness data from, for type 1 diabetes
    mellitus, 502
Natural history, of type 1 diabetes mellitus, **513–525**
        early immunization and, 519–520
        immune response profiles in, 520–521
        late immunization and, 520
        missing pieces in, 521
        prediction of vs., 514–519
        progression patterns in, 521
        summary overview of, 513, 521
Natural killer (NK) cells, in type 1 diabetes mellitus, nonobese diabetic mouse model vs.
    human, 542
Needle-like continuous glucose sensors, 612
Nephropathy, diabetic, 626, 630–634
        biochemical and molecular pathways of, 626–627
        chronic, 632
        management of, 632–634
        intensive blood glucose control for, 633
        intensive blood pressure control for, 633–634
        recommendations for, 576
    occurrence of, 630–631
    pancreas and islet transplantation impact on, 661–662
    screening for, 631–632
    stages of, 630–631
Nervous system complications, of type 1 diabetes mellitus. See *Neuropathy.*
Neural network algorithm, artificial/adaptive, for closed-loop systems, in type 1 diabetes
        mellitus management, 618–619
Neurogenic symptoms, of hypoglycemia, in type 1 diabetes mellitus, 642
Neuroglycopenic symptoms, of hypoglycemia, in type 1 diabetes mellitus, 642
        parenteral treatment of, 649–650
Neuropathy, diabetic, 626, 634–636
        biochemical and molecular pathways of, 626–627
        management of, 635–636
        autonomic neuropathy, 636
        peripheral neuropathy, 635–636
        recommendations for, 577
    occurrence of, 634
    pancreas and islet transplantation impact on, 661–662
    screening for, 634–635
Neutral protamine Hagedorn (NPH) insulin. See *NPH (neutral protamine Hagedorn)*
    insulin.
Nicotinamide, for type 1 diabetes mellitus, 530

Nocturnal hypoglycemia, with type 1 diabetes mellitus, 646–648
    aggressive glycemic therapy for, 647–648
Non–antigen-specific therapies, for type 1 diabetes mellitus, 530
Nonmedical costs, of type 1 diabetes mellitus, 500–501
Nonobese diabetic (NOD) mouse model, of type 1 diabetes mellitus, **541–561**
    genetics in, 548–552
        humanized mice for, 552
        insulin-dependent diabetes loci and, 541, 544–547, 549–551
    human similarities between, 541–542
    immunology and pathology comparisons, 542–543, 548
    intestinal microbiota alterations and, 566–567
    intestinal mucosal barrier–microbial interaction and, 566–567
    loci mapped in, 541, 544–547, 549–551
    preclinical trials and, 552–553
    summary overview of, 541, 553
NPH (neutral protamine Hagedorn) insulin, for type 1 diabetes mellitus, 575, 596
    in aggressive glycemic therapy, 647
    inpatient management of, 599, 603, 605
    perioperative management of, 604
    rapid vs. long acting, 575, 579
NPO status, with type 1 diabetes mellitus, insulin therapy and, 601–604
NRAMP1 gene, in type 1 diabetes mellitus, 549–551
Nursing/residential facility costs, of type 1 diabetes mellitus, 504–506
Nutrition therapy, for type 1 diabetes mellitus, medical, 585–586
        closed-loop systems and, 609, 619
    recommendations for, 576, 578
Nutritional factors, of type 1 diabetes mellitus development, 487
    microbial interactions with, 568–569
Nutritional insulin, 597–598

O

Onset age/month, of type 1 diabetes mellitus, birth month patterns related to, 486–487
    in nonobese diabetic mouse model vs. human, 542
Optimization-based approach, to closed-loop systems control, in type 1 diabetes mellitus
    management, 619
Oral self-treatment, of hypoglycemia, in type 1 diabetes mellitus, 649
Outpatient care costs, of type 1 diabetes mellitus, 504–506

P

Pancreas, artificial, components of, 610
    control algorithms for, 617–619
Pancreas after kidney (PAK) transplantation, for type 1 diabetes mellitus, history of, 655
    impact on secondary complications, 661–663
    problems with, 663–664
    survival rates with, 655–656
Pancreas transplantation alone (PTA), for type 1 diabetes mellitus, cellular function
    following, 658–661
    history of, 655
    impact on secondary complications, 661–663

    problems with, 663–664
    survival rates with, 655–658
Pancreatic cells, in type 1 diabetes mellitus, destruction of. See *Beta cell destruction;*
    Islet autoantibodies.
    function post-pancreas transplant, 658–661
Pathology/pathophysiology, of type 1 diabetes mellitus, environmental influences on.
    See *Environmental factors.*
        glucose counter-regulation and, 643–646
            autonomic failure associated with, 643, 645
                hypoglycemia-associated, 645–646
                risk factors for, 642, 646
            defective, schematic diagram of, 643, 645
                with unawareness, 643, 645
                    acknowledgment of, 646–647
            pancreas and islet transplantation impact on, 659–661
        intestinal microbial interactions and, with mucosal barrier, 566–568
            with nutrients, 568–569
        nonobese diabetic mouse model vs. human, 542–543, 548
Patient education. See *Education.*
Patient empowerment, for glycemic control, in type 1 diabetes mellitus, 647
Patient identification, for cost of illness analysis, of type 1 diabetes mellitus, 502–504
Patient survival rates, with pancreas transplantation, 657–658
Penetrance, in type 1 diabetes mellitus prediction, 515
Per capita summary, of total medical and indirect costs, of type 1 diabetes mellitus,
    507–508
Perioperative insulin, for type 1 diabetes mellitus, 601–604
Peripheral neuropathy, diabetic, biochemical and molecular pathways of, 626–627
    management of, 635–636
    occurrence of, 634
    screening for, 634–635
Peritoneal cavity, continuous subcutaneous insulin infusion into, 617
Pharmacodynamic profiles, of insulins and insulin preparations, 575, 579, 596
Pharmacokinetics, of insulin, 575, 579, 596–597, 643
Physician orders, for inpatient management, of insulin therapy, 605
Polymerase chain reaction (PCR), of intestinal microbiota, type 1 diabetes mellitus and,
    566–567
Porportional-integral-derivative (PID) algorithm, for closed-loop systems, in type 1 diabetes
    mellitus management, 618
Prandial insulin, 597–598
    in aggressive glycemic therapy, 647
    inpatient management of, 602
Preclinical trials, of type 1 diabetes mellitus, nonobese diabetic mouse model and, 552–553
Prediction, of type 1 diabetes mellitus, **513–525**
        combined biomarkers of, 518–519
        forensic, 516–518
            assay specificity and disease relevance in, 517–518
            quantifiable signals and diverse analytes requiring high-quality assays
                in, 516–517
            target or cognate autoantigens in, 517, 553
        genetic markers for, 514–516
            family history in, 514–515, 519

Prediction (*continued*)
      major genes in, 515–516
     natural history vs., 519–521
     summary overview of, 513, 521
Pregabalin, for diabetic peripheral neuropathy, 636
Preprandial insulin, recommended lag times for, 602
Prepubertal children, with type 1 diabetes mellitus, target glucose values for, 601
Presenteeism, with type 1 diabetes mellitus, 507–508
"Pre-type 1" diabetes, prevention strategies for, 527–530
Prevalence, of type 1 diabetes mellitus, 483
     lifetime costs and, 508
Prevention strategies, for beta cell destruction, in type 1 diabetes mellitus, glutamic
   acid decarboxylase 65 as, 530
      insulin as, 529–530
      intervention vs., 527–529
      using past lessons for future predictions, 534–536
  for continued glucotoxicity, closed-loop systems as, 619
  for diabetic nephropathy, 632–634
  for diabetic neuropathy, 634–635
  for diabetic retinopathy, 629
  for hypoglycemia, in type 1 diabetes mellitus, 646–649
      acknowledge the problem, 646–647
      aggressive glycemic therapy for, 647–649
      consideration of risk factors, 649
Primary care clinician, for type 1 diabetes mellitus management, 574
Probiotics, type 1 diabetes mellitus and, 568
Productivity costs, of type 1 diabetes mellitus, 506–508
Professional guidance, for glycemic control, in type 1 diabetes mellitus, 574, 585, 647, 649
Proinsulin, in islet autoimmunity, 519–520
Protein kinase C (PKC), vascular damage related to, in type 1 diabetes mellitus, 627
PTPN22 gene, in type 1 diabetes mellitus, 549, 551
Pumps, for insulin delivery. See *Insulin pump therapy.*

Q

Quality of life (QOL), with type 1 diabetes mellitus, insulin pump therapy and, 584–585
     insulin therapy and, 579–582
     nutrition therapy and, 586

R

Race/ethnicity, type 1 diabetes mellitus development and, 484–486
Radiofrequency (RF) signal, in continuous glucose monitors, 612
Rapid-acting insulins, for type 1 diabetes mellitus, 575, 579
     closed-loop delivery systems and, 617
     contemporary regimens for, 582–583
     inpatient management of, 598–599, 603
     pharmacodynamic profile of, 575, 579, 596–597
     preprandial, recommended lag times for, 602
Reactive oxygen species (ROS), mitochondrial, in type 1 diabetes mellitus, 550–551
Registered dietician (RD), for type 1 diabetes mellitus management, 574, 576, 585

Regular insulin, for type 1 diabetes mellitus, 575
    contemporary regimens for, 582–583
    non-traditional feeding and, 603
    pharmacokinetics and pharmacodynamics of, 575, 579, 596–597
Relative risk, in type 1 diabetes mellitus prediction, 514–515
Renal complications, of type 1 diabetes mellitus. See *Nephropathy.*
Retinopathy, diabetic, 626, 628–630
    biochemical and molecular pathways of, 626–627
    management of, 629–630
        recommendations for, 577
    occurrence of, 628
    pancreas and islet transplantation impact on, 661
    proliferative vs. nonproliferative, 629–630
    screening for, 629
    stages and development of, 628–629
Risk factors, for type 1 diabetes mellitus, and cardiovascular disease, 637
    and retinopathy, 630
    demographic, 484–486
    genetic markers of, 514–516
        autoantibodies combined with, 518–519
    other, 487
    stratification by islet autoantibody characteristics, 517–518
Rituximab, for type 1 diabetes mellitus, 531
RNA, messenger, in type 1 diabetes mellitus, 551
RNA interference (RNAi), in nonobese diabetic mouse model, of type 1 diabetes mellitus, 551, 553

S

School productivity, type 1 diabetes mellitus and, 506–507
SCL11A1 gene, in type 1 diabetes mellitus, 549
Screening, for diabetic nephropathy, 631–632
    for diabetic neuropathy, 634–635
    for diabetic retinopathy, 629
SEARCH for Diabetes in Youth study, 482–483
    glycemic control findings of, 488–489
    insulin therapy and, 582–583
    nutrition therapy and, 586
    race/ethnicity findings by age category, 485
    seasonality patterns and, 486–487
Seasonality, of type 1 diabetes mellitus onset and birth, 486–487
Self-management, of blood glucose, in type 1 diabetes mellitus, during inpatient stay, 601
        hypoglycemia thresholds for, 642–643
        oral glucose supplements for, 649
Self-monitoring of blood glucose (SMBG), for type 1 diabetes mellitus, 586–587
        aggressive glycemic therapy and, 647
Sensor, for continuous glucose monitoring. See *Subcutaneous (SQ) sensor.*
Sensory function, type 1 diabetes mellitus impact on, 634, 661. See also *Neuropathy.*
Sibling studies, of type 1 diabetes mellitus risk, 514–515
Simultaneous pancreas kidney transplantation (SPK), for type 1 diabetes mellitus, history of, 655

Simultaneous (*continued*)
    impact on secondary complications, 661
    survival rates with, 655–657
16S rRNA gene, intestinal microbiota and, in type 1 diabetes mellitus, 566
Skin problems, with continuous glucose monitors, 612
Slc11a1 gene, in type 1 diabetes mellitus, 549, 551
Sliding scale, for insulin therapy, 598
SQ sensor–SQ insulin delivery system, 610. See also *Closed-loop system.*
Standard order sets, for inpatient management, of insulin therapy, 605
Statistical life, of workers, in costs of type 1 diabetes mellitus, 501
Steroid-induced hyperglycemia, inpatient management of, 600, 603–605
Subcutaneous insulin administration, for type 1 diabetes mellitus, closed-loop system for,
    609–624. See also *Closed-loop system.*
    inpatient management of, 596, 598–602
        adjustment of, 601–602
        glycemic goals in, 599–601
        methods of, 598–599
        self-management of, 601
        transition from intravenous, 604–605
Subcutaneous (SQ) insulin delivery system. See also *Continuous subcutaneous insulin
    infusion (CSII).*
    for type 1 diabetes mellitus management, 610
Subcutaneous (SQ) sensor, for type 1 diabetes mellitus management, 610–612
    clinical pointers in use of, 613–614
    patient education on, 614–615
Superoxide-anion overproduction, type 1 diabetes mellitus complications related to, 627
Supply and demand, for pancreas and kidney transplantation, 664
Supply costs, of type 1 diabetes mellitus, 504–506
Support team, for glycemic control, in type 1 diabetes mellitus, 574, 585, 647, 649
Sympathoadrenal response, attenuated, to hypoglycemia, 643–646
Synergism, between intestinal microbiota and intestinal mucosa, 565–566

T

T cells, in type 1 diabetes mellitus, interventions based on, 531–532
        nonobese diabetic mice preclinical trials on, 552–553
    intestinal microbiota and, 568
    nonobese diabetic mouse model vs. human, 542
    risk prediction based on, 521
Target autoantigens, in type 1 diabetes mellitus, for therapeutic interventions, 532
    risk prediction based on, 517
        nonobese diabetic mice studies on, 553
Target values/ranges, in type 1 diabetes mellitus management, for cardiovascular disease
    prevention, 574, 576, 578
    for glycemic control, 574, 578
        for adults, 599–600
        for children, 600–601
        subcutaneous insulin adjustments and, 602
        with inpatient management, 599–601
    for hemoglobin A1c, 576, 578, 626
        by age group, 609–610

for lipid profile, 576, 578
in children, glucose values for, 601
   HbA1c goals for, 609–610
in critically ill patients, glucose values for, 599–600
T-cell receptor, in type 1 diabetes mellitus, nonobese diabetic mouse model vs.
  human, 548
Thyroid disease, with type 1 diabetes mellitus, 577
Tight glucose control (TGC), clinical trials of, 595–596
   closed-loop systems for, 619
Toll-like receptors (TLRs), intestinal microbiota and, in type 1 diabetes mellitus, 566–568
TPN, type 1 diabetes mellitus and, insulin therapy for, 602–603
Transplantation, for type 1 diabetes mellitus, beta cell, **655–667**. See also
  Beta cell transplantation.
   islet. See *Islet transplantation.*
   pancreas vs. kidney. See *Pancreas after kidney (PAK) transplantation; Pancreas*
     transplantation alone (PTA); Simultaneous pancreas kidney transplantation (SPK).
Transplantation sites, problems of, with pancreas and kidney transplantation, 664
Tricyclic drugs, for diabetic peripheral neuropathy, 635
Tube feedings, type 1 diabetes mellitus and, insulin therapy for, 601, 603
Twin studies, of type 1 diabetes mellitus risk, 514–515
Type 1 diabetes mellitus (T1D), beta cell destruction with, **527–539**
   intervention strategies for, anti-CD3 as, 531
     anti-CD20 as, 531
     anti-CD25 as, 531–532
     anti-thymocyte globulin as, 532–533
       granulocyte colony-stimulating factor with, 533
     cell therapies as, 533–534
     cytotoxic T-lymphocyte antigen-4 immunoglobulin as, 532
     mycofenolate mofetil as, 531–532
     prevention vs., 527–530
     using past lessons for future predictions, 534–536
   islet autoimmunity response and, 520
   prevention strategies for, glutamic acid decarboxylase 65 as, 530
     insulin as, 529–530
     intervention vs., 527–529
     using past lessons for future predictions, 534–536
  beta cell transplantation for, **655–667**
   cellular function following, 658–661
   complications of, 657–658
   graft survival rates of, 656–657
   history of, 655–656
   immunosuppressive drug problems with, 663
   impact on secondary complications, 661–663
   patient survival rates of, 657
   summary overview of, 665
   supply and demand problems with, 664
   transplantation site problems with, 664
  clinical course of, 488, 519–521
  complications of, **625–640**
   beta cell transplantation impact on, 661–663
   biochemical pathways of damage, 626–627

Type 1 (*continued*)
    blood sugar imbalances as. See *Hyperglycemia; Hypoglycemia.*
    cardiovascular disease as, 636–637
    costs of, 506
    macrovascular, 636–637
    metabolic memory and, 627–628
    microvascular, 628–636
    molecular pathways of damage, 626–627
    nephropathy as, 626, 630–634
    neuropathy as, 626, 634–636
    prevalence of, 489–490
    retinopathy as, 626, 628–630
    summary overview of, 625–626
  contemporary management of, **573–593**
    blood glucose monitoring in, 586–587
    cardiovascular risk factors and, 574, 576, 578
    glycemic control target ranges for, 574, 578
    goals of, 574
    historical background on, 573–574
    insulin analogues in, 574–582
    insulin pump therapy in, 583–585
    insulin regimens for, 582–583
    medical nutrition therapy in, 585–586
    multidisciplinary team in, 574
    routine health maintenance recommendations for, 574, 576–577
    summary overview of, 587
  description of, 595
  economics of, **499–512**
    cost of illness in, 500–509
      data availability for, 500–502
      methods for estimating, 500–501
      patient identification for, 502–504
    general evaluation components for, 500
    indirect costs in, 506–508
    lifetime costs in, 508–509
    medical costs in, 504–506
    summary overview of, 499–500, 509–510
  epidemiology of, **481–497**
    age and, 484
    clinical course trends, 488
    environmental factors, 487
      genetic risk markers and, 514–515
      islet autoimmunity and, 520–521
    gender and, 484
    genotype and, 486
    incidence of, 482–483
      temporal trends in, 483–484
    nutritional factors, 487
    prevalence of, 483
    prevalence of complications, 489–490
    race/ethnicity and, 484–486

    seasonality of onset and birth, 486–487
    summary overview of, 481–482, 490–491
    treatment and management trends, 488–489
hypoglycemia in, 490, **641–654**
    definition of, 642–643
    glucose counter-regulation and, pancreas and islet transplantation impact on,
        658–661
        pathophysiology of, 643–646
            autonomic failure associated with, 643, 645–646
                risk factors for, 642, 646
                defective, schematic diagram of, 643, 645
                    with unawareness, 643, 645
                        acknowledgment of, 646–647
        physiology of, 643–644
    impacts of, 642
    incidence of, 642
    limiting factor in glycemic control and, 641–642
    management of, 649–650
        insulin pump therapy and, 584
        long-acting insulins and, 579–581
        oral self-treatment, 649
        parenteral treatment, 649–650
        rapid-acting insulins and, 575, 580–581
        reduction of, 489–490
        reduction strategies in, 489–490
        sliding scale for insulin for, 598
        standard order sets for, 605
        summary of recommendations for, 650
        with inpatient insulin regimens, 595, 602
    minimizing risk of, 646–649
        acknowledge the problem, 646–647
        aggressive glycemic therapy for, 647–649
        consider conventional risk factors, 649
        consider HAAF risk factors, 649
    risk factors for, 646
        associated with autonomic failure, 642, 646
        conventional, 646
    symptomatic episodes of, 642
        pancreas and islet transplantation impact on, 658–661
inpatient management of, **595–608**
    adjusting insulin regimen for, 601–602
    children's insulin requirements for, 606
    discharge planning with, 606
    glucocorticoids and, 603–605
    insulin management fundamentals for, 597–598
    insulin orders for, 605
    insulin pharmacokinetics and pharmacodynamics in, 596–597
    intravenous insulin administration for, 597, 603–604
        transition to subcutaneous, 604–605
    perioperative insulin recommendations for, 604
    subcutaneous insulin administration for, 596, 598–602

Type 1 (*continued*)
        adjustment of, 601–602
        glycemic goals in, 599–601
        methods of, 598–599
        self-management of, 601
        transition from intravenous, 604–605
      summary overview of, 595–596, 606
      TPN and, 602–603
      tube feedings and, 601, 603
    insulin for. See also *Insulin entries.*
      contemporary management recommendations for, 574–585
      inpatient management of, **595–608**
    intestinal microbiome relationship to, **563–571**
      functions of, 564
      human superorganism and, 564–565
      microbiota alterations and, 566
      mucosal barrier–microbial interaction and, 566–568
      mucosal immunology and, 565–566
      nutrient interactions and immunity in, 568–569
      probiotics and, 568
      summary overview of, 563–564, 569
    management of, beta cell transplantation as, **655–667**. See also
      Beta cell transplantation.
      closed-loop system for, **609–624**. See also *Closed-loop system.*
      contemporary, **573–593**
      epidemiologic perspectives of, 488–489
      for beta cell destruction prevention, 527–529
      for hypoglycemia. See *Hypoglycemia.*
      glucose monitoring for. See *Blood glucose monitors/monitoring.*
      glycemic control in. See *Glycemic control.*
      inpatient, **595–608**
      insulin for. See *Insulin entries.*
      target HbA1c goals for, 609–610
    natural history of, **513–525**
      early immunization and, 519–520
      immune response profiles in, 520–521
      late immunization and, 520
      missing pieces in, 521
      prediction of vs., 514–519
      progression patterns in, 521
      summary overview of, 513, 521
    nonobese diabetic mice model of, **541–561**
      genetics in, 548–552
        insulin-dependent diabetes loci and, 541, 544–547, 549–551
      human similarities between, 541–542
      immunology and pathology comparisons, 542–543, 548
      loci mapped in, 541, 544–547, 549–551
      preclinical trials and, 552–553
      summary overview of, 541, 553
    prediction of, **513–525**
      combined biomarkers of, 518–519

forensic, 516–518
    assay specificity and disease relevance in, 517–518
    quantifiable signals and diverse analytes requiring high-quality assays in, 516–517
    target or cognate autoantigens in, 517, 553
    genetic markers for, 514–516
        family history in, 514–515, 519
        major genes in, 515–516
    natural history vs., 519–521
    summary overview of, 513, 521
  risk factors for, demographic, 484–486
    genetic markers of, 514–516
        autoantibodies combined with, 518–519
    other, 487
    stratification by islet autoantibody characteristics, 517–518
Type 2 diabetes mellitus (T2D), cost of illness analysis of, vs. type 1 diabetes mellitus, 502–504

U

Ultralente insulin, for type 1 diabetes mellitus, 579
Umbilical cord blood, for type 1 diabetes mellitus, 534
Unawareness, of hypoglycemia, in type 1 diabetes mellitus, 643, 645
        acknowledgment of, 646–647
        pancreas and islet transplantation impact on, 659
Urine ACR, in type 1 diabetes mellitus management, 578
Urine albumin excretion test, for diabetic nephropathy, 632

V

Vascular complications, of type 1 diabetes mellitus, 636–637
        biochemical and molecular pathways of, 626–627
        cardiovascular. See *Cardiovascular disease (CVD)*.
        macrovascular, 490
        metabolic memory and, 627–628
        microvascular. See *Microvascular diseases*.
Vision complications, of type 1 diabetes mellitus. See *Retinopathy*.
Vitamin D levels, type 1 diabetes mellitus and, intestinal microbial interactions related to, 568–569
    seasonality patterns related to, 487
VNTR class I alleles, in type 1 diabetes mellitus, 549
VWA2 gene, in type 1 diabetes mellitus, 549

W

Work compensation, in costs of type 1 diabetes mellitus, as indirect cost, 506–508
        mortality and, 501, 507–508
World Health Organization Multinational Project for Childhood Diabetes. See *DIAMOND Project*.

Moving?

Make sure your subscription moves with you!

To notify us of your new address, find your **Clinics Account Number** (located on your mailing label above your name), and contact customer service at:

Email: journalscustomerservice-usa@elsevier.com

800-654-2452 (subscribers in the U.S. & Canada)
314-447-8871 (subscribers outside of the U.S. & Canada)

Fax number: 314-447-8029

Elsevier Health Sciences Division
Subscription Customer Service
3251 Riverport Lane
Maryland Heights, MO 63043

*To ensure uninterrupted delivery of your subscription, please notify us at least 4 weeks in advance of move.

Printed and bound by CPI Group (UK) Ltd, Croydon, CR0 4YY

03/10/2024

01040445-0002